Understanding Labo Investigations

A Guide for Nurses, Midwives and Healthcare Professionals

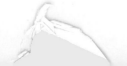

For Mary, Tom and Jon again

Understanding Laboratory Investigations

A Guide for Nurses, Midwives and Healthcare Professionals

Third Edition

Chris Higgins MSc FIBMS DMLM

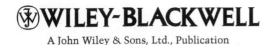

A John Wiley & Sons, Ltd., Publication

This edition first published 2013
© 2000 by Blackwell Science Ltd
© 2007 by Blackwell Publishing Ltd
© 2013 by John Wiley & Sons, Ltd

Wiley-Blackwell is an imprint of John Wiley & Sons, formed by the merger of Wiley's global Scientific, Technical and Medical business with Blackwell Publishing.

First published 2000
Second edition 2007
Third edition 2013

Registered Office
John Wiley & Sons, Ltd, The Atrium, Southern Gate, Chichester, West Sussex, PO19 8SQ, UK

Editorial Offices
9600 Garsington Road, Oxford, OX4 2DQ, UK
The Atrium, Southern Gate, Chichester, West Sussex, PO19 8SQ, UK
111 River Street, Hoboken, NJ 07030-5774, USA

For details of our global editorial offices, for customer services and for information about how to apply for permission to reuse the copyright material in this book please see our website at www.wiley.com/wiley-blackwell.

Library of Congress Cataloging-in-Publication Data

Higgins, Chris, FIBMS.
   Understanding laboratory investigations : a guide for nurses, midwives, and healthcare professionals / Chris Higgins. – 3rd ed.
      p. ; cm.
   Includes bibliographical references and indexes.
   ISBN 978-0-470-65951-9 (pbk. : alk. paper)
   I. Title.
   [DNLM: 1. Clinical Laboratory Techniques. QY 25]
   616.07′56–dc23
                                        2012031335
A catalogue record for this book is available from the British Library.

Wiley also publishes its books in a variety of electronic formats. Some content that appears in print may not be available in electronic books.

Cover image: courtesy of AJ Photo/Science Photo Library
Cover design by Workhaus

Set in 10/12.5 pt Sabon by SPi Publisher Services, Pondicherry, India

1   2013

CONTENTS

PREFACE

The purpose of this book is to help nurses to understand better how the work of clinical laboratories contributes to patient care. It is intended to answer the following questions:

- Why is this test being ordered on my patient?
- What sort of sample is required?
- How is that sample obtained?

And most importantly:

- What is the significance of the test result for my patient?

Answers to these questions must be based on an understanding of basic science. Care has been taken to introduce this science, which includes some basic biochemistry, physiology and anatomy, in a way which is accessible to all those with an interest in how the body works. Much will be familiar to nurses.

The format of the book is simple. After two introductory chapters (one of which emphasises the role of nursing staff in the process of laboratory testing), each chapter is devoted to consideration of a single test or group of related tests. Each of these chapters begins with some relevant biochemistry, physiology or anatomy to put the substance being measured (i.e. the test) in some physiological context. A consideration of the sample requirements follows, and finally interpretation of the test results. Wherever possible, patient pathology, symptoms and test results are related. Mock case histories are included at the end of each chapter to illustrate the practical clinical use of the test being discussed and give a human face to the science.

It is not possible in a book of this size to discuss all of the tests performed in clinical laboratories in this degree of detail, so it has been necessary to be selective. The tests discussed are the most commonly requested, and those which nurses are most likely to encounter. Taken together the tests discussed in this book account for around 70–80% of the total workload of clinical laboratories in the average district general hospital.

Although the primary audience for this book is nursing staff, it should be of interest to other healthcare workers and also students of biomedical sciences interested in pursuing a career in laboratory medicine.

The general format and philosophy of this book remains unchanged for this third edition but some revision has been necessary in the light of changing practice and new research. Significant additional features include a chapter on neonatal screening for disease, and discussion of some tests not considered in previous editions. These include the D-dimer test and the B-natriuretic peptide (BNP) test; inclusion of both is justified on the basis of their increasing clinical use.

In response to the welcome advice of reviewers, the number of mock case studies has been significantly increased and an attempt has been made to render the text more relevant to midwives and neonatal nurses.

Acknowledgements

Very special thanks to my son Jon who conceived and prepared the artwork for previous editions and willingly agreed to update it once again for this third edition. Also to my wife Mary for her continued support and patience.

Thanks too of course to everyone at Wiley-Blackwell involved in the production of the book, especially Magenta Styles for commissioning this edition and Catriona Cooper for assistance during preparation of the manuscript.

PART 1

Introduction

CHAPTER 1

INTRODUCTION TO CLINICAL LABORATORIES

Key learning topics
- The role of the nurse in patient testing
- The five sub-disciplines of clinical pathology
- Clinical laboratory staffing and costs

Patients may be subjected to many kinds of investigative procedure. These range in complexity from ward or clinic based measurements familiar to all nurses, such as determining body temperature, pulse and blood pressure, through monitoring of heart function by electrocardiographic (ECG) machines to body imaging techniques, such as X-ray, computed tomography (CT) and magnetic resonance imaging (MRI) scan. All of these require the presence of the patient; they are performed on the patient, if not by nurses, at least often in their presence.

In contrast, all the investigations described in this book are performed on samples removed from the patient. The remoteness of patients from the site of laboratory testing might engender the understandable though misguided perception that laboratory testing has little to do with nursing care. In fact an understanding by nursing staff of the work of clinical laboratories is important for several reasons.

Nurses are in a unique position to satisfy the need expressed by many patients for information about the tests that they are subjected to. Recent research[1] confirms the intuitive notion that patients want to understand the purpose of tests and significance of their test results. This may be to allay fears and anxieties among those who have never undergone such a test before, or it may simply reflect a right to know. Most laboratory tests are only minimally invasive but can only be done with a patient's implied informed consent. Of course many patients will express no interest, but some have questions that must be addressed.

Understanding Laboratory Investigations: A Guide for Nurses, Midwives and Healthcare Professionals, Third Edition. Chris Higgins.
© 2013 John Wiley & Sons, Ltd. Published 2013 by John Wiley & Sons, Ltd.

Nurses sometimes have responsibility for the collection and timely, safe transport of patient samples. It is vital that anyone collecting samples is aware of the importance of good practice during this pre-testing phase.

Nurses are frequently involved in the reception of laboratory test results. It is important that they are familiar with the terminology and format of laboratory reports and are able to identify abnormal results, particularly those that warrant immediate clinical intervention.

For many years nurses have performed limited testing of blood and urine samples (e.g. blood glucose and urine dipstick testing) in wards and clinics. With advances in technology, an ever increasing repertoire of tests can now be performed, within minutes, outside the laboratory in clinics and wards by nursing staff. This so called 'point of care testing' is particularly well established in intensive care, coronary care and emergency room settings where speed of analysis has proven benefit for patient care. It is important that nurses involved in the analysis of patient samples understand the pitfalls, limitations and clinical significance of this aspect of their work.

Traditionally, doctors have had sole responsibility for both requesting and interpreting laboratory test results, but the developing role of the clinical nurse specialist has required that some nurses become involved in both of these processes. In any case all

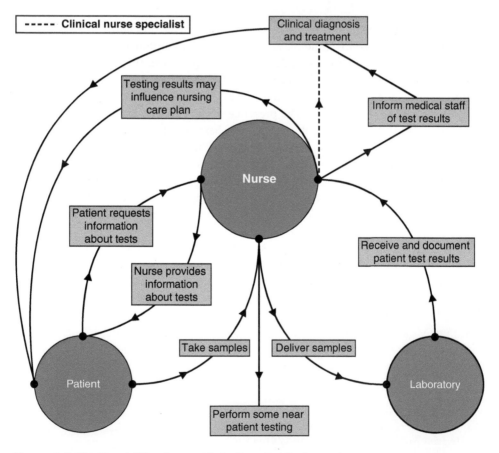

Figure 1.1 Nursing staff involvement in testing of patient samples.

qualified nursing staff members have to make judgements about how the results of laboratory tests might impact on the formulation of nursing care plans for their patients.

Finally, there are those nurses whose professional role requires especially detailed knowledge of the work of the laboratory as well as close co-operation with laboratory staff. These include haematology nurse specialists, blood transfusion nurse specialists, infection control nurses and diabetic nurse specialists. Figure 1.1 summarises the role of nursing staff in laboratory testing.

All the tests described in this book are performed – although, as has been made clear not exclusively so – in clinical pathology laboratories. The second part of this introductory chapter serves to describe in outline the work of the five sub-disciplines of clinical pathology. The range of samples tested is listed in Table 1.1.

Table 1.1 Range of samples used for laboratory investigation.

	Sample type
Chemical analysis	Usually blood or urine Less common: ● Faeces ● Cerebrospinal fluid (CSF): this is the fluid that surrounds the brain and spinal cord ● Pleural fluid: this is the fluid that surrounds the lungs in the pleural cavity and is only obtainable when there is abnormal accumulation, a condition called pleural effusion ● Ascitic fluid: this is the fluid that surrounds the abdominal organs in the peritoneal cavity and is only obtainable when there is abnormal accumulation, a condition called ascites
Haematological analysis	Usually blood only Less common: ● Bone marrow aspirate ● Bone marrow biopsy
Microbiological analysis	Common: ● Urine ● Faeces ● Sputum ● Swabs of any (potentially infected) accessible site including: throat, nose, eye, wound, vagina Less common: ● Cerebrospinal fluid ● Pleural fluid ● Vomit ● Skin scraping
Histopathological analysis	Tissue samples (biopsy) only
Cytopathological analysis	Urine Sputum Cellular material obtained by scraping the surface of organs or aspirating abnormal fluids (e.g. cysts)
Immunological analysis	Usually blood only

The clinical chemistry laboratory

(also known as chemical pathology, clinical biochemistry)
Clinical chemistry is concerned with the diagnosis and monitoring of disease by measuring the concentration of chemicals, principally in blood plasma (the non-cellular, fluid portion of blood) and urine. Occasionally, chemical analysis of faeces and other body fluids, for example cerebrospinal and pleural fluid, is useful.

Blood plasma is a chemically complex fluid containing many inorganic ions, proteins, carbohydrates, lipids, hormones and enzymes, along with two dissolved gases, oxygen and carbon dioxide. In health the concentration in blood of each chemical substance is maintained within limits that reflect normal cellular and whole body metabolism. Disease is often associated with one or more disturbances in this delicate balance of blood chemistry; it is this general principle that underlies the importance of chemical testing of blood for the diagnostic process. The range of pathologies in which chemical testing of blood and urine has proven diagnostically useful is diverse and includes disease of the kidney, liver, heart, lungs and endocrine system. Diseases that result from nutritional deficiency can be identified by chemical analysis of blood. The cells of some malignant tumours release specific chemicals into blood. Measurement of these so called tumour markers allows a limited role for the clinical chemistry laboratory in the diagnosis and monitoring of some types of cancer.

The safe and effective delivery of some drug therapies depends on measuring the blood concentration of those drugs. This is just one aspect of the broader monitoring of treatment role that the clinical chemistry laboratory serves.

Most chemical testing of blood and urine is performed on highly sophisticated, automated machinery. Modern clinical chemistry analysers can perform up to 1000 tests per hour; 20 or more different chemical substances can be measured simultaneously on these analysers using a single blood sample. Results of the most commonly requested tests, which include nearly all those discussed in this book, are usually available within 12–24 hours of receipt of the specimen. More rarely, requested tests may be performed just once or twice a week, and a small minority are only performed in specialist centres. Nearly all clinical chemistry laboratories provide an urgent 24 hour per day service for a limited and defined list of tests; results of such urgently requested tests can usually be made available within an hour.

Critically ill patients being cared for in intensive care units and emergency rooms often require frequent and urgent monitoring of some aspects of blood chemistry. In these circumstances blood testing is performed by nursing staff, using dedicated analysers sited close to the patient; this represents one aspect of point of care testing.

The haematology laboratory

Haematology is concerned principally with the diagnosis and monitoring of diseases that affect the number, size and appearance of the cellular or formed elements of blood. These are: the red blood cells (erythrocytes), the white blood cells (leucocytes) and platelets (thrombocytes). The full blood count (FBC) is probably the most frequently requested laboratory test and certainly the most frequently requested haematology test, reflecting the range of common and less common disorders which affect both the numbers and appearance of blood cells. It is in fact not one but a battery of tests.

Modern haematology analysers are able to process FBC tests at the rate of up to 400 samples per hour. The detailed information about the blood cells which these analysers provide has dramatically reduced the number of specimens that need to be examined under the microscope, but the microscope remains an essential tool to the haematologist for examination of bone marrow biopsy specimens and, in some circumstances, blood.

Apart from the cells in blood, haematology is also concerned with measurement of the concentration of some of the proteins present in blood plasma that are involved in the complex process of blood coagulation.

Disorders of blood in which haematology testing is vital include haematological malignancy (e.g. the leukaemias, Hodgkin's disease, myeloma), anaemia and diseases in which disturbances of blood coagulation result in an increased tendency to bleed (e.g. haemophilia) or an increased tendency for blood to coagulate within blood vessels (e.g. deep vein thrombosis). Some haematology tests including the FBC are useful in the diagnosis or clinical management of common, non-haematological diseases. For example, infectious disease is usually associated with an increase in the number of white blood cells. Anaemia is often a feature of kidney disease, chronic inflammatory disorders such as rheumatoid arthritis and some diseases that result from nutritional deficiency.

Many patients at risk of heart and blood vessel (cardiovascular) disease are prescribed medication that inhibits the process of blood clotting (coagulation). This anticoagulation therapy must be monitored by regular blood testing to prevent bleeding, a potentially dangerous side effect of such therapy.

Most haematology test results are routinely available within 12–24 hours. However if the need is clinically justified, results of some haematology tests, including FBC, can be made available within an hour, at any time of the day or night.

The clinical microbiology laboratory

Clinical microbiology is concerned with the diagnosis and monitoring of disease caused by infective agents, mostly bacteria but also viruses, fungi and parasitic worms. Much of the work involves isolation and identification of bacteria from many sorts of sample, including urine, sputum, faeces, blood, cerebrospinal fluid and swabs taken from a variety of infected sites. Bacteria can sometimes be seen by examining these specimens under the microscope, but more precise identification can only be made after culture, or 'growth' of bacteria on nutrient enriched media. One of the problems encountered by the microbiologist when dealing with clinical specimens is that many bacterial species are normally present in many sites around the body; indeed in some cases they are essential for normal health. The microbiologist must isolate those that are pathogenic (i.e. cause disease) from those that are normally present, and from any environmental bacterial contaminant introduced during sample collection. Some body fluids are normally sterile; these include blood, cerebrospinal fluid, and fluid aspirated from joints and the pleural cavity. Bacteria isolated from these sites are always pathogenic.

Having isolated and identified a species of pathogenic bacteria, the next step is to test the sensitivity of the organism to a range of antibiotics. This information helps in deciding which antibiotic therapy is likely to be most effective in eradicating the infection.

Blood testing plays an important and evolving role in detecting infections that are caused by organisms difficult to isolate by culture. During any infection the immune system produces specific antibodies directed at specific antigens present on the surface of the invading organism. A rising amount of the antibody in blood provides evidence of current infection.

Specific antigens present on the surface of microorganisms also provide a means of identifying infective agents. Testing blood for the presence of viral antigens is an important means of diagnosing viral infections such as those which cause hepatitis and acquired immune deficiency syndrome (AIDS).

Some microbiological investigation may take from several days to several weeks to complete; this delay is governed largely by the speed of bacterial growth in culture. Initial microscopical examination can be performed immediately on receipt of the specimen if clinically necessary, and results can usually be made available on the day the sample is received in an interim report.

Clinical microbiology laboratories operate a 24 hour service for the rare cases when urgent culture and microscopical examination of samples is necessary. These include suspected cases of immediate life threatening infections of blood (septicaemia) and central nervous system (meningitis).

Quite apart from their diagnostic role, hospital microbiology laboratories play an important role with infection control nurses in the monitoring and prevention of nosocomial infectious disease, that is infectious disease acquired by patients whilst in hospital – an ever present problem, which impacts on the working life of all nursing staff.

The blood transfusion laboratory

Blood transfusion is concerned with the provision of a safe supply of blood and blood products. In contrast to other pathology departments, blood transfusion has limited diagnostic function. In some senses its function more resembles a pharmacy, in that its main purpose is to supply therapeutic products. Transfusion of whole blood is very rarely practiced nowadays; rather specific components of whole blood are transfused. The most frequently transfused blood product is red cells, to correct anaemia and to replace blood lost during surgery or as a result of trauma or complication during childbirth. Much less commonly, the white cells of blood, platelets and the proteins present in blood plasma are therapeutically useful.

The National Blood Service (NBS) is responsible for the collection and supply of safe (disease free) donated blood products to hospital blood transfusion laboratories. Here, each donated unit of red cells must be tested for compatibility with the patient's blood before it can be transfused. The transfusion of incompatible blood products can have very serious health consequences and is potentially fatal. Advances in compatibility testing have ensured that compatible red cells can be made available for transfusion usually well within an hour of a patient's blood sample arriving in the laboratory; this service is available 24 hours a day.

The blood transfusion department also has an important specific diagnostic role for some forms of haemolytic anaemia, in which the body produces antibodies against its own red cells. One important aspect of this work is haemolytic disease of the newborn, a potentially fatal condition in which the red cells of the developing foetus are destroyed by antibodies present in the mother's blood. All pregnant women are routinely tested for the presence of such antibodies.

The histopathology laboratory

(also known as morbid anatomy, cellular pathology)
Histopathology, the oldest of all pathology disciplines, is concerned with the diagnosis of disease by microscopical examination of tissue samples (biopsies). The rationale for this approach is that disease processes, for example, malignancy, inflammation, infection etc., are characterised by specific changes at the tissue and cellular level, which are evident when tissue is viewed under the microscope. There are many ways of recovering tissue samples from the body. Tissue from the gastrointestinal tract, lungs and urinary tract are commonly sampled at the time of endoscopic examination. An endoscope is an instrument used to visually examine internal organs directly by fibre optics. The instrument includes small forceps which can be used to remove small pieces of tissue during the examination. Tissue may be taken during surgery by incision or excision biopsy. Incision biopsy is the removal of a sample cut from an area of diseased tissue, whereas excision biopsy involves removal of the whole area of diseased tissue.

Before transport to the laboratory, biopsy samples must be 'fixed' in a chemical fixative, usually formalin, to preserve structure. This process can take from a few hours to a whole day depending on the size of the specimen. In the laboratory 'fixed' specimens are impregnated with paraffin wax, allowed to harden and then cut into very thin sections just 3–5 μm thick. These wafer thin sections are then mounted on glass microscope slides and stained with chemicals, before examination under the microscope. The whole process from reception of specimen to issue of a histopathological report can take from one to four days depending on the size of the biopsy sample. Sometimes it is important to make a diagnosis very quickly, and in these circumstances a frozen section is performed. Tissue is 'fixed' immediately by freezing. This process allows tissue sections to be cut almost immediately the sample is removed from the patient. The sections are stained and examined under the microscope. This rapid technique allows a diagnosis of, for example, breast cancer to be made rapidly whilst the patient remains anaesthetized on the operating table. Armed with a laboratory report that confirms malignant disease, the surgeon can proceed immediately to surgical treatment.

Microscopical examination of tissue removed from the patient is probably most widely used in the diagnosis and staging of malignant disease in organs throughout the body. It is also used in the differential diagnosis of non-malignant disease of all body organs. It has a role in the diagnosis of connective tissue and skin disorders and in the early diagnosis of tissue rejection among patients who have received transplanted organs.

Clearly all histopathological tests are invasive, often requiring surgical intervention to recover samples. Both financial and patient safety consideration ensure that, unlike other laboratory investigations, histopathological investigations are reserved for those patients in whom there is a strong suspicion of serious disease. In many cases this suspicion will have been raised by the abnormal results of blood and urine tests performed in other pathology laboratories, so that histopathological examination of tissues can represent the final stage in laboratory diagnosis.

Finally, post mortem examinations to determine cause of patient death are conducted in the hospital mortuary, which is administratively part of the histopathology department.

Cytopathology

Cytopathology is a sub-discipline of histopathology. Whereas histopathology is concerned with microscopical examination of tissue samples, the focus of the cytopathologist is the cells that are normally exfoliated from the epithelial surface of organs. Sample recovery is less invasive than that required for histopathological investigation. Typically cells are scraped from the surface of organs such as the cervix, the mucosal surface of the duodenum and stomach and lungs. Cells can also be recovered by aspiration using a fine needle and syringe, from the pleural and peritoneal cavities, or from solid tumours, for example, in the breast. The cells are spread onto a glass microscope slide, fixed and stained and then examined under the microscope. Cytopathology is almost exclusively concerned with diagnosis of pre-malignant and malignant disease. The cervical smear test, used to screen all women for risk of cervical cancer, accounts for a large proportion of the workload of the cytopathology laboratory.

The immunology laboratory

Clinical immunology laboratories are concerned principally with blood testing for the diagnosis of autoimmune diseases, in which the body's normally protective immune system produces antibodies against its own tissue antigens. These self-reacting, destructive antibodies are called autoantibodies. The detection in blood of organ specific autoantibodies is helpful in the diagnosis of many diseases with an autoimmune component including coeliac disease, thyroid disorders, pernicious anaemia, systemic lupus erythematosus (SLE) and autoimmune disease of kidney and liver disease.

Laboratory staffing

Clinical laboratories are staffed by graduate trained biomedical scientists (BMS), who are responsible for the analysis of samples and the overall day to day management of the laboratory departments. They are helped in the analytical task by medical laboratory assistants (MLAs) who may have the additional responsibility of blood sample collection (phlebotomy) from patients. Cytoscreeners are a specially trained group whose work is confined largely to the examination of cervical smears.

Each laboratory department is headed by a medically qualified doctor of consultant status who has specialised in one area of laboratory medicine (in some cases a non-medically qualified clinical scientist fulfils this role). They provide consultancy for doctors and nurses on all aspects of laboratory medicine, so that they might advise both on the most appropriate laboratory investigation in particular cases, and the clinical significance of test results. Haematology consultants also have clinical responsibility for the care of patients suffering haematological disease (e.g. leukaemia). Medical consultants attached to clinical chemistry departments are often responsible for the clinical care of patients suffering diabetes and other metabolic and endocrine disorders, whilst a microbiology consultant advises doctors on the most effective use of antibiotic therapy and is responsible, with the control of infection nurse, for the formulation and implementation of the hospital control of infection policy.

Medically qualified histopathology consultants examine tissues prepared by biomedical scientists and make a histopathological diagnosis based on this examination. They provide diagnostic and prognostic advice to the medical team caring for cancer patients, although their clinical input is by no means confined to this patient group. They also perform all post-mortem (autopsy) examinations, with the assistance of an anatomical pathology technician.

Scope, workload and costs

The influential, government initiated Carter Review of Pathology Services[2,3] determined that 70–80% of all healthcare decisions regarding diagnosis and treatment are influenced by the results of laboratory tests. The Review provides the most reliable national data on pathology workload and costs. An estimated 500 million clinical biochemical tests and 130 million haematology tests are conducted each year in National Health Service (NHS) clinical laboratories across England. Additionally, 50 million microbiology requests are processed and 13 million histopathology slides along with 4 million cytology slides are examined. Demand for pathology testing rises at the rate of 8–10% per year. Primary care (GP) test requests account for around 40% of total laboratory workload, the rest is generated within hospitals (both inpatient and outpatient departments). Carter estimates the annual cost of NHS pathology services in England to be close to £2.5 billion, equivalent to 3.5% of the total NHS budget. The median (average) cost of a routine high-volume laboratory test – which describes nearly all of those discussed in this book – varies between hospitals and pathology discipline: clinical biochemistry (average: £1.00

per test, range: £0.50–2.80); haematology (average: £2.40 per test, range: £1.50–3.70); microbiology (average: £6.10 per test, range: £4.00–9.40) and histopathology (average: £48.10 per test, range: £21.40–73.40).

The modernisation of pathology services[4] – begun a decade ago and reflected in recommendations of the Carter Review – continues. The principal aim is to identify novel ways of delivering high quality pathology services that are responsive to patient needs and are cost effective. This has included an expansion of point of care testing, with nurses and other non-laboratory healthcare professionals becoming more involved in patient testing. The potential for economy of scale with centralisation of routine (non-urgent) pathology services in regional centres is receiving active consideration and in some hospitals pathology services have been rationalised so that haematology, blood transfusion and clinical biochemistry laboratories are combined to form one 'blood science laboratory'.

As in all other areas of patient care, successful clinical laboratory investigation depends on teamwork; nurses are important members of that team. Good communication between nursing and laboratory staff can help to ensure that resources consumed in delivery of pathology services are used to best effect for the patient.

References

1. Boyd, J., Hazy, J. and Sanders, S. (2007) Communicating and understanding laboratory tests: what matters? *Lab Medicine*, 38:680–84.
2. Department of Health (2006) Report of the review of NHS pathology services in England. Chaired by Lord Carter of Coles: an independent review for the Department of Health, HMSO (available on line: accessed May 2011).
3. Department of Health (2008) Report of the second phase of the review of NHS pathology services in England. Chaired by Lord Carter of Coles: an independent review for the Department of Health, HMSO (available on line: accessed May 2011).
4. Department of Health (2005) Modernising pathology: building a service responsive to patients, HMSO.

Useful Websites

www.ibms.org – website of the Institute of Biomedical Sciences – the professional organisation that represents biomedical scientists, the largest group of pathology laboratory staff.

www.rcpath.org – website of the Royal College of Pathologists – the professional organisation that represents pathologists, medically qualified laboratory staff.

www.acb.org.uk – website of the Association of Clinical Biochemistry – the professional organisation that represents non-clinical scientists working in clinical chemistry laboratories.

www.labtestsonline.org.uk – website for patients about clinical laboratory tests – includes a wealth of information about the work of pathology laboratories.

CHAPTER 2

SOME PRINCIPLES OF LABORATORY TESTING

Key learning topics

- The principles of patient sample collection
- Units of measurement used in clinical laboratories
- The concept of the normal (reference) range
- The concept of test sensitivity/specificity
- The concept of critical values
- Difference between (blood) plasma and (blood) serum

Laboratory investigation of patient samples is the sum of three distinct phases:

1. Pre-testing phase, which includes collection and transport of samples to the laboratory.
2. Analytical phase within the laboratory.
3. Post-testing phase, which includes communication and interpretation of test results as well as clinical response to test result in terms of patient management.

In this chapter some general principles relating to pre- and post-testing procedures are discussed.

Pre-testing procedures

It is difficult to over emphasise the importance of good practice during the pre-testing phase of laboratory investigation. The production of high quality, accurate results which are clinically useful depends as much on practice before the sample

Understanding Laboratory Investigations: A Guide for Nurses, Midwives and Healthcare Professionals, Third Edition. Chris Higgins.
© 2013 John Wiley & Sons, Ltd. Published 2013 by John Wiley & Sons, Ltd.

reaches the laboratory as it does on the analytical process within the laboratory. Aspects of the pre-testing phase that need to be considered are:

- The pathology request form.
- The timing of sample collection.
- Sampling technique.
- Collecting the right amount of sample.
- Sample containers and labelling.
- Safety during collection and transport of samples.

This chapter is concerned with principles only. The detail of pre-testing will be considered again under each test heading. However, it must be remembered that practice, although based on the principles in this book, does vary between laboratories. There is no real substitute for consultation with your local laboratory. Clinical pathology departments are now mandated to publish a manual – usually available online – for users (doctors and nurses) of local pathology services. Such user manuals provide the detail of local pre-testing procedures that should guide practice in this area.

Pathology request form

Each patient sample must be accompanied by the appropriate fully completed pathology request form, signed by the doctor or in some instances, where that responsibility has been delegated, the specialist nurse practitioner making the request. Attention to detail is particularly vital for blood transfusion requests. Most cases of incompatible blood transfusion are the result of documentation errors. All pathology request forms should include the following information set:

- Patient details, including: full name, date of birth and hospital number.
- Hospital ward/clinic or GP surgery.
- Nature of specimen (e.g. venous blood, urine, biopsy etc.).
- Date and time of sample collection.
- Name of test requested (e.g. blood glucose, full blood count).
- Clinical details (these should very briefly explain why the test is being requested and may include a suspected or provisional diagnosis or symptoms).
- Details of any drug therapy that might affect test analysis or interpretation.
- An indication, where relevant, of the urgency of the request.
- Some health authorities request details about budget cost centres.

Timing of sample collection

Whenever possible, samples should be taken to coincide with routine transport to the laboratory, so that they can be processed by the laboratory without undue delay. It is not good practice to leave samples for more than a few hours or overnight before sending them to the laboratory; in many cases the samples will be unsuitable for analysis. For a few biochemical tests, for example, blood hormone levels, it is vital that blood is sampled at a particular time of the day. For others (e.g. blood glucose) it is simply important to know what time the sample is collected. Some tests (e.g. blood gases) require that samples be processed immediately they are taken. Collection of these must be timed by prior agreement with the laboratory. Samples for microbiological investigation are best taken before antibiotic therapy is started, since antibiotics will inhibit the growth of bacteria in culture.

Sampling technique

Venous blood collection

Most blood tests are performed on venous blood collected by a technique known as venepuncture, using either a needle and syringe or, more commonly, an evacuated tube system (Figure 2.1).

- Patients may be anxious at the prospect of a venepuncture. A calm confident manner is important. Explain in simple terms what is involved and that mild discomfort or pain is usually felt as the needle is inserted.
- If there is a history of fainting during blood collection, take the sample with the patient lying down.
- When performing venepuncture on a patient receiving IV fluids, do not take blood from the arm used for IV administration. This avoids the risk of IV fluid contamination of the sample.
- Haemolysis (the rupture of red cells) during blood collection may render the sample unsuitable for analysis. This can occur if blood is forced at speed through narrow gauge needles or if the sample is shaken vigorously. When using syringe and needle technique, remove the needle before expelling blood into the sample container.
- Prolonged use of a tourniquet can affect laboratory results. Avoid the use of a tourniquet if possible and do not collect blood if tourniquet has been in place for more than one minute or two. Release the tourniquet and try the opposite arm.
- Although the cephalic or basilic vein in the forearm at the elbow is the usual preferred site, veins in the back of the hand or the foot provide alternative sites, for those with 'difficult' veins.

Capillary blood collection

Capillary blood can be recovered by a simple skin puncture with a sterile lancet, usually on the finger tip or, in the case of neonates and babies, the heel of the foot. It is useful if only very small sample volumes (less than 1 ml) are required. The technique can be performed by patients themselves and is routinely used, after training, by diabetic patients to obtain samples for self-monitoring of blood glucose concentration.

- The finger tip or heel is wiped with alcohol. A sterile lancet or autolet device is used to puncture the cleansed skin on the side of the finger tip or heel. Puncturing the ball of the finger tip is more painful.

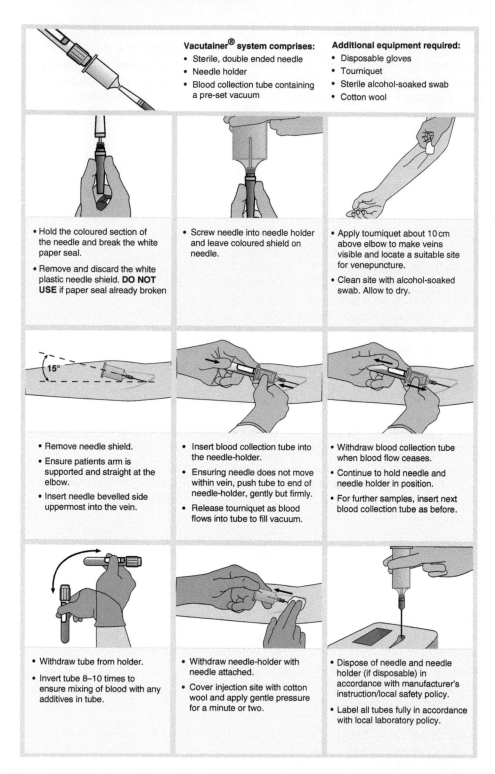

Vacutainer® system comprises:
- Sterile, double ended needle
- Needle holder
- Blood collection tube containing a pre-set vacuum

Additional equipment required:
- Disposable gloves
- Tourniquet
- Sterile alcohol-soaked swab
- Cotton wool

- Hold the coloured section of the needle and break the white paper seal.
- Remove and discard the white plastic needle shield. **DO NOT USE** if paper seal already broken

- Screw needle into needle holder and leave coloured shield on needle.

- Apply tourniquet about 10 cm above elbow to make veins visible and locate a suitable site for venepuncture.
- Clean site with alcohol-soaked swab. Allow to dry.

- Remove needle shield.
- Ensure patients arm is supported and straight at the elbow.
- Insert needle bevelled side uppermost into the vein.

- Insert blood collection tube into the needle-holder.
- Ensuring needle does not move within vein, push tube to end of needle-holder, gently but firmly.
- Release tourniquet as blood flows into tube to fill vacuum.

- Withdraw blood collection tube when blood flow ceases.
- Continue to hold needle and needle holder in position.
- For further samples, insert next blood collection tube as before.

- Withdraw tube from holder.
- Invert tube 8–10 times to ensure mixing of blood with any additives in tube.

- Withdraw needle-holder with needle attached.
- Cover injection site with cotton wool and apply gentle pressure for a minute or two.

- Dispose of needle and needle holder (if disposable) in accordance with manufacturer's instruction/local safety policy.
- Label all tubes fully in accordance with local laboratory policy.

Figure 2.1 Collection of venous blood with Vacutainer® system.

- Undue pressure to 'squeeze' blood out, can cause inaccurate results; blood must flow freely.
- Blood should be collected immediately into an appropriate container, designated for capillary samples and mixed gently by inversion.
- Pressure must be applied to the puncture site with a sterile gauze until blood flow ceases.

Arterial blood collection

The only test that requires sampling of blood from arteries is blood gases. The technique, which is more hazardous and painful than venepuncture, is described in Chapter 7.

Urine collection

Four kinds of urine collection are commonly made:

- A mid stream urine (MSU).
- A catheter specimen urine (CSU).
- An early morning urine (EMU).
- A 24 hour urine (i.e. all the urine passed during a 24 hour period).

The test requested determines which of these is appropriate. For most non-quantitative purposes, such as dipstick testing and microbiological testing, an MSU is necessary. This is a small 10–15 ml sample of urine collected part way through micturition, which can be collected at any time of the day. A CSU is the urine sample collected from a patient who has an indwelling urinary catheter. The detail of collecting an MSU and CSU for microbiological examination is provided in Chapter 21.

The first urine passed in the day, the so called EMU is the most concentrated and an EMU provides the best method of detecting substances in the urine which are present only in low concentration. An example of its use is pregnancy testing. The urine pregnancy test is based on detection of a hormone, human chorionic gonadotrophin (HCG), which is not normally detectable in urine, but is excreted in increasing concentration during the first few months of pregnancy. Early in pregnancy, the concentration is so low that unless a concentrated urine (i.e. an EMU) is used, the result may be falsely negative.

Sometimes it is useful to know exactly how much of a particular substance (e.g. sodium, potassium) is being lost from the body in urine, on a daily basis. Quantitation of this urinary loss can only be made by collecting all the urine passed during a 24 hour period. The detail of collecting a 24 hour urine is provided in Table 2.1.

Sputum, swab collection

All these specimens are destined for microbiological examination and the object is to sample only from infected sites, whilst avoiding bacterial contamination from other sites on the body or from the environment. For example, a sputum specimen is intended to reflect the environment of the respiratory tract, not the mouth. Saliva is not sputum. Sputum is best collected first thing in the morning and must be coughed

Table 2.1 Protocol for collection of 24-hour urine.

Clinical diagnosis or monitoring is occasionally aided by measurement of the rate of urinary excretion of a substance normally present in urine.

This requires collection of a timed (usually 24 hour) urine sample.

The validity of results of these tests depends crucially on an accurately timed sample; the object is to collect **ALL** urine passed during the 24 hour period.

- Obtain a 24 hour urine container for the test requested from the laboratory. Some tests require a container with an acid preservative. This may be a corrosive acid e.g. concentrated hydrochloric acid, so care must be taken.
- Label the bottle with patient details and date and time of start of urine collection.
- Explain to the patient that ALL urine passed during the 24 hour period must be saved.
- At a convenient time (usually 09.00) any urine in the bladder is voided and discarded.
- ALL the urine passed after 09.00 must be collected into the container.
- At 09.00 on the following day, the bladder is again emptied. This last sample must be added to the container. No urine passed after 09.00 on the second day should be added to the container.
- The urine collection, along with relevant test request form should be transported to the laboratory as soon as possible.

Notes: Sometimes a patient's 24-hour urine volume exceeds the 2 l capacity of the collection container. If this is the case a second container must be obtained to complete the collection. ALL the urine passed MUST be collected.

If the patient inadvertently discards some urine during the collection period, all the urine collected to that point must be discarded, a new container obtained and collection restarted.

The urine container should be stored in the ward sample fridge during the collection period.

up from the lungs. Washing out the mouth before sampling reduces the risk of salivary contamination. When collecting throat swabs it is important to ensure that the swab does not come into contact with the tongue or sides of the mouth. This can be avoided by use of a tongue depressor. The swab should be gently rubbed only over the area at the back of the mouth (pharynx) and tonsils, especially inflamed areas.

Wound swabs are obtained by sampling the affected site only, avoiding contact with surrounding normal skin or tissue. When collecting any microbiological specimen, it is important to minimise environmental contamination by using aseptic technique and replacing swabs back in sterile containers or transport medium immediately.

Tissue (biopsy) collection

A very brief reference to tissue sampling techniques necessary for histopathological examination has already been made in Chapter 1. Such sampling is always the responsibility of doctors and is beyond the scope of this book. Nurses are however involved in sampling of cervical cells for the cervical smear test (Chapter 24).

Collecting the right amount of sample

The amount of blood required for laboratory testing is governed largely by local laboratory equipment and is therefore a matter of local laboratory policy. In general, continuing technological advance serves to significantly reduce the amount of blood required for tests. The local laboratory user guide includes a list of tests with the minimum blood volume requirements. Anyone responsible for blood collection must be familiar with this local list. Some blood specimen bottles contain pre-weighed amounts of chemical preservatives and/or anticoagulants that determine the optimum volume of blood that the bottle should contain; this volume is stated on the side of the bottle. Erroneous results may occur if these blood volume instructions are not observed.

Whilst the volume of urine collected for MSU and CSU is not critical, it is vital, when collecting 24 hour urines, that all the urine passed in the collection period is collected, even if a second collection bottle is required.

In general, the size or amount of sample is important for successful isolation of bacteria. For example, it is more likely that bacteria will be isolated from a large specimen of sputum than a small specimen. Aspiration of pus with a needle and syringe is more likely to result in isolation of the causative organism than a swab of the pus. Falsely negative blood culture results can occur if insufficient blood is added to culture bottles.

Sample containers

Pathology laboratories supply a bewildering array of sample bottles and containers. Each container has specific uses; it is vital for accurate results that the correct container is used for the test requested. Guidance on this is contained within the local laboratory user manual.

The colour coded tops of blood sample containers indicate the chemicals, either in liquid or powder form, that they contain (Table 2.2). These chemicals serve two main purposes: prevention or acceleration of blood clotting; and preservation of blood cell structure or the concentration of some blood constituent. It is important that these chemicals are well mixed with the blood sample by repeated gentle inversion of the sample bottle.

A preservative may be necessary to preserve urine during collection of a 24 hour urine. The need for a preservative is determined by the substance in urine to be measured.

All sample containers for microbiological examination, for example, urine, swabs, blood culture bottles etc., are sterile and should not be used if seals are broken. Some bacteria will only survive outside the body if preserved in special transport media.

The structure of tissue samples is preserved by 'fixing' the tissue in formalin. Biopsy sample containers contain this preservative.

All sample containers must be fully labelled including patient's full name, date of birth and location (ward, clinic or GP). Laboratories receive many hundreds of specimens every day, which may include specimens from two or more patients with the same name. It is vital, if results are to find their way back to the correct patient records, that specimen labels accurately and fully identify the patient. Inadequately labelled specimens or labelled specimens that cannot be incontrovertibly linked to the accompanying pathology request card may be rejected by the laboratory, resulting in the need for the patient to be re-tested; an entirely avoidable waste of time and resources for both patient and staff.

Table 2.2 Some common additives present in blood collection tubes.

Additive	Purpose
Ethylenediaminetetraacetate (EDTA) – present as the potassium salt of this acid, i.e. K⁺-EDTA Colour code of tube top: lavender/purple	An anticoagulant that prevents blood from clotting by binding to and effectively removing the calcium present in blood (calcium is required for clotting to occur). EDTA also preserves the structure of blood cells. Principle use of EDTA tubes: full blood count (FBC) and some other haematology tests.
Heparin – present as the sodium or potassium salt of this acid, i.e. sodium or potassium heparin Colour code of tube top: dark green or orange	An anticoagulant that prevents blood from clotting by inhibiting the formation of thrombin from prothrombin. Principle use of heparin tubes: chemistry tests that require blood plasma.
Citrate – present as the sodium salt of this acid, i.e. sodium citrate Colour code of tube top: light blue	An anticoagulant that prevents blood from clotting by precipitating calcium, similar in action to EDTA. Principle use of citrate tube: coagulation study tests.
Oxalate – present as either the sodium or ammonium salt of this acid, i.e. sodium or ammonium oxalate Colour code of tube top: yellow or grey	An anticoagulant that prevents blood from clotting by precipitating calcium, similar in action to EDTA. Principle use of oxalate: used with sodium fluoride (see sodium fluoride entry) in tubes specifically for blood glucose measurement.
Sodium fluoride Colour code of tube top: yellow or grey	This is an enzyme poison that prevents continued metabolism of glucose by blood cells and thereby preserves blood glucose concentration. Principle use of sodium fluoride: used with oxalate in tubes specifically for blood glucose measurement.
Clot activator and gel Colour code of tube top: red or gold	This speeds up the blood clotting process and aids the separation of blood serum from blood cells. Principle use of clot activator/gel tubes: chemistry tests that require blood serum.

Safety during sample collection and transport

All laboratories have a locally written safety policy relating to the safe collection and transport of patient specimens, based on the premise that all patient specimens are potentially hazardous. Anyone involved in sample collection should be familiar with this policy. Among the many hazards that may be present in pathological specimens are viruses that cause AIDS and hepatitis, both of which can be transmitted by contact with infected blood. Tuberculosis can be transmitted by contact with infected sputum and gastrointestinal infections by contact with infected faeces. Good practice can have a major impact in reducing the risk to all staff and patients. The detail of good practice is included in the local safety policy. Some general points are included here.

- Disposable surgical gloves should be used during sample collection to reduce the risk of infection spread. Open sores offer an entry-point for microbial pathogens.
- Safe disposal of syringe and needles is vital. Needle stick injuries provide an excellent way of inoculating yourself with patient's blood, which may contain an infective virus.
- Leaking specimens present a major and surprisingly frequent potential hazard which can be prevented by the simple expedient of ensuring sample bottles are not overfilled and tops are well secured. Most clinical laboratories have a policy of discarding leaking specimens.
- Specimens should be transported in specially designed plastic bags which include a separate compartment for the accompanying pathology test request form.
- Specimen spillages should be dealt with in accordance with local policy.
- The use of additional protection (eye goggles, disposable gown) should be considered when collecting samples from patients known to be infected with HIV, or other blood transmissible virus e.g. those that cause viral hepatitis. Specimens from such patients should be clearly identified in some way according to locally agreed policy.

Topics relating to interpretation of laboratory results

The diversity of techniques used to examine patient samples results in many types of laboratory report. Anyone who has filed pathology reports in patient case notes will have noticed that test results may be expressed *quantitatively*, *semi-quantitatively* or *qualitatively*. All reports from the histopathology laboratory, for example, are qualitative; they take the form of highly technical written text, describing the appearance of tissue samples when viewed microscopically. The text will include a summary of the clinical significance of any deviations in appearance from that of normal tissue. Microbiological reports tend to be either qualitative or semi-quantitative. Text describes which pathogenic micro-organisms have been isolated from the sample, but the sensitivity of these micro-organisms to antibiotics tested is reported semi-quantitatively. In contrast, most reports from clinical chemistry and haematology laboratories are quantitative; they take the form of numerical results. As with any other numerical measurement (e.g. body weight, temperature, pulse rate), all quantitative results reported by clinical laboratories are defined by the unit of measurement.

Units of measurement used in clinical laboratories

Systeme international d'Unites (SI units)

Since the 1970s all units of scientific and clinical measurement in the UK have been based, wherever possible, on the SI system, devised in 1960. In the US non SI units continue to be used in the reporting of clinical laboratory results, so that care must be taken when interpreting laboratory results reported in US

Table 2.3 The seven basic SI units.

Basic SI unit	Measure of	Abbreviation/symbol
metre	length	m
kilogram	mass (weight)	kg
second	time	s
ampere	electric current	A
Kelvin	temperature	K
mole	amount of a substance	mol
candela	luminous intensity	cd

medical and nursing journals. Of the seven basic SI units (Table 2.3) only three are relevant to clinical laboratories. They are:

- the metre (m),
- the kilogram (kg),
- the mole (mol).

Although everyone is familiar with the metre as a unit of length and kilogram as a unit of mass or weight, the mole requires some explanation.

What is the mole (mol)?

The mole is defined as the quantity of a substance whose mass in grams is equal to its particle (i.e. molecular or atomic) weight. This is a useful measure because 1 mole of any substance contains the same number of particles, that is 6.023×10^{23}. This is known as Avogadro's number.

Examples

What is 1 mole of sodium (Na)?
Sodium is an element (single atom) whose atomic weight is 23.
Therefore 1 mole of sodium is 23 g of sodium

What is 1 mole of water (H_2O)?
Water is a molecule, composed of 2 atoms of hydrogen and 1 atom of oxygen.
The atomic weight of hydrogen is 1.
The atomic weight of oxygen is 16.
Therefore the molecular weight of water is $(2 \times 1) + 16 = 18$.
Therefore 1 mole of water is 18 g of water.

What is 1 mole of glucose?
A molecule of glucose is composed of:
  6 carbon atoms,
  12 hydrogen atoms,
  6 oxygen atoms.
The molecular formula of glucose is written $C_6H_{12}O_6$.

The atomic weight of carbon is 12.
The atomic weight of hydrogen is 1.
The atomic weight of oxygen is 16.
Therefore the molecular weight of glucose is

$$6 \times 12 = 72 \text{ plus}$$
$$12 \times 1 = 12 \text{ plus}$$
$$6 \times 16 = \underline{96}$$
$$180$$

Therefore 1 mole of glucose is 180 g glucose.

Thus 23 g of sodium, 18 g of water and 180 g of glucose all contain 6.023×10^{23} particles, either atoms in the case of sodium or molecules in the case of water and glucose. Knowing the molecular formula of any substance allows the use of mole as a unit of amount. For some molecular complex chemicals present in blood, for example, proteins, the precise molecular weight cannot be defined. The unit of amount (mole) cannot be used when measuring such substances; instead the kilogram is used.

Multiples and fractions of basic SI units

When the basic SI unit (metre, kilogram, or mole) is too large or too small for the measurement being made, it is convenient to use secondary units which are multiples or fractions of the basic unit. The SI system is decimal so that SI secondary units are expressed as powers of ten of the basic unit. Table 2.4 describes the most commonly used secondary SI units of length, mass (weight) and amount used in clinical and laboratory medicine.

Units for measuring volume

Strictly speaking the SI unit of volume should be based on the metre, that is cubic metre (m^3), cubic centimetre (cm^3), cubic millimetre (mm^3) etc.

However when the SI system was adopted for clinical measurements, it was decided to retain the litre as a measure of fluid volume because it was already in use and is almost exactly the same as $1000 \, cm^3$. In fact, 1 litre = $1000.028 \, cm^3$.

The litre (L or l) then is the basic 'SI' unit of volume. From this are derived the following secondary units of volume used in clinical and laboratory medicine:

decilitre (dL or dl) is 1/10 (one tenth or 10^{-1}) of a litre
centilitre (cL or cl) is 1/100 (one hundredth or 10^{-2}) of a litre
millilitre (mL or ml) is 1/1000 (one thousandth or 10^{-3}) of a litre
microlitre (μL or μl) is 1/1 000 000) (one millionth or 10^{-6}) of a litre

Note: 1 ml = $1.028 \, cm^3$

Units of concentration

Nearly all quantitative analysis of patient specimens involves determination of the concentration of a substance in blood or urine. Concentration is defined as the

Table 2.4 Secondary SI units of length, mass (weight) and amount used in laboratory medicine.

BASIC UNIT OF LENGTH – metre (m)

Secondary units

- centimetre (cm) is 1/100th (one hundredth or 10^{-2}) of a metre
  100 cm = 1 m
- millimetre (mm) is 1/1000th (one thousandth or 10^{-3}) of a metre
  1000 mm = 1 m   10 mm = 1 cm
- micrometre (μm) is 1/1 000 000 (one millionth or 10^{-6}) of a metre
  1 000 000 μm = 1 m   10 000 μm = 1 cm   1000 μm = 1 mm
- nanometre (nm) is 1/100 000 000 (one thousand millionth or 10^{-9}) of a metre
  1 000 000 000 nm = 1 m   10 000 000 nm = 1 cm   1 000 000 nm = 1 mm

BASIC UNIT OF MASS (WEIGHT) – kilogram (kg)

Secondary units

- gram (g) is 1/1000th (one thousandth or 10^{-3}) of a kilogram
  1000 g = 1 kg
- milligram (mg) is 1/1000th (one thousandth or 10^{-3}) of a gram
  1000 mg = 1 g   1 000 000 mg = 1 kg
- microgram (μg) is 1/000th (one thousandth or 10^{-3}) of a milligram
  1000 μg = 1 mg   1 000 000 μg = 1 g   1 000 000 000 μg = 1 kg
- nanogram (ng) is 1/1000th (one thousandth or 10^{-3}) of a microgram
  1000 ng = 1 μg   1 000 000 ng = 1 mg   1 000 000 000 ng = 1 g
- picogram (pg) is 1/1000th (one thousandth or 10^{-3}) of a nanogram
  1000 pg = 1 ng   1 000 000 pg = 1 μg   1 000 000 000 pg = 1 mg

BASIC UNIT OF AMOUNT – mole (mol)

Secondary units

- millimole (mmol) is 1/1000th (one thousandth or 10^{-3}) of a mole
  1000 mmol = 1 mol
- micromole (μmol) is 1/1000th (one thousandth or 10^{-3}) of a millimole
  1000 μmol = 1 mmol   1 000 000 μmol = 1 mol
- nanomole (nmol) is 1/1000th (one thousandth or 10^{-3}) of a micromole
  1000 nmol = 1 μmol   1 000 000 nmol = 1 mmol   1 000 000 000 nmol = 1 mol
- picomole (pmol) is 1/1000th (one thousandth or 10^{-3}) of a nanomole
  1000 pmol = 1 nmol   1 000 000 pmol = 1 μmol   1 000 000 000 pmol = 1 mmol

amount or mass (**weight**) of a substance that is contained in a specified **volume** of fluid. Units of concentration then comprise two elements; the unit of amount or mass (weight) and the unit of volume. For example, if we weigh out 20 g (mass) of salt and dissolve it in 1 l (volume) of water we have a solution of salt whose concentration is 20 g per litre. In this case the unit of mass (weight) is the gram and the unit of volume is the litre and the SI unit of concentration is gram per litre or g/L. Where the molecular weight of the substance being measured is precisely defined, as it is for many of the blood born chemicals measured in clinical laboratories, the mole (unit of amount) is used.

The 'real' examples given here demonstrate some of the variety of units used in the chemical analysis of blood.

Examples

What does the result **'plasma sodium 144 mmol/L'** mean?

Every litre of blood plasma contains 144 mmol of sodium, that is (144×23) mg or 3.3 g.

What does the result **'plasma albumin 23 g/L'** mean?

There are 23 grams of albumin in every litre of blood plasma.

What does the result **'plasma iron 9 µmol/L'** mean?

Every litre of blood plasma contains 9 micromoles of iron, that is (9×0.055) mg or 0.5 mg.

What does the result **'plasma B12 300 ng/L'** mean?

There are 300 ng or 0.0000003 g of the vitamin B12 in every litre of blood plasma.

Units of cell count

Much haematology testing involves counting the concentration of cells in blood. Here the unit of amount is the number of cells and the unit of volume is again the litre. Healthy individuals have between 4 500 000 000 000 (i.e. 4.5 million million) and 6 500 000 000 000 (i.e. 6.5 million million) red cells in every litre of blood. The unit of red cell count is the number of million million cells there are in 1 l of blood, expressed in short notation as 10^{12} per litre or 10^{12}/L. This allows the use of manageable numbers so that in normal practice we might say a patient has a red cell count of 5.3. This does not of course mean the patient has only 5.3 red cells; rather in every litre of blood, the patient has 5.3 million million red cells. There are far fewer white cells than red cells in blood and this is reflected in the unit of the white cell count, which is 10^{9}/L or the number of thousand million cells in every litre of blood.

The reference (normal) range

When making any clinical measurement, for example weighing a patient or measuring pulse rate, results are interpreted by reference to what is normal. The same is true of tests performed on patient samples.

All quantitative tests have a reference range recorded alongside patient test results to aid interpretation. Biological variation determines that just as there is no clear cut demarcation between normal and abnormal height and weight, there is no clear cut demarcation between normal and abnormal concentration of any constituent of blood and urine. The use of the term reference range in preference to normal range is recognition of this limitation. Reference ranges are constructed by measuring the substance in question in a large population of apparently healthy 'normal' individuals.

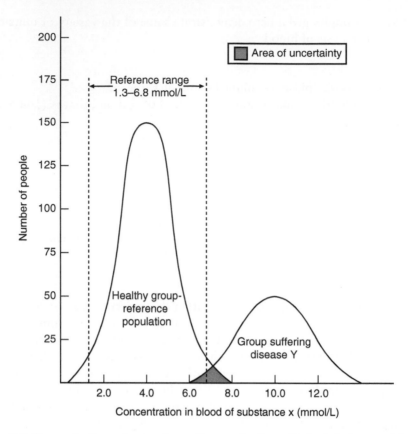

Figure 2.2 Demonstrating reference (normal) range for theoretical substance x and the overlap in blood concentration of x among healthy individuals and those suffering theoretical disease y (see text for explanation).

The graph in Figure 2.2 describes the results of measuring the concentration of hypothetical substance X in the blood of a large population of apparently healthy individuals (the reference population), and those with a hypothetical disease Y.

Since the blood concentration of substance X is usually raised in those suffering disease Y, it is used as a blood test to confirm the diagnosis among those with symptoms of Y. From the graph it can be seen that the concentration of X among apparently healthy individuals ranges from 0.3 to 8.0 mmol/L. The chance that a particular result is normal diminishes the further that result is away from the average or mean result of the reference population, in this case 4.0 mmol/L. The extreme ends of the range *may* represent abnormality. To take account of this, all reference ranges are conventionally constructed by excluding the results of 2.5% of the reference population, whose results lie at either end of this 'normal' range. By definition then, a reference range is the range in concentration of 95% of the reference (healthy) population. Hence in this case the reference range is 1.3–6.8 mmol/L. Using this reference range we can identify those who are suffering disease Y. Clearly there is a high degree of certainty that patients with a blood X concentration of more than 8.0 mmol/L are suffering disease Y, and that those with a concentration of less than 6.0 mmol/L, are not. However there is a grey area of uncertainty for those whose blood levels lie between 6.0 and 8.0 mmol/L. The poor discriminating power near the limits of a reference range is very typical of quantitative laboratory tests and should always be taken into account when interpreting laboratory test result.

For example, supposing the local reference range for serum sodium is 135–145 mmol/L, there is no doubt that a sodium concentration of 125 mmol/L is abnormal and may require treatment. By contrast an isolated sodium concentration of 134 mmol/L, although clearly outside the reference range, has no particular significance. Remember by definition 5% (i.e. 1 in 20) of the healthy population have a result outside the limits of a reference range.

Factors that affect the reference range

Various quite normal physiological factors may need to be taken into account when interpreting laboratory test results. Test results may be affected by:

- Age of the patient.
- Sex of the patient.
- Pregnancy.
- Time of the day the sample was collected.

For example, blood urea concentration rises with age and blood hormone levels are different among adult males compared with adult females. Pregnancy can affect the results of laboratory tests of thyroid function. Blood glucose levels fluctuate throughout the day. Alcohol and many drugs can affect blood test results in a variety of ways. The precise nature and extent of these physiological and drug effects will be considered in more detail as each test is discussed.

Harmonisation of reference ranges

Reference ranges vary depending on the particular analytical techniques used by laboratories. Historically, laboratories used different analytical techniques and consequently had to publish their own reference ranges. In recent years these analytical differences have diminished for many tests. This has enabled an ongoing project, started in 2007 and supported by the Department of Health[2,3], that aims to harmonise reference ranges for as many tests as possible. This means that for an increasing number of tests all UK hospital laboratories are using, or will soon be using, the same reference range. Throughout this book the reference ranges quoted will be the agreed harmonised reference range or, if that has not yet been agreed, an approximation of the reference range used in all laboratories. When interpreting any individual patient result, it is important to use only the reference range published by the laboratory that produced the test result.

Sensitivity and specificity

The sensitivity and specificity of a diagnostic test defines just how reliable that test is in making or excluding the diagnosis it is intended for. The ideal diagnostic test is 100% sensitive and 100% specific. A test that is 100% sensitive identifies all those with the disease – there are no false negatives, and one that is 100% specific is never positive in those without the disease – there are no false positives. To illustrate the concept consider pregnancy testing. Suppose a pregnancy test has a quoted sensitivity of 99.5% and specificity of 99.7%. This means that if 1000 pregnant women were submitted for the test, in 995 cases the result would be correctly positive but in five cases the result would be falsely negative. If 1000 non-pregnant women were submitted for the test 997 would be correctly negative but there would be three false positive results. In practice no laboratory test is 100% sensitive and 100% specific for a particular diagnosis but of course the closer to this ideal, the more reliable and useful is the test in making that diagnosis.

Critical values

When a patient test result lies outside the reference range, it is useful for nursing staff to know if the result warrants immediate clinical intervention. Should medical staff be informed urgently of this test result? The concept of critical values (inappropriately sometimes called 'panic' values) is intended to help with this area of decision making. A critical value has been defined as 'a pathophysiological state at such variance with normal as to be life-threatening, unless something is done promptly and for which some corrective action could be taken'[3]. Not all tests warrant critical values but, where appropriate throughout this book, suggested critical values for each test will be recorded alongside reference range values. As with reference ranges, critical values are determined by local laboratories; just as it is important to use locally published reference ranges in the interpretation of actual patient test results, so too nurses should follow local protocol relating to critical values.

Difference between serum and plasma

Throughout this book reference will be made to blood serum (or simply serum) and blood plasma (or simply plasma). Before leaving this chapter it is important to clarify what these terms mean.

Blood is composed of cells (red cells, white cells and platelets) suspended in a liquid, which is essentially an aqueous (water) solution of many different inorganic and organic chemicals. It is this liquid which is analysed in most clinical chemistry and some haematological blood tests. The first step for all these tests is to separate and remove the liquid part from the cells. In physiology texts the liquid is called plasma.

Case history 1

On the second day following elective surgery, Alan Howard, a 46 year old man, was feeling unwell. Blood was taken for a range of chemical tests and a full blood count (FBC). Among the results phoned back to the ward were the following:

Plasma Sodium	135 mmol/L	(reference range 135–145)
Plasma Potassium	8.0 mmol/L	(reference range 3.5–5.2)
Plasma Bicarbonate	28 mmol/L	(reference range 25–35)
Plasma Urea	5.5 mmol/L	(reference range 2.5–6.6)
Plasma Calcium	1.10 mmol/L	(reference range 2.35–2.75)

The FBC results were normal. Realising that the potassium and calcium results were critical values, the patient's named nurse immediately informed the surgical house officer, who took a second sample. Twenty minutes later the laboratory telephoned back with an entirely normal set of results. It transpired that the person who had taken the first sample had overfilled the full blood count bottle and tipped blood into the bottle for chemistry tests to bring the level in the full blood count bottle down to the right mark on the label.

Question

How did this cause the abnormal potassium and calcium results?

Discussion of case history

Blood for a full blood count must be prevented from clotting. This is achieved by the presence in the sample tube of a chemical anticoagulant namely the potassium (K^+) salt of **e**thylene**d**iamine**t**etr**a**acetate (or more manageably, K^+-EDTA). This is an anti-coagulant which works by chelating (effectively removing) calcium from blood. (Calcium is essential for the normal clotting process.) The addition of K^+-EDTA, whilst preventing blood from clotting, has two incidental effects: it raises the potassium concentration and reduces calcium concentration. The small volume of blood that was tipped into the bottle for U&E contained sufficient K^+-EDTA to markedly reduce calcium concentration and increase potassium concentration. This case history demonstrates that a K^+-EDTA sample of blood is unsuitable for potassium and calcium estimation, and provides a graphic illustration of one of many ways in which poor sampling technique can adversely affect laboratory results. In this case the abnormal results were actually incompatible with life and therefore easily identified. Less dramatic changes, which may remain undetected and therefore potentially more dangerous, can be caused by poor practice at the time of sample collection and transport.

An alternative name is serum. The essential difference between serum and plasma is the sample tube into which blood is collected. If blood is collected into a plain tube containing no additive or a tube containing a chemical gel that accelerates the clotting process, the blood will clot and the liquid recovered is serum. By contrast if blood is collected into a tube containing an anticoagulant the whole blood sample remains fluid (does not clot). The fluid that remains when cells have been removed from this sample is called plasma. With some important exceptions, most notably tests of blood coagulation, the results from testing either plasma or serum are virtually the same; in these circumstances it is a matter of local laboratory preference which is used.

References

1. Pathology harmony website www.pathologyharmony.co.uk.
2. Berg, J. and Lane, V. (2011) Pathology harmony; a pragmatic and scientific approach to unfounded variation in the clinical laboratory, *Annals Clin Biochem*, 48:195–7.
3. Emancipator, K. (1997) Critical values – ascp practice parameter, *Am J Clin Pathol*, 108: 247–53.

Further reading

Lavery, I. and Smith, E. (2008) Venepuncture practice and the 2008 nursing & midwifery code, *Br J Nursing*, 17: 824–8.

McCallk, R. and Tankersley, C. (2011) *Phlebotomy Essentials* (5th edition) Lippinicott Williams & Wilkins.

Narayanan, S. (2000) The preanalytical phase. An important component of laboratory medicine, *Am J Clin Pathol*, 113: 429–52.

Shah, V. and Tadido, A. (2005) Neonatal blood sampling, available on the web at: http://www.acutecaretesting.org

Sharma, P. (2009) Preanalytical variables and laboratory performance, *Indian J Clin Biochem*, 24:109–10.

Skales, K. (2008) A practical guide to venepuncture and blood sampling, *Nursing Standard*, 22: 29–36.

PART 2

Clinical Biochemistry Tests

CHAPTER 3

BLOOD GLUCOSE AND HbA1c

Key learning topics

- Function of glucose as an energy source
- Hormone regulation of blood glucose concentration
- Defining normal and abnormal blood glucose
- Diabetes and diabetic ketoacidosis
- Using blood glucose to diagnose diabetes
- Using blood glucose and HbA1c to monitor diabetes
- Non-diabetic causes of raised blood glucose
- Causes and effects of reduced blood glucose

The most significant reason for measurement of the concentration of glucose in blood is diagnosis and monitoring of diabetes mellitus (known commonly as simply diabetes). This is a common chronic metabolic disease, most often associated with obesity, that represents a major and ever growing health problem in the UK, and around the world. Close to 2.9 million people in the UK (4.7% of the total population) are diagnosed with diabetes; an estimated further 850 000 have diabetes but remain undiagnosed[1]. Recent study[2] suggests that by 2035 there will be over 6.25 million diabetic patients in the UK (8.6% of projected total population). Current annual cost to the NHS of diabetes is estimated at £10 billion (10% of total NHS spending); this is forecast to rise to £16.9 billion by 2035[2].

As we shall see, abnormality in blood glucose concentration is not confined to those suffering diabetes. This chapter also includes consideration of another test, HbA1c, which is used for monitoring the effectiveness of diabetes treatment.

Understanding Laboratory Investigations: A Guide for Nurses, Midwives and Healthcare Professionals, Third Edition. Chris Higgins.
© 2013 John Wiley & Sons, Ltd. Published 2013 by John Wiley & Sons, Ltd.

Normal physiology

The carbohydrate present in the food we eat accounts for around 60% of our dietary requirement. In the gastrointestinal tract, complex food carbohydrates (starches) are digested by enzymes to simple molecules, for absorption to the blood stream. These simple molecules are the monosaccharides: glucose, fructose and galactose. Of these, glucose is by far the most abundant, representing on average around 80% of absorbed monosaccharides. Once inside the body most of the fructose and galactose is converted to glucose. Nearly all of our dietary carbohydrate then is converted to glucose. Most cells in the body also have mechanisms for converting non-carbohydrates (fats and proteins) to glucose when demand for glucose is high and supply is low (starvation).

Why is glucose important?

Glucose can only function within cells, where it is the major source of energy. In every cell of the body this energy is realised by the metabolic oxidation of glucose to carbon dioxide and water. In the process the energy contained within glucose is used to form the energy rich compound adenosine triphosphate (ATP) from adenosine diphosphate (ADP). The energy contained within ATP in turn is used to drive the many chemical reactions within the cell that are needed for it to remain viable and fulfil its function (Figure 3.1).

The oxidation of glucose, with resulting generation of energy rich ATP occurs in two major cellular metabolic pathways (Figure 3.2). They are the glycolytic pathway (sometimes called simply glycolysis or the Embden-Meyerhof pathway after the two scientists who first described it) and the Krebs cycle (alternative name tricarboxylic acid cycle). The process begins with the glycolytic pathway, in which glucose is converted (oxidised) via 13 separate enzymic reactions to the tri-carboxylic acid, pyruvate. The fate of pyruvate depends on the relative amount of tissue oxygen. In normally oxygenated tissue, pyruvate is converted to a substance called acetyl CoA which enters the Krebs cycle and joins (condenses) with another tri-carboxylic acid, oxaloacetic acid to form citric acid. In a further nine enzymic reactions, citric acid is converted back to oxaloacetic acid for condensation with more acetyl CoA generated by glycolysis.

Oxidation of one molecule of glucose in the glycolytic pathway yields two molecules of pyruvate and eight molecules of ATP. Further oxidation of the two molecules of pyruvate generated by glycolytic pathway in Krebs cycle yields a further 30 molecules of ATP. So in total, oxidation of one molecule of glucose to CO_2 and H_2O yields 38 molecules of energy rich ATP.

In the absence of sufficient oxygen, glucose can be converted to pyruvate by the glycolytic pathway, but pyruvate cannot enter Krebs cycle. Instead it is converted to lactate (lactic acid). Accumulation of lactic acid in the blood occurs in any illness (usually critical illness) in which, for any number of reasons, oxygen delivery to tissue cells is compromised. This accumulation of lactic acid is a direct result of anaerobic glycolysis (i.e. glycolysis in tissues with relative oxygen deficiency).

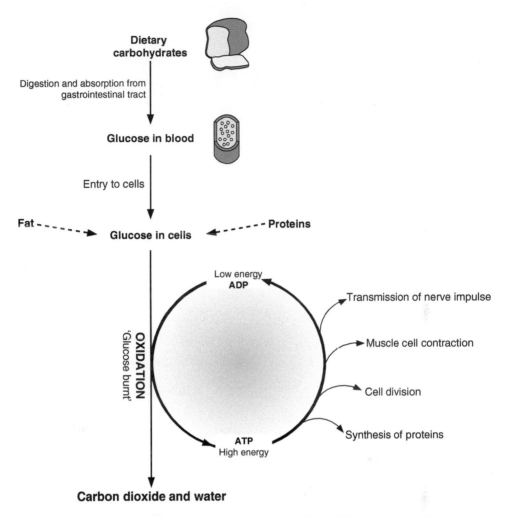

Figure 3.1 Glucose has central metabolic role within cells providing energy for the chemical reactions required for cells to function.

Importance of maintaining normal blood glucose concentration

Unlike other tissues, the brain is unable to manufacture or store glucose and is dependent on a ready supply of glucose in blood for its energy requirements. The maintenance of a minimum amount of glucose in blood is essential for normal brain function. Blood glucose concentration above around 4.0 mmol/L ensures this function. It is equally important however to ensure that blood glucose concentration does not rise too high. Glucose is an osmotically active substance. This means that as the concentration of glucose in blood rises its osmotic effect tends to draw water out of surrounding cells leaving them relatively dehydrated. In order to combat this potentially lethal effect on cells, the kidneys compensate by excreting glucose in urine when blood levels rise above a certain concentration called the renal threshold (usually around 10.0–11.0 mmol/L). However, in doing this, the

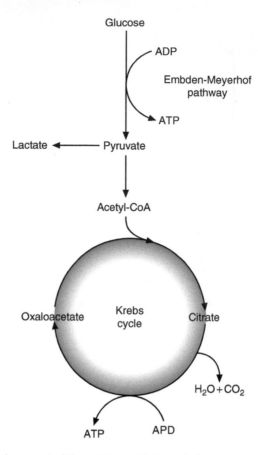

Figure 3.2 Simplified account of the cellular oxidation of glucose.

valuable energy resource which glucose represents, is lost from the body. For good health then, blood glucose concentration must not rise above a maximum level, or the body's most significant energy resource will be lost in urine, but it must not fall too low either, or brain function will be threatened.

Glucose can be stored

Although all cells require glucose for energy, the demand may vary between cells and will vary at different times of the day. For example, muscle cell demand will be highest during exercise and lowest during sleep. Cellular demand for glucose does not always coincide with meals when glucose is available and there is therefore a need to store dietary glucose until it is required. Most cells in the body can store limited amounts of glucose but three sorts of tissue mainly serve this function:

- liver,
- muscle,
- fat (adipose tissue).

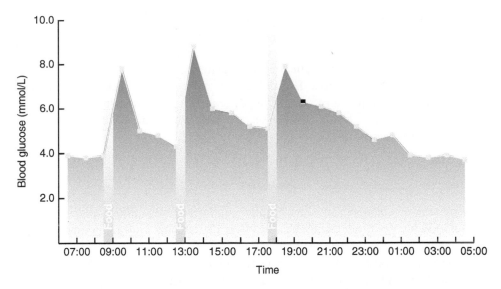

Figure 3.3 Typical variation of blood glucose concentration throughout the day.

The cells of these organs are able to remove glucose from blood and store it when demand is low or supply is high (immediately after meals). Between meals when glucose is in short supply glucose is mobilised from these stores.

Liver and muscle cells store glucose as the polymer molecule glycogen, which is effectively many glucose molecules joined together. The enzymic process by which glycogen is formed from glucose in these cells is called glycogenesis. The reverse process called glycogenolysis allows glucose to be recovered from this store and occurs in response to a falling blood glucose concentration. Glucose can be taken up by fat cells and converted by a process called lipogenesis to triglyceride, a fat, and stored in this form. Triglyceride can be mobilised from fat stores to provide energy by a process known as lipolysis, but this will only occur after glycogen stores are depleted. In this way glycogen provides short-term storage of glucose and fat provides long-term storage of glucose.

How is blood glucose concentration maintained within the normal range?

Despite the considerable variation in glucose intake and utilisation throughout the day, blood glucose concentration never usually rises above around 8.0 mmol/L or falls below around 3.5 mmol/L. Figure 3.3 describes typical normal daily fluctuation.

Immediately after a meal blood glucose concentration rises as glucose derived from food is absorbed from the gut. The cells of the body take up this glucose; some is utilised to satisfy current energy requirement and any excess is stored as glycogen in liver and muscle cells, or as fat (triglyceride) in adipose tissue. As a consequence of this movement of glucose from blood to cells, blood glucose concentration falls between meals. However in order to maintain minimum blood glucose concentration between meals, glucose is mobilised from hepatic glycogen stores. If necessary glucose may also be manufactured within cells from non-carbohydrate sources such as protein, by a process called gluconeogenesis.

Both the uptake of glucose from blood by cells and the metabolic pathways involved in blood glucose regulation (glycogenesis, glycogenolysis etc.) are under the overall control of hormones, the secretion of which are governed in turn by blood glucose concentration.

Hormonal control of blood glucose concentration

The pancreatic hormones insulin and glucagon are the most important for regulating blood glucose levels. Insulin has the effect of reducing blood glucose levels by:

- Promoting uptake of glucose by cells from blood (the uptake of glucose by cells of the liver and central nervous system is independent of insulin).
- Promoting the cellular metabolism (oxidation) of glucose to pyruvate (glycolysis).
- Increasing formation of glycogen from glucose in liver and muscle (glycogenesis).
- Increasing formation of triglyceride from glucose in adipose cells (lipogenesis).
- Inhibiting production of glucose from non-carbohydrate sources (gluconeogenesis).

Insulin is synthesised in, and secreted by the beta (β) cells of the pancreas in response to rising blood glucose concentration, and operates by binding to insulin receptors present on the surface of insulin sensitive cells. The normal hormonal response to rising blood glucose depends then on:

- adequate amount of insulin and therefore normally functioning pancreatic β cells; and
- adequate and functioning insulin receptors on the surface of insulin sensitive cells.

Without either of these, blood glucose concentration continues to rise.

Glucagon is an insulin antagonist hormone synthesised in, and secreted from, the alpha (α) cells of the pancreas in response to a falling blood glucose concentration. In direct contrast to the action of insulin, glucagon has the effect of raising blood glucose levels by:

- Increasing hepatic production of glucose from glycogen (glycogenolysis).
- Increasing production of glucose from non-carbohydrate sources (gluconeogenesis).

To recap, rising blood glucose concentration stimulates the pancreas to secrete insulin. By its various effects, insulin reduces blood glucose concentration. Falling blood glucose levels induces glucagon secretion, which prevents further blood

Table 3.1 Hormones involved in regulating blood glucose concentration.

Hormone	Site of production and release to blood	Released to blood in response to	Effect on blood glucose concentration
Insulin	Pancreas (β-cells)	Raised blood glucose concentration	Reduces blood glucose concentration
Glucagon	Pancreas (α-cells)	Reduced blood glucose concentration	Increases blood glucose concentration
Epinephrine (adrenaline)	Adrenal glands (adrenal medulla)	Stress	Increases blood glucose concentration
Cortisol	Adrenal glands (adrenal cortex)	Reduced blood glucose concentration and/or stress	Increases blood glucose concentration
Growth hormone	Anterior pituitary gland	Reduced blood glucose concentration and/or stress	Increases blood glucose concentration

glucose reduction. Continuous synergy of these two opposing hormonal effects ensures that blood glucose concentration is maintained within normal limits.

Three further hormones are secreted in response to a low blood glucose concentration and also in response to stress. They are: cortisol, synthesised by the adrenal cortex; epinephrine (formerly known as adrenalin), synthesised by the adrenal medulla; and growth hormone, secreted by the anterior pituitary. These all have the effect of increasing blood glucose concentration. There are then four hormones, glucagon, cortisol, epinephrine and growth hormone, that serve to prevent blood glucose concentration falling too low, but only insulin prevents blood glucose concentration from rising too high. This reflects the prime importance of maintaining adequate minimal level of glucose in blood for normal brain function. Table 3.1 provides a summary of the hormones involved in blood glucose regulation.

Laboratory measurement of blood or plasma glucose

Patient preparation

If the test is to determine fasting blood glucose, no food should be taken for at least 12 hours prior to blood sampling; otherwise no particular patient preparation is necessary.

Timing of sample

Blood glucose concentration varies throughout the day, highest at around 1 hour after the main meal of the day and lowest first thing in the morning before food; correct interpretation demands that the time be recorded on the specimen. Samples may be random (without reference to time of food), fasting (sample taken after an overnight 12 hour fast) or 2 hour post-prandial (sample taken 2 hours after a meal).

Sample requirement

Around 2 ml venous blood is collected into a special tube (most often grey or yellow top), containing the glucose preservative sodium fluoride and an anticoagulant, potassium oxalate. Fluoride is an enzyme poison that effectively prevents continued red cell glycolysis, and therefore preserves glucose concentration. Anticoagulant prevents the sample from clotting. The blood should be mixed with these chemicals by gentle inversion. Glucose may be measured directly on the whole blood sample, or on plasma recovered from the blood sample.

Reference range

Fasting blood glucose	3.5 – 5.0 mmol/L.
Random blood glucose	3.5 – 8.0 mmol/L.
Two hour post-prandial glucose	at 2 hours after food, glucose levels should be falling toward normal fasting concentration.

[Note: Plasma glucose results are between 10–15% higher than those derived from whole blood.]

Terms used in interpretation of results

Normoglycaemia	normal blood or plasma glucose concentration.
Hyperglycaemia	raised blood or plasma glucose concentration.
Hypoglycaemia	low blood or plasma glucose concentration.

Critical values

Blood glucose <2.2 mmol/L or >25.0 mmol/L. Severe hypoglycaemia, particularly among neonates, is associated with the risk of convulsions, coma and permanent brain damage. Severe hyperglycaemia may signal ketoacidosis or hyperosmolal (nonketotic) coma; these are acute life threatening complications of diabetes.

Causes of abnormal blood glucose

Abnormality of blood glucose concentration (either hyper- or hypoglycaemia) is almost always the result of too little or too much of one of the hormones required for normal regulation of blood glucose concentration. The most significant cause of hyperglycaemia by far is diabetes mellitus.

Diabetes mellitus

Diabetes mellitus – which must be distinguished from diabetes insipidus, a quite separate and much rarer disease – is the name given to a group of disorders that are characterised by hyperglycaemia, due to an absolute or relative deficiency of

Table 3.2 Major features that distinguish Type 1 and Type 2 diabetes.

Type 1 diabetes	Type 2 diabetes
Less common (accounts for 10–15% of total diabetic population)	More common (accounts for 85–90% of total diabetic population)
Usually diagnosed in childhood (peak age at diagnosis 10–14 years)	Usually diagnosed in adults over the age of 40 years. Prevalence increases with age beyond 40 years. Increase in child obesity has driven the emergence of Type 2 diabetes in childhood, once a very rare occurrence
Little or no insulin production	Insulin production normal or may be increased
Genetic factors less significant	Genetic factors more significant – very often a family history
Patients typically not obese – may be thin	Obesity common and a significant causative risk factor
Ketoacidosis is a common presenting feature at diagnosis and can occur after diagnosis	Ketoacidosis – rare
Absolute requirement for insulin	No absolute requirement for insulin in the short term – treatment usually based on tablets (hypoglycaemic agents) that reduce blood glucose concentration. Insulin treatment may eventually become necessary

insulin. Glucose accumulates in blood for two main reasons. Firstly, glucose present in blood cannot enter cells (except those of the liver and brain) in the absence of an effective insulin response. Secondly, hepatic production of glucose from glycogen (glycogenolysis) is inappropriately increased by insulin deficiency.

Primary diabetes is classified on clinical and aetiological grounds to one of two main types. Type 1 diabetes, which accounts for around 10–15% of the total diabetic population, results from selective autoimmune destruction of the insulin producing β cells of the pancreas. These people have an absolute insulin deficiency and require daily injections of exogenous insulin for survival. Type 2 diabetes is much more common, accounting for around 85–90% of the diabetic population. Here the primary problem is not insulin deficiency but lack of insulin effect (sometimes called insulin resistance); the cellular response to normal physiological insulin levels is defective. Type 2 diabetes is strongly linked to obesity and this link largely accounts for the increasing prevalence of diabetes among adults and the recent emergence of Type 2 diabetes in children, once an extremely rare occurrence. Some of the distinguishing features of Type 1 and Type 2 diabetes are highlighted in Table 3.2.

Pregnancy is associated with a number of hormonal changes that predispose to diabetes. Depending on the population studied, as well as the criteria adopted for diagnosis, between 1% and 14% of women become temporarily diabetic during their pregnancy; the prevalence of this complication of pregnancy is increasing[3]. When diabetes is diagnosed during pregnancy it is called gestational diabetes. The

Table 3.3 Most common causes of secondary diabetes.

Primary disease	Underlying pathology	Hormone affected	Effect on blood glucose
Acromegaly (gigantism)	Tumour of the pituitary gland	Increased growth hormone production	INCREASE blood glucose
Cushing's disease/ syndrome	Overactivity of the adrenal cortex	Increased cortisol production	INCREASE blood glucose
Phaeochromocytoma	Tumour of the adrenal medulla	Increased epinephrine production	INCREASE blood glucose
Haemochromatosis	Accumulation of iron in the pancreas – β-cell damage	Decreased insulin production	INCREASE blood glucose
Chronic pancreatitis	Inflammation of the pancreas – β-cell damage	Decreased insulin production	INCREASE blood glucose

diagnosis does not apply to those women with Type 1 or Type 2 diabetes who subsequently become pregnant. In most cases of gestational diabetes, the abnormality disappears at the end of the pregnancy. However women with a history of gestational diabetes have a significantly greater than normal lifelong risk of developing Type 2 diabetes; a recent follow up study found that close to 20% develop Type 2 diabetes within nine years of their pregnancy[4]. All women with a history of gestational diabetes should be offered lifelong regular (annual) fasting blood glucose testing to screen for Type 2 diabetes.

In addition to Type 1, Type 2 and gestational diabetes, there is a fourth group of diabetic patients whose diabetes is caused by some underlying, quite separate disease or by the action of some drugs (most notably steroids). This very small subset of the total diabetic population are said to be suffering secondary diabetes. Successful treatment of the underlying disease or withdrawal of an offending drug cures diabetes in such cases. Causes of secondary diabetes are listed in Table 3.3.

Whether the disease be primary diabetes (i.e. Type 1 or Type 2), gestational diabetes or much more rarely secondary diabetes, all untreated diabetic patients have a raised blood glucose. A consistently normal blood glucose concentration excludes the diagnosis.

Signs and symptoms of diabetes

So long as blood glucose concentration remains within normal limits, urine contains no detectable glucose. However as blood glucose concentration rises above the renal threshold, which for most people (i.e. diabetics and non diabetics), is between 10 and 12 mmol/L, glucose begins to be lost in urine. By its strong osmotic effect, glucose draws water with it, causing polyuria (increased urine volume) and potential dehydration. This stimulates thirst centres in the brain to increase fluid intake. By these mechanisms severe hyperglycaemia causes five classical signs or symptoms of untreated diabetes:

- Glucose excreted in urine (glycosuria).
- Increased urination, often at night (polyuria, nocturia).
- Thirst.
- Increased fluid intake (polydipsia).
- Dehydration (only if compensatory increased fluid intake is not sufficient to replace fluid lost in urine).

Type 2 diabetes has a long sub-clinical period during which hyperglycaemia is not sufficiently severe to cause symptoms, or perhaps mild symptoms may go unrecognised. A diagnosis is often made quite by chance when a raised blood glucose or glycosuria is discovered during a general health screen or investigation of some apparently unrelated medical problem. Diabetes is associated with increased risk of some bacterial and fungal infections, for example, skin abscess or boils; urinary tract infection; candida infection of the penis (balanitis); and female genital tract (vaginitis). Such infections may be the first sign of Type 2 diabetes.

The autoimmune damage to pancreatic cells that causes Type 1 diabetes begins in the very early years and accumulates over many years until the resulting insulin deficiency is sufficient to cause clinical signs, usually in late childhood years or early adolescence. Onset is usually acute and the first evidence of diabetes among this group may be diabetic ketoacidosis, an acute and life threatening metabolic disturbance that results from severe insulin deficiency.

Diabetic ketoacidosis

In the absence of insulin, glucose cannot enter cells and an alternative energy source is required for cells to survive and function. Such an alternative is provided for by the stored fat (triglyceride) in adipose tissue. Many of the symptoms of diabetic ketoacidosis are a result of mobilisation of fat to provide energy in the absence of intracellular glucose. Incidentally, the mobilisation of fat as a source of energy is a quite normal physiological response to starvation, when dietary glucose is absent and glycogen stores are exhausted.

The first step in realising the potential energy in fat is enzymic splitting of triglyceride (lipolysis) to release constituent fatty acids. Fatty acids are transported from adipocytes via blood to all the cells of the body, where they are utilised as an energy source. In the liver, fatty acids are oxidised. The products of this oxidation are two keto-acids (acetoacetate and 3-hydroxybutyrate) and acetone, collectively called ketones. Normally these products of fat metabolism would be metabolised further. However in diabetic ketoacidosis, the rate of their production outstrips the rate of their metabolism and they accumulate in blood and are excreted in urine. Some acetone is excreted by the lungs and can be smelt on the breath of a patient in ketoacidosis. Accumulation of keto-acids in blood overwhelms the normal homeostatic mechanisms that maintain normal blood pH, with development of metabolic acidosis (see Chapter 7).

Increased respiration (hyperventilation) to promote removal of carbon dioxide from the blood, thereby restoring normal blood pH is a normal compensatory mechanism in metabolic acidosis. This is clinically evident as a deep sighing respiration (Kussmaul breathing) in patients with ketoacidosis. To summarise then, in addition to symptoms already mentioned due to hyperglycaemia – glycosuria, polyuria, thirst, polydipsia and dehydration – patients in diabetic ketoacidosis also:

- Have ketones in blood and urine (ketonaemia, ketouria).
- Have the smell of acetone on their breath.
- Have a metabolic acidosis (low blood pH).
- Hyperventilate (exhibit Kussmaul breathing).
- Are usually hypotensive due to severe fluid and electrolyte loss in urine and vomit (vomiting is common in diabetic ketoacidosis).

Without treatment, patients have decreasing level of consciousness and can eventually lapse into coma. Low blood volume consequent on fluid loss threatens normal perfusion of the kidney, so that acute kidney disease (renal failure) may occur if blood volume is not restored immediately.

Laboratory diagnosis of diabetes

Criteria for laboratory diagnosis of diabetes are based on expert recommendations made in 1997[5] and reviewed by the World Health Organisation (WHO) in 2006[6].

Diabetes is confirmed if a single fasting blood glucose is greater than 6.1 mmol/L (plasma glucose 7.0 mmol/L) or random blood glucose is greater than 10.0 mmol/L (plasma glucose 11.1 mmol/L) on at least two occasions. If a patient has symptoms strongly suggestive of diabetes but fasting or random glucose concentration is not sufficiently high to make the diagnosis, a glucose tolerance test (GTT) is indicated.

Glucose tolerance test

Principle: the GTT involves measuring blood glucose before and after ingestion of a standard (75gm) glucose dose, on a fasted patient.

Patient preparation: for at least three days prior to the test, patients must be on a normal carbohydrate diet (i.e. > 150 g/day). The test is conducted in the morning following an overnight fast of at least 12 hours. The patient may have free access to water. Smoking on the morning of the test should be prohibited.

Test protocol: blood is sampled for fasting glucose estimation and 75 g of glucose dissolved in 300 ml water administered by mouth (a more palatable alternative is 353 ml of Lucozade). Two hours later, a second blood sample is taken for glucose estimation.

Interpretation: the normal response to a glucose load is an initial increase in blood glucose, which stimulates insulin secretion. This in turn reduces blood glucose so that at two hours, glucose concentration has returned to near fasting levels. In both Type 1 and 2 diabetes, blood glucose remains high. Table 3.4 describes how the results of a GTT are used to make or exclude a diagnosis of diabetes.

Table 3.4   Interpretation of glucose tolerance test results.

	Fasting plasma glucose (mmol/L)	Plasma glucose (mmol/L) at 2hrs after 75g glucose
Diabetes	Equal to or greater than 7.0 (6.1)	Equal to or greater than 11.1 (10.0)
Impaired glucose tolerance	Less than 7.0 (6.1)	7.8–11.1 (6.7–10.0)
Impaired fasting glycaemia	6.1–7.0 (5.3–6.1)	
Normal	Less than 5.5 (4.9)	Less than 7.8 (6.7)

Note: Figures in parentheses should be used for interpretation if blood glucose rather than plasma glucose is measured.

The term impaired glucose tolerance is reserved for those patients whose results do not indicate diabetes but which nevertheless are abnormal. Such patients are at increased risk of diabetes and should be re-tested annually. Adoption of a healthy lifestyle (diet, exercise) and normalisation of body weight and blood pressure, where indicated, can prevent progression of impaired glucose tolerance to Type 2 diabetes.

Antenatal screening for gestational diabetes

Gestational diabetes is invariably asymptomatic and so can only be identified by blood glucose screening. Current UK recommendations[7] are that the glucose tolerance test be used to screen pregnant women for gestational diabetes at 24–28 weeks of pregnancy, but only for selected women with any one of the following four high risk factors:

- Obesity – BMI > 30 kg/m.
- Previous large baby – birth weight > 4500 g.
- Family history of diabetes.
- High risk ethnicity (Asian, African, Hispanic).

There are no internationally agreed diagnostic criteria for gestational diabetes as there are for diagnosis of diabetes outside of pregnancy. Currently in the UK, gestational diabetes is diagnosed if glucose tolerance testing reveals fasting plasma glucose is equal to or greater than 7.0 mmol/L or 2 hour plasma glucose is equal to or greater than 7.8 mmol/L.

The Hyperglycaemia Adverse Pregnancy Outcome (HAPO) study has recently revealed that even the most mild degree of hyperglycaemia threatens the health of mother and baby, a notion that had previously been regarded as controversial. Results of this study have prompted a fresh look at diagnostic criteria and formulation of international guidelines[8] that recommend all pregnant women be screened at 24–28 weeks using the glucose tolerance test, and that gestational diabetes be diagnosed if fasting plasma glucose exceeds only 5.1 mmol/L (rather than 7.0 mmol/L); or 1 hour plasma glucose exceeds 10.0 mmol/L; or 2 hour plasma glucose exceeds 8.5 mmol/L. In the US, this recommended policy has already been adopted[9] and now all pregnant women in the US are offered a glucose tolerance test at their first antenatal visit to screen for pre-existing but undiagnosed Type 2 diabetes. If this test is normal a second test at 24–28 weeks is offered to screen for gestational diabetes. In the UK, recommended policy is currently under review in the light of the new evidence from the HAPO study and the proposed international guideline.

It is estimated that close to one in five pregnant women (rather than the current one in 20) would be diagnosed with gestational diabetes if the new diagnostic criteria are adopted.

Monitoring diabetic treatment

Patients with Type 1 diabetes have a lifelong need for daily insulin injections supplemented by dietary manipulation. For those with Type 2 or gestational diabetes, a combination of dietary manipulation and oral hypoglycaemic (glucose lowering) tablets is usually sufficient, though some may require insulin injections eventually.

Whatever the treatment, the principle objective is to maintain blood glucose concentration as close as is possible to that of the non-diabetic healthy population. Normalisation of blood glucose concentration not only removes the acute symptoms and complications of diabetes, such as dehydration, polyuria, thirst and ketoacidosis, but also significantly reduces the risk of the devastating long-term complications of diabetes: kidney disease (diabetic nephropathy), loss of vision (diabetic retinopathy), nerve damage (diabetic neuropathy) and cardiovascular disease[10,11,12]. So far as gestational diabetes is concerned, normalisation of blood glucose reduces the associated risks of hyperglycaemia to mother and baby that include: maternal hypertension and pre-eclampsia/eclampsia; large baby (foetal macrosomia) and consequent need for Caesarean delivery; neonatal jaundice; neonatal hypoglycaemia; and respiratory distress syndrome.

Striving to reduce blood glucose concentration to that of the non-diabetic population is associated with increasing risk of hypoglycaemia, an acute and dangerous consequence of diabetic over treatment. A careful balance has to be maintained.

The target of ideal control for Type 1 diabetes has been defined by the National Council for Clinical Excellence (NICE) as pre-prandial blood glucose concentration maintained in the range 4–8 mmol/L and post-prandial blood glucose concentration <10.0 mmol/L for children and <9.0 mmol/L for adults[13]. Diabetic patients, particularly those requiring insulin therapy, are often encouraged to self-monitor their blood glucose concentration regularly.

Patient self monitoring – blood glucose
A range of hand held blood glucose meters designed for use by diabetic patients in their home is commercially available. All have a similar mode of operation and allow measurement of blood glucose concentration from a single drop of capillary

blood, displaying a digital readout of within a minute or two. Poor technique can cause erroneous results. Adequate training and a continuing quality control programme are essential for results of optimum accuracy and precision. This requires co-operation between patients, diabetic nurse specialist and laboratory staff. The following points need to be borne in mind:

- Blood must be sampled from a clean, dry finger or ear lobe.
- Whatever the sampling device used for pricking the finger, it must result in free blood flow and not be dependent on squeezing the finger unduly, which can cause falsely low results. Warming the finger can increase blood flow.
- Blood must be dropped on (not smeared or spread) and must cover the entire reagent pad. False low results can occur if only part of the reagent pad is covered.
- The reagent contained in strips can deteriorate so strips must be stored in accordance with manufacturers' instructions. They must not be used once the printed expiry date has passed.

Quality control is essential. Some systems are internally calibrated. All systems should be tested at regular intervals using an external quality control solution of known blood glucose concentration. This confirms continuing reliability of both glucose meter and patient's analytical expertise.

Patient self monitoring – urine testing

Before methods for the estimation of blood glucose concentration outside the laboratory were available, diabetic patients monitored blood glucose concentration by testing urine for the presence of glucose. The test is performed using one of several commercially available urine glucose test strips that are, in principle, similar to those used for measuring blood glucose. A colour change on dipping the strip in urine indicates the presence of glucose. The test is semi-quantitative, so that increasing intensity of the colour change reflects increasing concentration of glucose in urine. A positive result indicates that at some time since the bladder was last emptied, blood glucose rose above the renal threshold, which is usually between 10 and 12 mmol/L. Since the renal threshold varies, and may be as low as 6.0 mmol/L, urine testing is a relatively crude indicator of blood glucose concentration. Furthermore it is unable to distinguish hypoglycaemia from normoglycaemia; the test is negative in both instances. Despite these limitations urine glucose testing continues to be used by a minority of diabetic patients to monitor blood glucose control.

Glycosylated haemoglobin (HbA1c)

This test is the most reliable way of assessing long-term blood glucose control and current guidelines suggest all diabetic patients should be offered this test every two to six months[13,14].

In health around 7% of the oxygen carrying protein haemoglobin contained in red blood cells has a glucose molecule attached and is said to be glycosylated. The actual amount of glycosylated haemoglobin (HbA1) is dependent on the concentration of blood glucose that red cells are exposed to during their 120 day life. At any one moment the amount of HbA1 reflects the mean (average) blood glucose concentration during the preceding two to three months, and provides a reliable retrospective view of blood glucose control. HbA1 is composed of three fractions (HbA1a, HbA1b and HbA1c). Of these HbA1c is quantitatively the most significant, accounting for nearly all glycosylated haemoglobin; this is the fraction measured in laboratories.

A 2.5 ml sample of venous blood collected into a bottle containing the anticoagulant EDTA (usually lavender/purple top) is required. No particular patient preparation is necessary and the sample can be taken at any time of day.

Interpretation of HbA1c results

[Units of measurement – prior to 2009 HbA1c results were universally expressed as a percentage (%) of total haemoglobin; that remains the case in the US. But in the UK and the rest of Europe HbA1c results are now expressed as mmol per mol of total haemoglobin (mmol/mol). The relationship between the two units of measurement are described in the following equation: HbA1c (%) = HbA1c (mmol/mol) ÷ 10.929 + 2.15]

Non-diabetic reference range HbA1c 28–42 mmol/mol (4.7–6.0%)
Diabetes HbA1c >48 mmol/mol (>6.5%)

National guidelines[13,14] define target HbA1c <59 mmol/mol for the generality of patients with Type 1 and Type 2 diabetes. Some patients with Type 2 diabetes, who are at higher than normal risk of cardiovascular disease, benefit from tighter blood glucose control and have a lower target of <48 mmol/mol. HbA1c above 60 mmol/mol represents increasingly poor blood glucose control and consequent increasing risk of suffering the long-term complications of diabetes. The estimated mean blood glucose concentration[15] over the preceding two to three months for a patient with an HbA1c of 59 mmol/mol is around 9.3 mmol/L; the equivalent figure for a patient with an HbA1c of 48 mmol/mol is around 7.7 mmol/L.

The HbA1c test is used to monitor the effectiveness of diabetes treatment. Over the 40 years since the test was first introduced to diabetic care there has been increasing level of interest in the notion that it could also be used to diagnose diabetes. In 2011 the test was finally approved for this purpose in the US; the finding of an HbA1c equal to or greater than 6.5% (48 mmol/mol) is sufficient evidence to make a diagnosis of diabetes in the US[9]. UK authorities have not yet approved the use of HbA1c for diagnosis of diabetes; the test is only used to monitor treatment. It seems likely that in the not too distant future UK authorities will follow the US lead and approve the HbA1c test for diagnosis as well as monitoring of diabetes[16].

Hyperglycaemia in the non-diabetic

A raised blood glucose does not necessarily indicate diabetes. A transient increase in blood glucose concentration often accompanies acute stress because epinephrine, a hormone produced in response to stress, is one of those that tend to increase blood glucose. An example of this mechanism is the transient hyperglycaemia that often accompanies myocardial infarction but any severe stress (e.g. trauma, surgery, critical illness) may be associated with raised blood glucose. For this reason critically ill patients requiring intensive care represent a patient group particularly prone to hyperglycaemia. What distinguishes these stress-related causes of hyperglycaemia from diabetes is their transitory nature. As the illness or trauma that precipitated the stress resolves, blood glucose concentration soon returns to normal. A landmark study, in 2001, provided evidence that correction of this transient hyperglycaemia with intensive insulin therapy improves the chances of surviving critical illness. Since then, aiming to ensure, with the use of insulin therapy if necessary, that blood glucose does not rise too much above 8.0 mmol/L has become a standard of care in the intensive care unit for all patients (both diabetic and non-diabetic).

Finally administration of IV fluids containing glucose and a range of drugs (e.g. corticosteroids, phenytoin, thiazide and loop diuretics) may cause increase in blood glucose concentration.

Hypoglycaemia

Hypoglycaemia is often defined as blood glucose concentration less than 2.2 mmol/L, although symptoms may occur at higher concentration (up to 3.0 mmo/L) Since the brain is dependent on an adequate supply of glucose in blood, low levels cause neuroglycopaenia, that is reduced glucose within the brain and throughout the central nervous system. Hypoglycaemia also stimulates synthesis and release of the insulin-antagonist hormones including the adrenal hormone, epinephrine, to increase blood glucose. It is a combination of neuroglycopaenia and increased epinephrine secretion which causes symptoms of hypoglycaemia

Signs and symptoms of hypoglycaemia

Those due to raised levels of circulating epinephrine may include:

- Feeling of hunger.
- Palpitations.
- Sweating.
- Fainting.
- Tremor.
- Feeling of anxiety.

Those due to reduced glucose in cells of the brain (neuroglycopaenia) may include:

- Lethargy.
- Headache.
- Confusion.
- Apparent drunkenness (unsteady gait, slurred speech).
- Convulsions.

Untreated, severe hypoglycaemia results in coma and (rarely) permanent brain damage. The condition is potentially fatal.

Causes of hypoglycaemia

Inappropriately high level of insulin is usually the cause, and diabetes related treatment (insulin, hypoglycaemic drugs) is by far the most common cause of hypoglycaemia. Striving to maintain normal blood glucose by non-physiological means (i.e. diabetic treatment modalities) is inevitably associated with risk of hypoglycaemia. Inadequate food intake after insulin dose and excessive exercise without insulin dose reduction represent two ways in which a diabetics lifestyle, when not matched well with insulin dose, can lead to hypoglycaemia. Diabetic patients learn to recognise the early symptoms of hypoglycaemia and take the appropriate action to raise blood glucose concentration. However with repeated episodes, this 'awareness of hypoglycaemia' is lost and in this circumstance blood glucose continues to fall to levels that precipitate the more serious neuroglycopaenic symptoms (convulsions and coma).

Hypoglycaemia among non-diabetics may be due to insulinoma (a rare tumour of the β cells of the pancreas) in which the normal control of insulin secretion is lost. The cells of the tumour continue to secrete insulin despite falling blood glucose.

A deficiency of any of the three hormones that increase blood glucose concentration and oppose the action of insulin may precipitate hypoglycaemia. For example, in Addison's disease the cells of the adrenal gland that normally produce cortisol are destroyed, and the resulting cortisol deficiency may precipitate hypoglycaemia.

The liver plays a central role in regulating blood glucose levels; this function remains intact during mild to moderate liver disease but hypoglycaemia may be a feature of severe liver disease. Alcohol is metabolised in the liver and inhibits the process of liver gluconeogenesis, which provides glucose during starvation. Alcoholics who are not eating adequately during a period of binge drinking are particularly at risk of hypoglycaemia for this reason.

Hypoglycaemia may be a feature of the neonatal period, particularly among premature babies. Babies born to diabetic mothers including those with gestational diabetes are at increased risk during the hours following birth. However there is often no identifiable cause. A very small minority of babies with hypoglycaemia, on further investigation, turn out to have an inherited (genetic) deficiency of one of the many enzymes involved in carbohydrate or fat metabolism. One of these conditions, called medium chain Acyl-CoA dehydrogenase deficiency (MCADD), is screened for at birth and discussed in Chapter 23.

Case history 2

Mrs Bishop is a slightly anxious 25 year old mother of two whose older brother has recently been diagnosed as suffering Type 2 diabetes. Mrs Bishop has read that diabetes runs in families and decides to test her urine for the presence of glucose, using her brother's urine test strips. A positive result convinces her that, although she feels well, she has diabetes. She goes to see her GP, who takes blood for glucose estimation. The random blood glucose result is well within the reference range at 6.2 mmol/L but, despite attempts at reassurance, Mrs Bishop remains convinced she has diabetes. Her concern is fuelled by two subsequent urine tests that are also positive for glucose. Her GP suggests a glucose tolerance test. The results of this were: fasting plasma glucose 4.8 mmol/L and plasma glucose, 2 hours after ingesting 75 g glucose, 7.5 mmol/L.

Questions

(1) Is Mrs Bishop right to be concerned?
(2) Does she have diabetes?
(3) What is the significance of the positive urine test for glucose?

Discussion of case history 2

(1) Mrs Bishop is justified in her concern, it is possible to inherit a predisposition to diabetes; in around a third of Type 2 diabetes cases there is a family history of the condition. Furthermore the presence of glucose in urine is a presenting feature of diabetes. The lack of symptoms is not an argument against the diagnosis. Many cases are discovered before symptoms develop, when blood or urine is tested for occupational or insurance health examinations.

(2) However, the results of Mrs Bishop's glucose tolerance test are entirely normal (see Table 3.4) and the diagnosis can be excluded on the basis of these results.

(3) Glycosuria, the presence of glucose in urine, usually only occurs when blood glucose concentration is high and is therefore suggestive of diabetes. The renal threshold is the blood glucose concentration above which glucose is detectable in urine. Normally this is around 10–12 mmol/L. For some people however, the renal threshold is significantly lower and glucose may appear in urine at normal blood glucose concentration. Mrs Bishop is among this group. The term 'renal glycosuria' is used to describe this entirely benign defect of kidney function. Although the finding of glucose in urine should never be ignored, it does not necessarily indicate diabetes.

Case history 3

Evan is a 19 year old student currently in his second year at university. He was diagnosed with Type 1 diabetes six years ago following urgent admission to hospital in a state of ketoacidosis. His plasma glucose on admission was 28.3 mmol/L. Evan's diabetes was generally well controlled throughout his early teenage years whilst at home, and he has suffered no further episodes of diabetic ketoacidosis. He now attends a local diabetic clinic in his university town. At his most recent appointment blood was sampled for random glucose estimation and HbA1c. Blood glucose was 7.8 mmol/L and HbA1c was 83 mmol/mol.

Questions

(1) What is the purpose of this blood testing?
(2) What do the results indicate? – is there any cause for concern?

Discussion of case history 3

(1) The purpose of these blood tests is to monitor the effectiveness of Evan's current insulin treatment regime and lifestyle choices in maintaining blood glucose concentration as close as is possible to that of the non-diabetic (healthy) population. This is important because raised blood glucose (hyperglycaemia) may precipitate the acute life-threatening complication, diabetic ketoacidosis, that brought him to hospital six years ago. Prolonged hyperglycaemia also significantly increases the risk that Evan may in later years suffer any one of several chronic complications of diabetes: renal failure (diabetic nephropathy); loss of vision (diabetic retinopathy); nerve damage (diabetic neuropathy), that might lead to necessary limb amputation; and cardiovascular disease (heart attack/stroke).

Blood glucose estimation alone only informs about blood concentration at the time blood was sampled. HbA1c is more informative because it is a measure of the mean (average blood glucose) over the preceding two to three months.

(2) Evan's blood results are somewhat conflicting; the blood glucose result is within the target for Type 1 diabetes, indeed is consistent with healthy non-diabetic status; by this measure his diabetes is well controlled. His HbA1c result however exceeds the target (<59 mmol/mol) for optimal glucose control. Using a novel, somewhat controversial, calculation based on HbA1c measurement[15] it is possible to determine that Evan's mean blood glucose during the previous two to three months was in the region of 12.8 mmol/L, which is well in excess of target blood glucose. His HbA1c result indicates diabetes is not well controlled.

It seems likely that Evan took special care to ensure that his blood glucose was within healthy limits for the hospital appointment but that overall, the scrupulous attention to insulin dosing, diet and exercise that ensured continuing good glucose control whilst at home has in recent months been somewhat lacking. This is not uncommon among young diabetics freed from the discipline of home life. Evan may benefit from sympathetic counselling aimed at emphasising the risk to his long-term health of continuing poor blood glucose control.

References

1. Diabetes UK (2011) Diabetes in the UK 2011/2012: Key statistics on diabetes, available at the Diabetes UK website: http://www.diabetes.org.uk/Documents/Reports/Diabetes-in-the-UK-2011-12.pdf.
2. Hex, N., Bartlett, C., Wright, D. et al. (2012) Estimating the current and future costs of type 1 and type 2 diabetes in the United Kingdom, including direct health costs and indirect societal and productivity costs, *Diabetic Medicine*, 29: 855–62.
3. Theodoraki, A., Baldweng, S. (2008) Gestational diabetes, *Br J Hosp Med*, 69: 562–67.
4. Feig, D., Zinmann, B., Wang, X. et al. (2008) Risk of development of diabetes mellitus after diagnosis of gestational diabetes, *CMAJ*, 179: 229–34.
5. Expert Committee on Diagnosis and Classification of Diabetes Mellitus (1997) Report of the Expert Committee on diagnosis and classification of diabetes mellitus, *Diabetes Care* 20: 1057–8.

6. International Diabetes Federation (2006) Definition and diagnosis of diabetes mellitus and immediate hyperglycemia: report of a WHO/IDF consultation, World Health Organisation.
7. National Institute for Health and Clinical Excellence NICE (2008) Diabetes in pregnancy: management of diabetes and its complication from pre-conception to the postnatal period (*Clinical Guideline 63*), RCOG Press.
8. International Associations of Diabetes and Pregnancy Study Groups (2010) International Associations of Diabetes and Pregnancy Study Groups recommendations on the diagnosis and classification of hyperglycemia in pregnancy, *Diabetes Care*, 33: 676–82.
9. American Diabetes Association (2011) Executive summary: standards of medical care in diabetes-2011, *Diabetes Care*, 34(1): S4–S10.
10. Diabetes Control and Complications Trial Research Group (DCCT) (1993) The effect of intensive treatment of diabetes on the development and progression of long term complications of diabetes, *New Eng J Med*, 329: 977–86.
11. UK Prospective Diabetes Study (UKPDS) group (1998) Intensive blood-glucose control with sulphonylureas or insulin compared with conventional treatment and risk of complication in patients with type 2 diabetes (UKPDS 33), *Lancet*, 352: 837–53.
12. Diabetes Control and Complications Trial Research Group (DCCT) (2005) Intensive diabetes treatment and cardiovascular disease in patients with type 1 diabetes, *New Eng J Med*, 353: 2643–53.
13. National Institute for Clinical Excellence NICE (2004) Type 1 diabetes: diagnosis and management of type 1 diabetes in children, young people and adults (*Clinical Guideline 15*), National Institute for Clinical Excellence.
14. National Collaborating Centre for Chronic Conditions (2008) Type 2 diabetes: national guideline for management in primary and secondary care (update), Royal College of Physicians.
15. Nathan, D. Kuenen, J., Borg, G. et al. (2008) Translating the A1C assay into estimated average glucose values, *Diabetes Care*, 31: 1473–78.
16. Day, A. (2012) HbA1c and diagnosis of diabetes. The test has finally come of age, *Ann Clin Biochem*, 49: 7–8.

Further reading

Cryer, P. (2008) The barrier of hypoglycemia in diabetes, *Diabetes*, 57: 3169–75.
Dineen, S., Heller, S. et al. (2010) Diabetes (Part 1), *Medicine*, 38: 589–638.
Dineen, S., Heller, S. et al. (2010) Diabetes (Part 2), *Medicine*, 38: 639–92.
Dungan, K., Braithwaite, S. et al. (2009) Stress hyperglycaemia, *Lancet*, 373: 1798–807.
Hawdon, J. (2008) NICE guidance for neonatal care after diabetes in pregnancy, *Infant*, 4:154–8.
Kielzel, M. and Marsons, L. (2009) Recognizing and responding to hyperglycaemic emergencies, *Br J Nursing*, 18: 1094–8.
Milic, T. (2008) Neonatal glucose homeostasis, *Neonatal Network*, 27: 203–07.

Useful websites

www.diabetes.org.uk
www.diabetes.nhs.uk

CHAPTER 4

PLASMA/SERUM SODIUM AND POTASSIUM

Key learning topics

- Maintaining normal sodium and water balance
- Maintaining normal potassium balance
- Poor blood sampling/transport can affect plasma potassium
- Causes and effects of raised plasma/serum sodium
- Causes and effects of reduced plasma/serum sodium
- Causes and effects of raised plasma/serum potassium
- Causes and effects of reduced plasma/serum potassium

The most frequently requested blood chemistry test is Urea and Electrolytes (U&E). This is not one but five tests performed simultaneously on the serum or plasma recovered from one sample of blood. These tests are: serum or plasma concentration of sodium, potassium, bicarbonate, urea and creatinine. The first three are electrolytes, that is positively or negatively charged ions in solution. This chapter focuses on the positively charged ions (cations), sodium (Na^+) and potassium (K^+). Bicarbonate, a negatively charged ion (anion), is considered in Chapter 7. Urea and creatinine are the subject of Chapter 5.

Physiology – sodium and water balance

[Note: An understanding of sodium and water balance requires outline knowledge of kidney function and the process by which urine is formed from filtered blood. This topic is not addressed here but in Chapter 5, and readers may wish to refer there for clearer understanding of some aspects of this section.]

Sodium is required for nerve cell conduction and bone formation but the principle physiological significance of sodium is that sodium concentration of extracellular fluid determines its volume, which in turn determines blood volume

Understanding Laboratory Investigations: A Guide for Nurses, Midwives and Healthcare Professionals, Third Edition. Chris Higgins.
© 2013 John Wiley & Sons, Ltd. Published 2013 by John Wiley & Sons, Ltd.

and thereby blood pressure. This function of sodium reflects the interrelatedeness of sodium and water metabolism. As will become clear monitoring water intake and output (fluid balance) is as important as measuring sodium concentration for elucidating cause and monitoring treatment of abnormal plasma sodium concentration.

Distribution of body water

Around 60% of human body weight is water; for an average adult weighing 70 kg this represents close to 40 L of water. Approximately 26 L is contained in the totality of cells within the body, this is called the intracellular fluid (ICF), and 14 L is outside cells and called the extracellular fluid (ECF). The ECF comprises approximately 3.5 L of plasma, the fluid (non-cellular) part of blood contained within the vascular system, and 10.5 L of interstitial (or extravascular) fluid, which fills the microscopical space between tissue cells (Figure 4.1).

It is vital for health that both the total amount of water in the body and its distribution between these compartments is constant. The passage of water across cell membranes, that is between the ECF and ICF, is dependent on the osmolarity on either side of the cell membrane; so long as this is equal, water will not pass and the volumes of each compartment are maintained. In health both plasma (ECF) osmolarity and ICF osmolarity is maintained within the range 280–295 mOsmol/kg.

How does sodium determine ECF volume?

The osmolarity of any solution is determined by the total concentration of dissolved solutes. Because they are present in relatively high concentration in body fluids (i.e. ECF and ICF), compared with other solutes, sodium and potassium are the major determinants of ECF and ICF osmolarity respectively. Figure 4.2 describes the distribution of electrolytes between the ECF and ICF.

Within cells, the predominant cation is potassium; here there is relatively low concentration of sodium. By contrast, the ECF has a high concentration of sodium and relatively low potassium concentration; these differing electrolyte concentrations on either side of the cell membrane must be maintained by active transport. This active transport is achieved by the so called sodium–potassium pump (Figure 4.3), an energy requiring system present in the membrane of all cells that continuously 'pumps' sodium out of cells as potassium is 'pumped' in.

Without such active transport, sodium and potassium would diffuse passively across cell membranes until concentrations of ECF and ICF were equal. The active transport of sodium out of cells ensures its high concentration in the ECF, and therefore its predominant effect on osmolarity of the ECF. Since osmolarity determines the distribution of water between the ICF and ECF, and sodium concentration is the principal determinant of ECF osmolarity, it follows that plasma (i.e. ECF) sodium concentration is a major determinant of ECF volume and therefore blood volume.

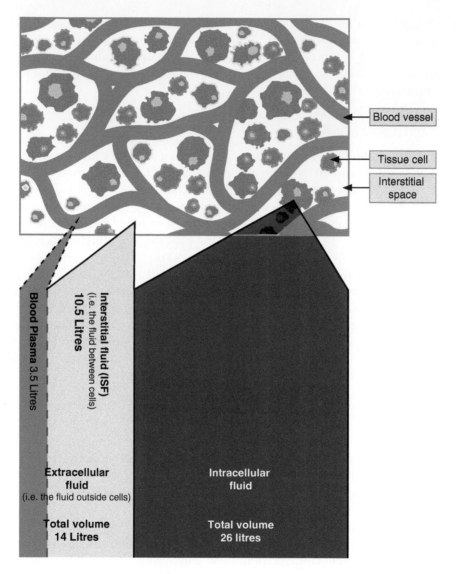

Figure 4.1 Distribution of water in adult (body weight approx. 70 kg)

Control of water balance

To avoid dehydration or overhydration, water intake and output must be the same. A minimum urine volume (i.e. water loss) of 500 ml per day is required for excretion of the waste products of metabolism by the kidneys. To this must be added the water lost via the lungs in expired air (around 400 ml), via the skin in sweat (around 500 ml) and in faeces (around 100 ml). Thus a minimum of 1500 ml of water is normally lost from the body each day. Approximatley 400 ml of water is produced by the body each day, a by-product of cellular metabolism. To maintain normal balance then, a minimum intake of around

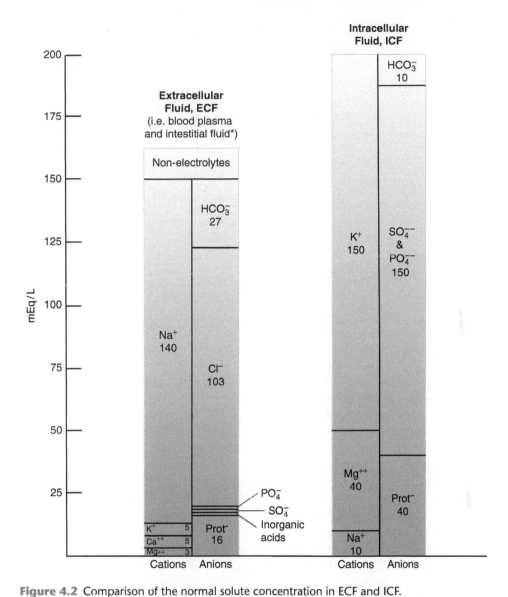

Figure 4.2 Comparison of the normal solute concentration in ECF and ICF.
Notes: 1. mEq/L = mmol/L for monovalent ions (e.g. sodium, Na and Potassium, K) but mEq/L must be divided by 2 to convert mmol/L for divalent ions (e.g. Calcium, Ca and Magnesium, Mg).
2. Figures for ECF refer specifically to blood plasma; interstitial fluid very similar except it has lower protein and higher chloride concentration.

1100 ml is required. In practice, fluid intake is greater than this minimum, but the kidneys are easily able to excrete an increased volume of water, to balance intake. In fact on average most people excrete 1200–1500 ml of urine every day, and the kidneys have the capacity to produce a urine volume far in excess of this, if required.

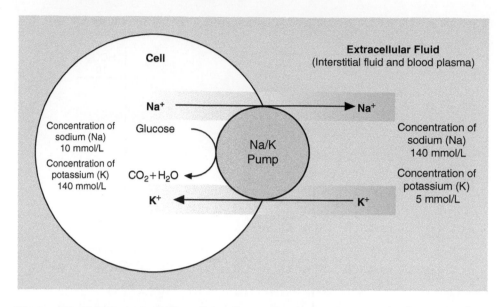

Figure 4.3 Maintenance of differential sodium and potassium concentration between cells and surrounding extracellular fluid.

Water intake and urine loss is controlled by plasma osmolarity. If, for example, water is being lost from the body without adequate replacement, the ECF volume decreases and osmolarity rises. This causes water to pass from cells into the ECF, restoring ECF volume and osmolarity to some extent. This internal movement of water can however only be a short-term corrective as cells become relatively dehydrated. More water is required.

The normal response to this water deficit is described in Figure 4.4. As blood with plasma of high osmolarity passes through the hypothalamus in the brain, specialised cells called osmoreceptors sited there respond to increased osmolarity with two simultaneous outcomes: the thirst response is invoked; and the pituitary gland secretes the antidiuretic hormone, arginine vasopressin (AVP). Thirst of course induces increased water intake. AVP conserves body water by its action on the kidney; specifically it increases water reabsorption to blood from the distal tubules and collecting ducts of the kidney. The result of AVP action is excretion of concentrated urine of relatively low volume. The net effect of this dual response is more water in the ECF and restoration of normal plasma osmolarity.

Conversely, if fluid (water) is drunk in excess of current requirement, ECF osmolarity falls and osmoreceptors remain unstimulated. Consequently there is no sensation of thirst and no AVP secretion/action. The net effect is that dilute urine of relatively high volume is excreted, and the effective water overload is corrected; normal plasma osmolarity is restored.

It must be remembered that around 8000 ml of water is secreted into the gastrointestinal tract each day as saliva, gastric juice, bile, pancreatic and intestinal juice.

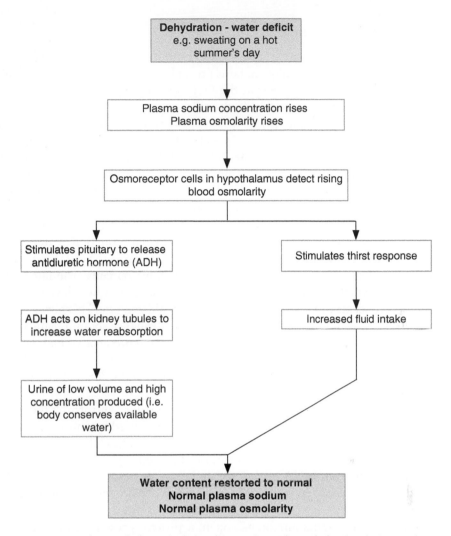

Figure 4.4 Normal water balance is dependent on intact hypothalamic–pituitary axis: adequate ADH, thirst response and renal function.

In health 99% of this water is reabsorbed from the gastrointestinal tract and just 100 ml is lost in faeces each day. However, failure to conserve the water contained in these secretions – evident symptomatically as diarrhoea and/or vomiting – can result in severe water imbalance. Maintenance of normal water balance is dependent then on:

- An intact thirst response, which requires consciousness.
- A normally functioning hypothalamus and pituitary gland.
- Normally functioning kidney.
- Normally functioning gastrointestinal tract.

Control of sodium balance

Just as health demands a balance between water intake and loss, the same is true of sodium. A human adult normally contains around 3000 mmol of sodium, most of which, as we have seen, is present in the ECF (i.e. blood plasma and interstitial fluid) at a concentration of around 140 mmol/L.

A minimum of 10 mmol/day is lost in urine, sweat and faeces and this must be replaced to remain in balance. In fact, we ingest far more than this minimum: the average diet contains on average 100–200 mmol/day, mostly as salt flavouring (a teaspoon of table salt contains 100 mmol sodium). Excess sodium is excreted by the kidneys, in urine. It is kidney regulation of sodium excretion that ensures normal sodium balance, despite wide variation in intake.

Most (90–95%) of the sodium filtered at the glomerulus is reabsorbed to blood during passage of the ultrafiltrate through the proximal convoluted tubule and ascending limb of Henle. By the time the ultrafiltrate arrives in the distal convoluted tubule just 5–10% of sodium filtered at the glomerulus remains. The fate of this sodium, that is whether it is excreted in urine or reabsorbed to blood, is dependent on the blood concentration of the adrenal hormone, aldosterone. This hormone acts on the cells of the distal tubule and collecting duct to enhance sodium reabsorption in exchange for potassium or hydrogen ions. Thus in the presence of high levels of aldosterone most of the remaining sodium in the distal tubule is reabsorbed; if aldosterone concentration is low no more is reabsorbed and urine of relatively high sodium concentration is excreted.

Aldosterone secretion by the adrenal cortex is controlled in turn by the renin–angiotensin system (Figure 4.5). Renin is an enzyme produced by and secreted from the cells of the juxtaglomerulus of the kidney when blood flow through the glomerulus is reduced. Since the rate of blood flow through the kidneys (indeed any organ) is dependent on blood volume and therefore sodium concentration, it follows that renin is secreted from the kidneys when plasma sodium concentration is falling.

Renin enzymically splits angiotensinogen, a protein present in blood; one of the products is a small peptide of ten amino acids called angiotensin I. A second enzyme derived predominantly from the lungs, called angiotensin converting enzyme (ACE) then splits two amino-acids from angiotensin I. The remaining eight amino-acid peptide is the hormone angiotensin II. This hormone has two important effects:

- It causes capillary blood vessels to narrow (a process called vasoconstriction), increasing blood pressure, and thereby increasing renal blood flow.
- It stimulates the cells of the adrenal cortex to synthesise and secrete aldosterone, the effect of which as described here is reabsorption of sodium, and thereby restoration of normal plasma sodium.

Two additional hormones, atrial natriuretic peptide (ANP) and brain natriuretic peptide (BNP) released by the cells of the heart in response to atrial and ventricular

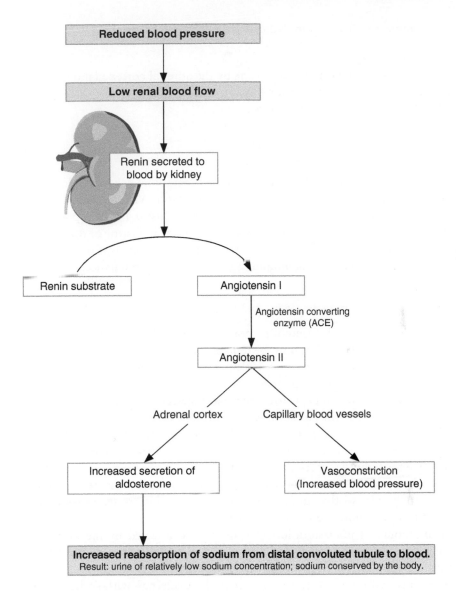

Figure 4.5 Renin–angiotensin system.

stretch, have an antagonistic effect to that of aldosterone. The effect of rising blood levels of ANP and BNP is reduced sodium reabsorption from the distal tubule and excretion of urine with relatively high sodium concentration.

Around 1500 mmol of sodium is excreted into the gastrointestinal tract along with water every day (as already discussed). Normally all – save around 10 mmol which is excreted in faeces – is reabsorbed to blood. Failure of gastrointestinal sodium reabsorption inevitably leads to potential sodium deficit, which becomes real if renal compensation is incomplete.

To summarise then sodium balance is chiefly dependent on:

- Normal kidney function.
- Appropriate secretion of aldosterone by the adrenal cortex gland (which in turn is dependent on an intact renin–angiotensin axis).
- Normal gastrointestinal function.

Normal physiology – potassium

Potassium is required for the action of many metabolic enzymes, electrical transmission of nerve impulses and muscle contraction. Virtually all of the body's 3000 mmol of potassium is contained within cells. Just 0.4% is in plasma where it can be measured, so that plasma potassium is a poor indicator of total body potassium. The maintenance of normal plasma potassium concentration, which is essential for health, depends on maintaining overall potassium balance.

Normal control of potassium balance

A minimum of around 40 mmol of potassium is lost from the body every day in urine, faeces and sweat. This must be replaced in order to maintain balance. Normal dietary intake is of the order of 100 mmol/day, obtained from citrus fruits and bananas, leafy vegetables, potatoes and bread. The kidneys ensure that sufficient potassium is excreted in urine to match that ingested. As with sodium, most of the potassium filtered at the glomerulus of the kidney is reabsorbed in the first (proximal) part of the kidney tubule. Fine regulation occurs in the distal part of the tubule and collecting ducts. Potassium can be either secreted from blood into the tubule in exchange for sodium ions, or reabsorbed to blood at this point. As has already been made clear sodium–potassium exchange is enhanced by the renin–angiotensin-aldosterone axis, so that under the influence of aldosterone, as sodium is reabsorbed to blood, potassium is lost in urine.

The amount of potassium lost in urine is also affected by the kidneys' role in maintaining the pH of blood within normal limits. One of the mechanisms for preventing blood becoming too acidic is renal excretion of excess hydrogen ions in urine. This hydrogen ion excretion occurs by exchange with sodium ions in the distal tubule. This means that in acidosis less sodium is available for exchange with potassium and consequently relatively less potassium is excreted in urine. As will become clear, there are other ways in which potassium balance is affected by disturbance in acid-base balance.

Around 60 mmol of potassium is normally secreted into the gastrointestinal tract every day but most is reabsorbed; just 10 mmol/day is lost in faeces. Potassium deficit can occur if this gastrointestinal reabsorption is defective.

Movement of potassium across cell membranes
As already described the high concentration of ICF potassium and low concentration of ECF (plasma) potassium is maintained by the sodium–potassium pump.

Increased and decreased activity of this pump can have profound effect on the plasma potassium concentration, as potassium shifts between the ECF and ICF. In addition, since hydrogen ions compete with potassium for exchange across the cell membranes, disturbances of acid base-balance may affect the plasma potassium concentration. An abnormal increase or decrease in plasma potassium concentration does not necessarily mean an overall body deficit or excess, it may simply reflect a shift of potassium into or out of cells.

Maintenance of a normal plasma potassium level is dependent then on:

- Adequate dietary intake of potassium.
- Normal renal function.
- Normal gastrointestinal tract function.
- Normal production of aldosterone by adrenal glands.
- Maintenance of normal acid-base balance.
- Normal action of the sodium–potassium pump.

Laboratory measurement of sodium and potassium

Patient preparation

No particular patient preparation is necessary. Sodium and potassium are frequently requested on patients receiving fluids intravenously. Sampling blood from an arm into which IV fluid is being administered may cause errors and should be avoided.

Timing of sample

Blood may be sampled at any time for sodium and potassium but as these estimations may be made more than once a day on the same patient, it is important to record the time the sample was collected.

Sample requirements

Around 3–5 ml of venous blood is required. Measurement may be made on the serum or plasma recovered from a blood sample. If local policy is to use serum then blood must be collected into a collection tube without anticoagulant. Plasma estimation requires collection into a tube containing the anticoagulant lithium heparin. No other anticoagulant is suitable for sodium and potassium estimation.

Poor technique during blood collection may cause damage to the membrane of blood cells (haemolysis), resulting in erroneously high potassium concentration. This is because potassium is present at such high concentration within cells compared with plasma (Figure 4.2). Damage to (red and white) blood cells, that is haemolysis, results in a massive influx of potassium (and other cell contents) from cells into plasma. Haemolysis has relatively little effect on plasma/serum sodium concentration because its concentration in cells is low, compared with that of plasma. Haemoglobin, released from haemolysed red cells, changes the colour of plasma/serum from straw coloured to red, providing laboratory staff with a means of identifying haemolysed samples. Haemolysis may occur if blood is forced at pressure through syringe needles, if blood is shaken violently or frozen. It is a common occurrence if there has been any difficulty in sampling blood. Haemolysed samples are unsuitable for potassium analysis, although some modern analysers have the capacity to measure the degree of haemolysis, allowing a rough estimate of the 'true' plasma potassium concentration of haemolysed samples.

Some sodium and potassium analysers including those sited in intensive care units or recovery rooms allow immediate analysis on whole blood without the need to separate serum or plasma. Blood must be collected into a syringe or bottle containing the anticoagulant lithium heparin. There is no way of knowing if such samples are haemolysed.

Effects of storage

When blood is removed from the body, the available energy source, glucose required for normal maintenance of the sodium pump is soon used up and the sodium–potassium pump begins to fail. At this point potassium begins to leak from cells into plasma and sodium passes from plasma into cells. As with haemolysis, the effects are greater for potassium and erroneously high plasma/serum potassium levels are seen in samples left for more than a few hours. Blood for potassium estimation must be transported to the laboratory within an hour or so. Samples are best left at room temperature during any delay in transport. Blood left for more than three hours before transport to the laboratory is unsuitable for potassium analysis.

Interpretation of results

Reference range

Plasma/serum sodium   133–146 mmol/L
Serum potassium   3.5–5.3 mmol/L
(plasma potassium is slightly lower than serum potassium)

Critical values

Plasma/serum sodium   <120 mmol/L or >160 mmol/L
Plasma/serum potassium   <2.5 mmol/L or >6.0 mmol/L

Terms used in interpretation

Hyponatraemia reduced plasma/serum sodium concentration, i.e. sodium <133 mmol/L

Hypernatraemia raised plasma/serum sodium concentration, i.e. sodium >146 mmol/L

Hypokalaemia   reduced plasma/serum potassium concentration, i.e. potassium
                <3.5 mmol/L
Hyperkalaemia   raised plasma/serum potassium concentration, i.e. potassium
                >5.3 mmol/L

Causes of hyponatraemia

As we have seen sodium and water metabolism are inextricably linked. Plasma/
serum sodium concentration is dependent on two variables; the amount of sodium
in blood plasma (ECF) and the amount of water in blood plasma, that is (ECF)
volume. Hyponatraemia, the most common electrolyte abnormality occurring in
15–30% of hospitalised patients[1], may develop if sodium is lost from the body in
excess of water (sodium depletion) or if there is an abnormal excess of water relative to sodium (sodium dilution). Hyponatraemia can also be classified according
to clinical impression of the patients ECF volume status as: hypovolaemic
hyponatraemia (volume depleted, water deficit); hypervolaemic hyponatraemia
(increased volume, water excess); or euvolaemic hyponatraemia (normal volume,
no significant water excess or deficit).

In general hyponatraemia is much more commonly due to disturbance of the
mechanisms involved in maintaining water balance than in those involved in maintaining sodium balance. Hyponatraemia thus does not necessarily indicate sodium
deficiency and can occur in those who have sufficient sodium and even an excess of
sodium.

Sodium depletion

Abnormal losses of both sodium and water via the gastrointestinal tract occur during vomiting and diarrhoea, from skin during profuse sweating or as a result of
burns. Haemorrhage represents a loss of both sodium and water. The effect that
these losses have on serum sodium concentration depend on the sodium concentration of the fluid lost compared with that of plasma. Excessive vomiting, diarrhoea
or sweating are generally associated with predominant water deficiency and therefore a tendency for plasma/serum sodium to rise. However, if these conditions are
treated with fluid relatively deficient of sodium (i.e. hypotonic solutions),
hyponatraemia may develop. This is a common cause of hyponatraemia.

Fluid lost during extensive burns and during haemorrhage has the same concentration as that of serum and in these cases, despite being sodium depleted, patients have a
near normal sodium concentration. However, hyponatraemia may again develop if the
fluid used to replace losses is, relatively to plasma, deficient of sodium (hypotonic).

Excessive loss of sodium in urine is the cause of the hyponatraemia that often
accompanies diuretic therapy and contributes to the hyponatraemia seen in renal
failure.

The hormone aldosterone regulates sodium loss in urine. A deficiency of the
hormone results in increased inappropriate losses of sodium in urine. Addison's
disease is characterised by destruction of the adrenal gland; the resulting deficiency
of aldosterone causes hyponatraemia.

Sodium dilution

Mild hyponatraemia is a frequent finding among any population suffering disease (the mean sodium concentration of hospital in-patients is 3–5 mmol lower than a control population in good health). The sick cell syndrome is thought to be the cause of this non-specific mild hyponatraemia frequently seen in generalised illness. The sick cell is one in which reduced cellular energy causes an abnormal increase in cell membrane permeability. This allows a slight abnormal shift of water from the ICF to the ECF, effectively diluting plasma sodium. This transient slight fall in serum sodium concentration usually requires no treatment and resolves as the underlying illness is treated.

Untreated diabetes mellitus is often associated with hyponatraemia. Glucose is an osmotically active substance. If, as is the case in diabetes, blood glucose concentration increases, then plasma osmolarity too increases. Water passes from cells to plasma to correct osmolality, thereby diluting sodium. This tendency to hyponatraemia in diabetes is compounded by the sodium loss in urine which accompanies the osmotic diuresis, as excess glucose is excreted in urine.

The importance of the antidiuretic hormone, AVP for renal regulation of water loss has already been discussed. The syndrome of inappropriate antidiuretic hormone (SIADH) results in abnormal retention of water, with dilution of sodium and therefore hyponatraemia. SIADH may complicate the course of many serious pathologies, including some lung cancers, infectious disease of the lungs, head injury, brain tumours and Guillain-Barré syndrome. Some drugs can also precipitate SIADH.

Water and sodium excess is a feature of oedema, accumulation of fluid in the interstitial space. Such fluid accumulation occurs in liver disease (cirrhosis), cardiac failure and chronic kidney disease. Despite increased total body sodium, water excess predominates in oedema with resulting hyponatraemia. Sodium replacement therapy is of course not indicated for this subset of hyponatraemic patients who have more than sufficient sodium but are retaining abnormal amounts of water. The causes of hyponatraemia are summarised in Table 4.1.

Causes of hypernatraemia

Hypernatraemia is much less common than hyponatraemia. Although excess sodium can cause hypernatraemia, relative water depletion is more often the cause.

Excess sodium

Hypernatraemia may occur during over vigorous sodium replacement therapy among patients with sodium depletion.

Uncontrolled secretion of aldosterone by a tumour of the adrenal gland is the cause of sodium retention of Conn's syndrome (primary hyperaldosteronism). The kidneys respond to high plasma sodium by excreting less water; this tends to restore plasma sodium concentration towards normal but is usually insufficient and slight hypernatraemia is a common finding in Conn's syndrome.

Excess cortisol (another hormone which affects renal loss of sodium), a feature of Cushing's syndrome, has a similar effect.

Table 4.1 Causes of abnormal plasma/serum sodium and potassium.

Causes of reduced plasma/serum sodium (hyponatraemia)

- Heart failure
- Cirrhosis
- Diabetic ketoacidosis
- Acute kidney disease (acute renal failure)
- Chronic kidney disease (chronic renal failure)
- Syndrome inappropriate antidiuretic hormone (SIADH)
- Addison's disease
- Diuretic therapy
- Fluid replacement therapy

Causes of increased plasma/serum sodium (hypernatraemia)

- Chronic kidney disease (chronic renal failure)
- Failure of thirst response due to unconsciousness, head trauma
- Conn's syndrome/disease
- Cushing's syndrome/disease
- Diabetes insipidus
- Over vigorous sodium replacement therapy
- Lithium therapy

Causes of reduced plasma/serum potassium (hypokalaemia)

- Diuretic therapy
- Severe or chronic diarrhoea/vomiting
- Alkalosis
- Conn's syndrome/disease
- During treatment of diabetic ketoacidosis
- Bartter's syndrome
- Inadequate potassium intake (starvation)
- Purgative abuse
- Liquorice abuse

Causes of increased plasma/serum potassium (hyperkalaemia)

- Chronic kidney disease (chronic renal failure)
- Acidosis (including diabetic ketoacidosis)
- Severe tissue damage (e.g. rhabdomyolysis, trauma, major surgery)
- Cytotoxic drug therapy for haematological malignancy
- Addison's disease
- Excessive potassium replacement therapy
- Poor specimen collection/handling (e.g. blood cells haemolysed, delayed transport to laboratory)

Water deficit

Despite maintenance of normal amounts of sodium, hypernatraemia will develop if water output in urine, sweat, faeces and expired air exceeds water intake. Inability of the kidneys to retain water may cause hypernatraemia in chronic kidney disease. Abnormal loss of fluid of relatively low sodium concentration is a feature of protracted vomiting, diarrhoea and sweating. All result in hypernatraemia if fluid intake is not increased to replace losses.

The thirst response is essential for adequate water intake. A minimum loss of water from the body each day is inevitable. Under normal circumstances the thirst response ensures that we take sufficient water to replace these losses. Unconscious patients and those who have sustained head injury involving damage to hypothalamic thirst centres within the brain are at increased risk of water depletion and therefore hypernatramaemia, because they have no effective thirst response.

The ability of the kidneys to conserve water when necessary by excreting urine of low volume and high concentration is dependent on adequate amounts of AVP (see Figure 4.4). A deficiency of AVP, or in some cases lack of AVP effect on the kidney tubules, is the cause of diabetes inspidus. This syndrome results in water depletion as urine of inappropriately high volume and low concentration is excreted. Failure of the pituitary to secrete AVP can be due to damage to the hypothalamus or the pituitary (e.g. head injury, neurosurgery). Some rare invasive tumours of the hypothalamus and pituitary can cause diabetes insipidus. Infections of the central nervous system (meningitis and encephalitis) sometimes precipitate diabetes insipidus.

In some types of diabetes insipidus, AVP production and secretion are normal, but the kidney tubules are unable to respond normally. This so called nephrogenic diabetes insipidus can be inherited, or precipitated by the action of some drugs (lithium, used in the treatment of manic depressive disorders is the most widely documented).

The principle causes of hypernatraemia are summarised in Table 4.1.

Causes of hypokalaemia

Although hypokalaemia can be a feature of chronic starvation, for example, in anorexia nervosa, inadequate potassium intake is a rare cause of hypokalaemia. Most cases are the result of increased losses from the body. Increased loss of potassium in urine is an unwanted side effect of some diuretic drugs (e.g. frusemide, Lasix). Diuretic therapy is probably the most common cause of hypokalaemia. Potassium supplements may need to be prescribed for patients receiving diuretic therapy.

The adrenal cortex hormone aldosterone regulates potassium excretion in urine. Excess aldosterone causes abnormally high urinary losses of potassium with resulting hypokalaemia and is a feature of Conn's syndrome, in which there is excessive aldosterone secretion by an adrenal tumour. Raised levels of aldosterone in part accounts for the severe hypokalaemia that occurs in those with the rare inherited condition Bartter's syndrome, and in a similar condition precipitated by liquorice abuse!

Like sodium, potassium can be lost in abnormally high amounts from the gastrointestinal tract; for example, severe acute diarrhoea and the chronic diarrhoea associated with purgative (laxative) abuse can result in sufficient potassium to be lost from the body to cause hypokalaemia. Vomiting is not usually associated with significant potassium depletion except in the specific case of pyloric stenosis, in which the projectile vomiting of acid contents of the stomach causes alkalosis.

Hypokalaemia may be caused not by loss of potassium from the body but by a shift of potassium from the ECF into cells. Such an abnormal shift occurs for one of two reasons: increased activity of the sodium–potassium pump or if there is a hydrogen ion deficit, that is raised blood pH (alkalosis). In the first case, potassium passes into cells in exchange for sodium; in the second, potassium passes into cells in exchange for hydrogen ions (to correct ECF pH). The pancreatic hormone insulin increases the activity of the sodium–potassium pump, so that a shift of potassium from ECF to cells occurs during insulin therapy for diabetic ketoacidosis. This contributes to the hypokalaemia that often occurs as diabetic ketoacidosis is treated. Incidentally this action of insulin is used therapeutically to reduce plasma potassium in those with severe hyperkalaemia, whatever the cause.

The passage of potassium from ECF to cells in exchange for hydrogen ions is a feature of alkalosis and is the reason for the hypokalaemia of pyloric stenosis. This tendency to hypokalaemia during alkalosis is potentiated by increased renal excretion of potassium as hydrogen ions are conserved to in an attempt to raise blood pH. Other causes of alkalosis that may be associated with hypokalaemia are considered in Chapter 7.

The causes of hypokalaemia are summarised in Table 4.1.

Causes of hyperkalaemia

Excessive intake of potassium during treatment with potassium supplements to correct potassium depletion may cause hyperkalaemia but is very rarely the sole cause. Reduced renal excretion of potassium is the more common mechanism. As kidneys fail they lose the ability to excrete potassium in urine; chronic kidney disease is the most common cause of hyperkalaemia and hyperkalaemia is usually a feature of acute kidney injury.

Autoimmune destruction of the adrenal glands, that is Addison's disease, results in a deficiency of aldosterone, the hormone which regulates renal excretion of potassium. The hormone deficiency results in reduced potassium excretion and therefore hyperkalaemia.

Most of the human body's potassium is contained within cells; widespread damage to cells results in release of potassium into the ECF. For example, severe trauma may result in hyperkalaemia, as may the massive cell destruction associated with cytotoxic therapy for the treatment of leukaemia and the widespread skeletal muscle cell destruction that characterises the usually trauma-related syndrome rhabdomyolysis. This tendency to hyperkalaemia due to tissue destruction will be potentiated by any degree of renal dysfunction.

Potassium passes from cells into the ECF in exchange for hydrogen ions if blood is abnormally acidic. For this reason acidosis is often associated with hyperkalaemia. The causes of acidosis are outlined in Chapter 7. Special mention however is made here of the acidosis associated with untreated diabetes.

Untreated diabetic ketoacidosis is usually associated with hyperkalaemia although whole body potassium is depleted. Potassium depletion occurs due to increased urinary losses of potassium during the osmotic diuresis caused by urinary excretion of glucose. This potassium depletion is masked however by movement of potassium out of cells into the ECF, due to acidosis, and dehydration consequent on the massive amounts of water lost during the osmotic diuresis. Although severely depleted of potassium, serum levels are normal or high. The potassium depletion soon becomes apparent as the acidosis and dehydration are corrected; hypokalaemia develops as potassium returns to cells and rehydration is effected.

It is as well to emphasise the possibility that a raised potassium level might be due solely or partially to poor practice during collection, storage and transport of specimens (see sample collection).

The causes of hyperkalaemia are summarised in Table 4.1.

Consequence of abnormal plasma/serum sodium potassium concentration

Signs and symptoms of hyponatraemia

The clinical effect of low serum sodium depends on the cause, the magnitude of the abnormality and rapidity of onset. Mild hyponatraemia (130–133 mmol/L) is not usually associated with symptoms, but most patients with a plasma sodium of less than 125 mmol/L will experience some symptoms; these will be more severe if the decrease is rapid (within 24–48 hours). As we have seen, most cases of severe hyponatraemia are due to relative water excess. Symptoms result from over hydration of cells; the cells of the brain are particularly sensitive to this water excess and neurologic symptoms predominate. Headache, lethargy, mental depression and confusion may develop. Severe hyponatraemia (plasma sodium <115 mmol/L), particularly of rapid onset, is associated with convulsions and coma; if left untreated severe hyponatraemia can be fatal.

If hyponatraemia is accompanied by significant water depletion, as in say late Addison's disease, symptoms of low ECF volume (circulatory shock) predominate; these include reduced blood pressure, tachycardia and dizziness. If, on the other hand, hyponatraemia is accompanied by significant water excess, symptoms associated with increased ECF volume predominate; these include weight gain, oedema, hypertension and breathlessness on exertion (pulmonary oedema).

Signs and symptoms of hypernatraemia

Most cases of hypernatraemia result from a water deficit of both the ECF and ICF. Rapidity of changes increases the severity of symptoms, which are essentially those of dehydration: thirst, dry mouth, difficulty in swallowing and red swollen tongue. Cerebral cell dehydration causes neurological symptoms including confusion and lethargy, increased neuromuscular activity (twitching) and eventually coma. Like hyponatraemia, severe hypernatraemia can be fatal.

Signs and symptoms of hypokalaemia

Symptoms of hypokalaemia do not usually arise until potassium concentration falls below 3.0 mmol/L. But when they do arise symptoms are related to the function of potassium in transmission of nerve impulses to muscle.

Muscular weakness associated with general lethargy is the most common symptom. Constipation due to impaired muscle tone of the gastrointestinal tract may be a problem. Muscular paralysis may occur in patients with severe hypokalaemia (plasma potassium <2.5 mmol/L).

Cardiac muscle is frequently affected resulting in cardiac arrhythmias including tachycardia and sinus bradycardia. Severe hypokalaemia can result in ventricular fibrillation and cardiac arrest. Electrocardiographic (ECG) examination is frequently indicated for patients with hypokalaemia; typical ECG changes include: prominent U waves; decreased amplitude and broadening of T waves; and S-T segment depression. The toxic effects of digoxin therapy are potentiated by hypokalaemia. Metabolic alkalosis (discussed in Chapter 7), which can accompany hypokalaemia, may result in symptoms of tetany.

Signs and symptoms of hyperkalaemia

Hyperkalaemia may be accompanied by vague feelings of muscle weakness, not as pronounced as those that are characteristic of hypokalaemia. Affected patients may be apathetic or even confused. Slurred speech is occasionally evident. The most significant effect of hyperkalaemia however is life-threatening changes in cardiac muscle contraction (cardiac arrhythmias). As serum potassium rises above 7.0 mmol/L there is a real risk of cardiac arrest and sudden death. Electrocardiograph (ECG) examination is indicated for all patients with hyperkalaemia; characteristic ECG changes associated with hyperkalaemia include: tall, peaked T waves; low or missing P waves; and broadening of the QRS complex. Urgent potassium lowering therapy is indicated for patients with moderate/severe hyperkalaemia.

Case history 4

Mark Andrews is a healthy 22 year old athlete who represents his US college at a high level in inter-collegiate American style football. After a particularly intense training session, he reported to the team doctor complaining of muscle cramps. The doctor diagnosed dehydration and ordered IV fluid replacement therapy. Over a period of five hours Mark received 5 L of hypotonic saline in 5% dextrose; a further 3 L of fluid was taken by mouth. Within an hour or so of receiving the IV fluids, Mark appeared acutely ill and was admitted to the emergency room at his local hospital in a confused and disoriented state, unable to follow the simplest of instructions. He was having trouble breathing. Blood was taken for U&E; among the results the laboratory reported was:

Serum sodium 121 mmol/L.

Questions

(1) Is the serum sodium low, normal or raised?
(2) Could the sodium result explain Marks clinical state?
(3) Why were IV fluids administered?
(4) What would be the principle of treatment in this case?

Discussion of case history 4

(1) The serum sodium is significantly reduced. Mark was hyponatraemic on admission.

(2) Most cases of hyponatraemia including the one under discussion are due not to a deficit of sodium but to fluid (water) excess. Because the sodium is effectively diluted in this water excess, this form of hyponatraemia is referred to as 'hypervolaemic hyponatraemia'. The excess water in the ECF results in a shift of water from ECF across cell membranes so that cells become relatively overhydrated or water logged.

The cells of the brain are particularly sensitive to this excess water; the symptoms of confusion and lack of mental agility are due to the excess water in the cells of Mark's brain. Accumulation of water in the lungs results in pulmonary oedema, the cause of Mark's breathlessness.

(3) Hypotonic saline (i.e. a salt solution with a sodium concentration less than that of plasma) was administered to correct the fluid deficit (dehydration) that was assumed to have occurred during training. The fluid replacement was clearly over vigorous in this case.

(4) When Mark was admitted he simply had too much water in his body. The principle of treatment is water restriction and diuretic therapy to increase the rate of water loss via the kidneys, that is increase urine volume.

Case history 5

David Allsop, a 20 year old apprentice tree surgeon, was admitted to the emergency department of his local hospital having sustained horrific hand injuries while operating a chainsaw. During an eight hour long operation his complex wounds, which included severed tendons and nerves, were debrided and repaired. Within hours of the operation David's condition worsened quite unexpectedly. He became increasingly confused, agitated and eventually unresponsive. As his mental status deteriorated, there was also evidence (reducing blood pressure, increased heart rate) of severe and worsening haemodynamic instability that prompted emergency admission to intensive care. Here, examination of his fluid balance chart revealed very high urine output (4.3 L during the five hours since his operation) and, after volume of administered IV fluids was taken into account, an estimated water deficit of close to 8 L. Questioning of David's mother revealed that David had recently developed an apparent need to drink copious amounts of water, and had to urinate frequently. He was now, she reported, in the habit of getting up several times in the night to urinate and satiate his thirst. On the basis of this revelation, and clinical evidence of severe water deficit, a tentative diagnosis of diabetes insipidus was made and later confirmed. With appropriate treatment David soon made a full recovery.

In the emergency department before going for surgery, blood was sampled from David for U&E; this test was repeated on admission to intensive care. The plasma sodium results reported were:

Plasma sodium (pre-op) 144 mmol/L
Plasma sodium (5 hrs post-op) 189 mmol/L

Questions

(1) Are these results abnormal – do they indicate normotraemia, hypontraemia or hypernatraemia?

(2) Considering David's water balance and clinical condition do you think he was normovolaemic, hypovolaemic or hypervolaemic on admission to intensive care? How is this helpful in interpreting plasma sodium concentration?

(3) Would you have expected David's plasma osmolarity to be normal, raised or reduced at the time he was admitted to intensive care?

(4) Why might David's mental status have deteriorated so dramatically?

(5) Diabetes inspidius is characterised by deficiency of a hormone, what is that hormone and what is its function? How does deficiency lead to the curiously excessive thirst and urination described by David's mother?

(6) Why is diabetes insipidus sometimes diagnosed, as in this case, after surgery?

Discussion of case history 5

(1) Prior to surgery David's plasma sodium was within the reference range – he was normonatraemic at this stage. On admission to intensive care however he was suffering severe acute hypernatraemia. Acute indicates onset was within hours. The term chronic hypernatraemia is used to describe hypernatraemia that develops more slowly over a period of several days or weeks. Hypernatraemia of the severity evident in David's case is potentially fatal and requires urgent treatment.

(2) David had a severe water deficit – he was hypovolaemic. This deficit was reflected in the signs of clinical shock (in this case hypovolaemic shock), such as tachycardia, severe hypotension that prompted his admission to intensive care. Disturbances of sodium metabolism are classified according to whether there is water deficit (hypovolaemia), water excess (hypervolaemia) or neither water excess nor deficit (euvolaemia). David was suffering severe acute hypovolaemic hypernatraemia. Because his raised plasma sodium was due to water deficit rather than sodium excess, it was best corrected with fluid containing no sodium (e.g. 5% dextrose), or hypotonic fluid.

(3) Plasma (ECF) sodium concentration is the principle determinant of plasma (ECF) osmolarity. In cases of severe hypernatraemia plasma osmolarity is also markedly raised.

(4) David's deteriorating mental status was due principally to dehydration of brain cells that inevitably occurs if plasma sodium and plasma osmolarity rises. Water passes from cells to the ECF because of the higher osmolarity of ECF compared with ICF. The cells of the brain are particularly sensitive to dehydration, especially if it develops rapidly (acutely) as in David's case.

(5) Diabetes insipidus is characterised by a deficiency of the pituitary hormone arginine vasopressin (AVP). This hormone, which is antidiuretic in action, is essential for maintaining normal water balance; it regulates the amount of water lost from the body in urine. A deficiency results in inappropriate increased loss of water in urine. As a consequence of this excessive water loss and resulting rise in plasma osmolarity, the thirst mechanism is almost constantly invoked. David's mother had reported three classical features of diabetes insipidus: polyuria (excessive urine production), nocturia (waking through the night in order to urinate) and polydipsia (excessive thirst).

(6) Patients with undiagnosed, untreated diabetes insipidus are dependent on the thirst response and resulting increased fluid intake to compensate for inappropriate water loss in urine. During surgery David was unconscious and therefore unable to experience or respond to thirst. It was the lack of compensatory water intake that lead to the severe water deficit (dehydration) and resulting hypernatremia that threatened his survival.

References

1. Upadhay, A., Jaber, B. et al. (2006) Incidence and prevalence of hyponatremia, *Am J Med*, 119 (1): S30–S35.

Further reading

Bhattacharjee, D. and Page, S. (2010) Hypernatraemia in adults: a clinical review, *Acute Medicine*, 9: 60–5.

El-Sherif, N. and Turitto, G. (2011) Electrolyte *disorders and arrhythmogenesis*, *Cardiology Journal*, 18: 233–45.

Marshall, W. and Bangert, S. (2008) Water, sodium and potassium. In: *Clinical Chemistry*, 6th edn. pp. 15-44, Mosby: London.

Reddy, P. and Mooridan, A. (2009) Diagnosis and management of hyponatraemia in hospitalised patients, *Int J Clin Pract*, 63: 1494–508.

Scales, K. and Pilsworth, J. (2008) The importance of fluid balance in clinical practice, *Nursing Standard*, 22: 50–7.

Schaefer, T. and Wolford, R. (2005) Disorders of potassium, *Emerg Clin North Amer*, 23: 723–47.

CHAPTER 5

PLASMA/SERUM UREA AND CREATININE; AND e-GFR

Key learning topics

- Urine production – the concept of glomerular filtration rate (GFR)
- Metabolic production of urea and creatinine
- Urea and creatinine as markers of renal disease
- Non-renal causes of increased plasma urea
- Estimating GFR from plasma creatinine concentration
- Use of eGFR in identifying and staging chronic kidney disease

Measurement of the serum or plasma concentration of urea and creatinine are included in the most commonly requested profile of blood chemistry, 'urea and electrolytes' (U&E). They are both tests of kidney function, though plasma creatinine is the more specific in this regard. Estimated glomerular filtration rate (e-GFR) is a calculated parameter based on plasma creatinine concentration that is now recommended for diagnosis and monitoring of chronic kidney disease (CKD), a common slowly progressive condition that currently affects close to 10% of the adult UK population[1]. Diabetes, hypertension, obesity and advancing age are the major risk factors that predispose individuals to CKD. With an ever ageing population, and increasing prevalence of both diabetes and obesity, CKD is a major and growing health problem in the UK and other developed countries around the world. eGFR allows early identification, long before symptoms develop; medical intervention at this stage can prevent or slow progression of CKD as well as reduce the risk of the cardiovascular disease (hypertension, heart attacks, strokes) that CKD can be associated with.

Understanding Laboratory Investigations: A Guide for Nurses, Midwives and Healthcare Professionals, Third Edition. Chris Higgins.
© 2013 John Wiley & Sons, Ltd. Published 2013 by John Wiley & Sons, Ltd.

Normal physiology

Formation of urine by the kidneys – what is GFR?

As the site of production of the hormones renin, erythropoietin and calcitriol – that regulate respectively blood pressure, red blood cell production and absorption of dietary calcium from the gut, – the kidneys have significant and disparate endocrine function. But the principle function of the kidneys is formation of urine from filtered blood.

Urine is the vehicle for excretion of many unwanted or toxic products of metabolism (including urea and creatinine) as well as substances (e.g. sodium, potassium, hydrogen ions) that are essential to life but present in quantity surplus to the body's immediate needs. By their ability to vary over wide limits the amount, chemical composition and pH of urine, the kidneys serve a major role in maintaining constant volume, chemical composition and pH of both blood and the fluid within all tissue cells. This constant internal environment is essential for normal cell function; life depends upon it. Thus urine is not just a vehicle for excretion; its formation has life-preserving homeostatic significance.

The two kidneys are located one on either side of the vertebral column at the level of the two lowest ribs, partially projecting below the rib cage. They are deep within the abdominal cavity in the small of the back. Adult kidneys are around 12 cm long and each is supplied with blood via its own single renal artery that branches directly from the main vessel (the aorta) descending from the heart. Blood leaves each kidney via a single renal vein that drains directly to the inferior vena cava, one of two major vessels that convey blood back to the heart.

The functional unit of the kidney – where urine is formed – is the nephron (Figure 5.1) a tiny tubular structure whose length is measured in millimetres. There are around 1 million nephrons in each kidney. The nephron comprises two distinct elements: the glomerulus and the renal tubule. The glomerulus is a knot of blood capillaries conveying arterial blood that has flowed from the renal artery via multiple sub-dividing smaller bore vessels to the smallest (arterioles), and finally into the glomerulus. This knot of tiny blood vessels (capillaries), the glomerulus, is sited in a round, 'globular' structure called Bowman's capsule, which forms the first part of the renal tubule, called the proximal renal tubule.

Formation of urine begins at the glomerulus. Net filtration pressure within the capillary bed (due principally to arterial blood pressure) forces water and all other blood borne substances of medium and low molecular weight (including urea and creatinine) to pass from blood flowing through the glomerulus into the Bowman's capsule. The process is called glomerular filtration and the fluid formed, which is the precursor of urine, is called the glomerular filtrate. The glomerulus is not sufficiently permeable to allow the passage of blood cells or large molecular weight proteins into Bowman's capsule so that the glomerular filtrate is essentially protein-depleted blood plasma.

The rate at which this filtrate is formed by the totality of nephrons is the glomerular filtration rate (GFR). In health the GFR is around 125 ml/minute or 180 L per day. If there were no way of reabsorbing the product of glomerular filtration, the whole of the blood volume (around 5–6 L) would be lost within a few hours!

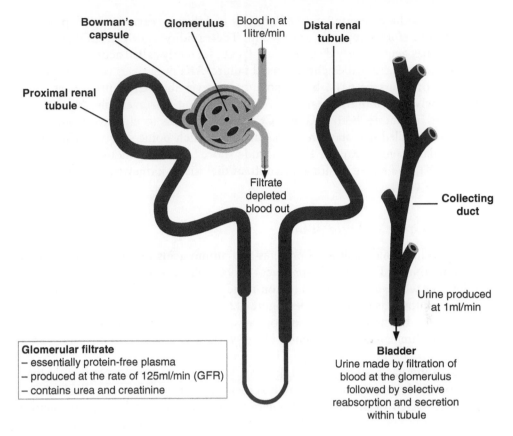

Figure 5.1 A nephron – the functional unit of the kidney.

In fact the composition and volume of the glomerular filtrate is greatly modified as it passes from the Bowman's capsule through the length of each renal tubule. Around 80% of the filtered water and essential constituents of blood, for example, electrolytes, amino acids, glucose etc., are reabsorbed back into the blood during passage through the proximal renal tubule. There is further capacity for some substances to be reabsorbed to blood and secreted from blood into the tubule during final regulation of urine composition in the distal renal tubule. The exact amount of water, electrolytes and nutrients reabsorbed depends upon the body's requirement at the time, but urine, the final product of first filtration, then tubular reabsorption and secretion, is produced at the rate of around 1 ml/minute, that is 1.5 L/day. The urine produced by each nephron flows into a system of collecting ducts which coalesce, thereby connecting all nephrons to the ureter, the muscular tube that propels urine from the kidney to the bladder.

Clinical significance of GFR

The glomerular filtration rate (GFR) is a parameter of prime clinical importance because it defines kidney function. All those with loss of kidney function, whatever its cause, have reduced GFR. There is good correlation between GFR and severity of kidney disease, and GFR begins to fall very early in development of CKD, long before symptoms are evident. The rapidity at which GFR decreases distinguishes acute kidney disease/injury (AKI), formerly called acute renal failure, from CKD, formerly called chronic renal failure. AKI progresses very rapidly over a matter of hours or days, but is potentially reversible; CKD progresses much more slowly over months, years or even decades, but is irreversible. Although by no means inevitable, both AKI and CKD may progress to effective renal failure (sometimes called end-stage renal disease), at which point survival depends on renal replacement therapies. These include short-term continuous dialysis in the case of AKI, and either life-long intermittent dialysis or kidney transplantation, in the case of CKD.

What are urea and creatinine?

Normal cellular metabolism of proteins and amino acids results in production of ammonia (NH_3). This toxic by-product of metabolism is transported in the blood to the liver where it is converted to non-toxic urea by a series of enzyme mediated reactions known as the urea cycle (Figure 5.2).

Urea itself has no metabolic function; as a waste product of normal metabolism it must be eliminated from the body. Once synthesised in the liver it is transported via the blood to the kidney where it is excreted in urine.

Creatinine has a similar fate. Like urea it is a waste product of metabolism, more precisely muscle metabolism; it is formed from a substance called creatine that is involved in producing the energy required for muscle cell contraction. Creatinine is released to blood from muscle cells and transported to the kidneys where it is excreted in urine along with urea. If the ability of the kidneys to excrete urea and creatinine is compromised, they accumulate in blood; the plasma concentration of both rises. Of the two tests, plasma creatinine concentration is the most reliable marker of kidney function in part because, as will become clear, increase in plasma urea concentration is not confined to those individuals suffering kidney disease; it is a less specific marker of renal disease.

Renal handling of urea and creatinine

Both urea and creatinine are filtered from blood at the glomerulus. Since both are waste products of metabolism there is no reason for either to be reabsorbed. However a very small proportion of filtered urea is reabsorbed to blood and this tendency to reabsorption is greater if the urea concentration of the filtrate is particularly high. No creatinine is reabsorbed, but a small amount of that appearing in urine (5–10%) is secreted from blood into the tubule. Notwithstanding these two minimal effects, the amount of urea and creatinine excreted in urine and therefore the amount remaining in blood is dependent on the glomerular filtration rate; as GFR falls, so does urea and creatinine excretion. As excretion falls, blood levels rise.

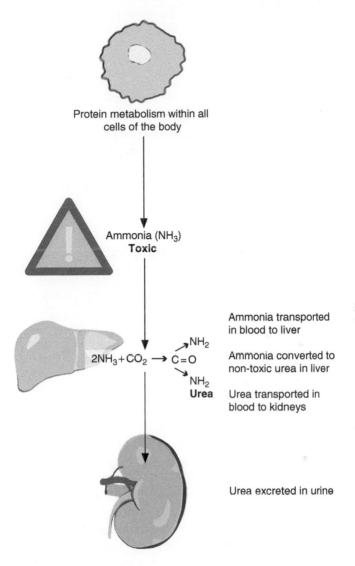

Figure 5.2 Production and fate of urea.

Laboratory measurement of plasma/serum urea and creatinine

Patient preparation

Ideally, patients should be on a meat free diet during the 24 hours prior to creatinine measurement, because cooked meat is a potential source of exogenous creatinine. It is important for most accurate assessment of kidney function that only the creatinine produced within the body is measured.

Timing of sample

Blood may be sampled at any time of the day.

Sample requirements

These two tests are usually performed as part of the U&E screen. Around 5 ml of venous blood is required for U&E. Measurement may be made on either the serum or plasma recovered from a blood sample. If local policy is to use serum then blood must be collected into a collection tube without anticoagulant. Plasma estimation requires collection into a collection tube containing the anticoagulant lithium heparin.

Effects of storage

Unlike the other parameters measured in a U&E profile, urea and creatinine concentration remains stable when blood is stored for up to 24 hours at room temperature.

Interpretation of results

Approximate reference ranges

Plasma/serum urea concentration   2.5–7.8 mmol/L
Plasma/serum creatinine concentration   55–105 µmol/L

[Note: There are gender and age differences for plasma/serum creatinine because concentration depends on total muscle mass. In general plasma concentration among females and the elderly, who have relatively low muscle mass, tends to be at the lower end of the reference range whereas that for non-elderly adult males (i.e. those with greatest muscle mass) tends to be at the high end of the reference range.]

Old age is associated with physiological deterioration in renal function, so that urea increases very gradually with increasing age. The tendency for creatinine concentration to increase due to reduced renal excretion in old age is offset by decreased production due to age related reduction in muscle mass.

Critical values

Plasma/serum urea   > 28.0 mmol/L
Plasma/serum creatinine   > 450 µmol/L

Causes of reduced plasma/serum urea concentration

- Pregnancy is normally associated with an increased GFR and therefore increased rate of urea excretion; pregnant women typically have lower plasma/serum urea concentration than non-pregnant women.

- Low protein diet. Urea synthesis is a function of amino acid and protein metabolism, which in turn is affected by dietary intake of proteins. Those on a low protein diet synthesise less urea than those on a normal diet.
- Liver disease. Urea synthesis occurs in the liver. Although this function is not usually affected in mild to moderate liver disease, liver failure is associated with decreased urea synthesis and as a consequence accumulation in blood of oxic ammonia.

Causes of a reduced plasma/serum creatinine

- Pregnancy is associated with increased GFR and therefore increased excretion of creatinine.
- Creatinine is produced by muscle cells. Any disease associated with significant decrease in muscle mass (e.g. muscular dystrophy, severe malnutrition) may result in abnormally low plasma creatinine concentration.

Causes of an increased plasma/serum urea and creatinine concentration

Renal causes

Both plasma urea and plasma creatinine concentration are raised if glomerular filtration rate (GFR), that is renal function, is significantly reduced. The glomerulus is analogous to any other filtration system where the rate of filtration depends on three factors:

- The rate at which the liquid (blood in this case) to be filtered is presented to the filter.
- The patency of the filter (a 'blocked' filter will result in a slower filtration rate).
- Any opposing pressure on the other side of the filter, reducing filtration rate.

Extending this analogy to the many causes of renal disease allows a simplified classification of renal disease to pre-renal (reduced blood flow to kidneys), renal (damage to the filter itself) and post-renal (obstruction to urine flow) renal disease. Table 5.1 describes such an approach emphasising that a low GFR and therefore raised concentration of urea and creatinine is a feature of all causes of renal dysfunction.

These tests provide no information about the cause of renal dysfunction. However they are good markers of renal disease progression, because as renal function (GFR) falls, both urea and creatinine concentration rise.

It is important to emphasise that a normal urea and creatinine concentration does not exclude early chronic kidney disease, because concentration of both urea and creatinine only begin to rise reliably above the reference range after considerable loss of renal function. Figure 5.3 illustrates this point; plasma urea and creatinine concentrations remain within their respective reference range until the GFR has fallen to around 40 ml/minute, less than 50% of its normal value.

Table 5.1 A classification of some common causes of renal disease – irrespective of the cause GFR is reduced.

Pre-renal renal disease	Renal disease	Post-renal renal disease
Reduced GFR due to reduction in blood volume being presented for filtration. Kidneys structurally normal (at least initially) but functionally compromised.	Reduced GFR due to disease related damage to 'filter' (glomerulus). In simplistic terms 'blocked filter'. Kidney structurally damaged and therefore functionally compromised.	Reduced GFR due to blockage on the distal side of the nephron opposing filtration pressure. Kidneys structurally normal but functionally compromised.
Causes: Any condition that results in marked reduction in blood volume or blood pressure: • Major haemorrhage (e.g. trauma/ surgery) • Significant salt and water depletion (e.g. protracted vomiting/diarrohea, extensive burns) • Reduced cardiac output (cardiac arrest) • Septic shock These causes develop acutely and give rise to acute kidney injury (AKI).	Causes: • Diabetic nephropathy • Glomerulonephritis (inflammation/infection) • Polycystic kidney disease • Gout • Chronic hypertension • Toxic damage (drugs/heavy metals) With exception of toxic damage these causes of renal disease are slowly progressive and give rise to chronic kidney disease (CKD).	Causes: Any condition that obstructs urine flow: • Renal/ureteric stones • Benign prostate enlargement • Tumours (e.g. carcinoma of bladder, carcinoma of prostate) Post-renal renal disease may give rise to both AKI and CKD.

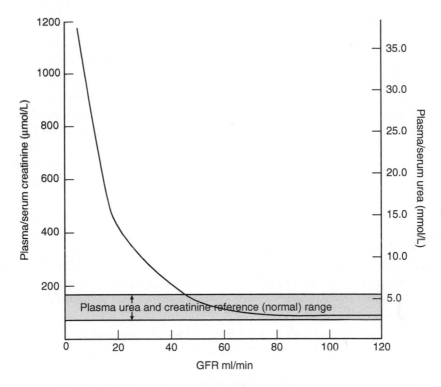

Figure 5.3 Relationship between glomerular filtration rate (GFR) and plasma concentration of urea and creatinine. Note plasma concentration of urea and creatinine remains normal until GFR is reduced by more than 50%.

Although a marked increase in urea concentration (i.e. a level greater than around 10 mmol/L) always indicates renal damage, a slight to moderate increase in urea (around 7.8–10 mmol/L) may be the result of some other pathology. In these cases plasma creatinine remains within the reference range. A marginally raised urea accompanied by an equivalent rise in creatinine indicates renal dysfunction. A marginally raised urea accompanied by a normal plasma creatinine concentration result is likely to be due to non-renal causes.

Non renal causes of raised urea

- Diet rich in protein. Urea synthesis is increased among those on a high protein diet.
- Chronic starvation is accompanied by increased protein catabolism as the body uses its energy reserves for survival; increased protein catabolism results in increased urea synthesis.
- Gastrointestinal bleeding from ulcers, malignant tumours etc. is associated with increased protein absorption (blood within the gut is effectively a protein rich meal!) and therefore increased urea synthesis.
- Dehydration. The amount of urea reabsorbed into the blood by the kidney tubules after glomerular filtration is increased in those who are dehydrated.

Estimated glomerular filtration rate (eGFR)

Although plasma concentrations of urea and creatinine reflect GFR – that is to say, as GFR decreases plasma concentrations rise – neither is a direct measure. No increase in concentration above the reference range of either may occur until around 50% of kidney function is lost (that is GFR is reduced by 50%), so that they are poor indicators of early asymptomatic CKD. This limitation of plasma urea and creatinine measurement is not a problem in the context of AKI because progression is so rapid that GFR is reduced below 50% in all cases; the finding of both plasma urea and creatinine values within the reference range is thus sufficient evidence to exclude a diagnosis of AKI, but is clearly not sufficient evidence to exclude a diagnosis of CKD.

Ideally, for investigation of CKD renal function would be assessed by direct measurement of GFR. Although it is quite possible to measure GFR accurately, methods are technically complex, expensive and not suited for routine use. An estimation of GFR is provided by the creatinine clearance test, which involves measurement of plasma creatinine and the creatinine concentration of a sample recovered from a 24 hour urine sample. The creatinine clearance test, which was routinely used to estimate GFR until fairly recently, has many shortcomings, not the least of which is the necessity to collect a 24 hour urine. The test has now been largely abandoned. In its stead GFR is now estimated by calculation using the following Modification of Diet in Renal Disease (MDRD) formula based on plasma creatinine concentration, age, gender and ethnicity:

$$\text{e-GFR (ml/min)} = 186 \times [\text{plasma creatinine} \times 88.4]^{-1.154} \times \text{age in years}^{-0.0203}$$

[Multiply result by 0.0742 if female and by 1.21 if Black-African]

The MDRD formula was devised and first validated by study in 1999[2]; a number of studies since have confirmed that it provides a more accurate estimate of GFR than the old creatinine clearance test. Additionally, it is far more convenient, allowing at no extra cost an eGFR to be recorded alongside all plasma creatinine results, a policy that is now recommended in national guidelines[3] and adopted by most clinical laboratories.

Table 5.2 provides details of interpretation of e-GFR and the way in which eGFR is used to diagnose and stage CKD. The guidelines advise that plasma creatinine should be measured and e-GFR calculated every 3–12 months for all those with established CKD (frequency depending on severity of disease). In addition they advise annual measurement for all those at high risk of CKD (Table 5.3).

Improving the accuracy of e-GFR

It must be emphasised that the MDRD formula only provides an estimate of GFR. It is not suitable for estimating GFR in the context of acute kidney injury, although as already discussed this limitation is not important because plasma creatinine alone or in combination with plasma urea is sufficient for diagnosis and monitoring of AKI. A more significant limitation of the MDRD formula is that it tends to underestimate renal function in those with a normal or near normal eGFR (i.e. in the

Table 5.2 Using eGFR to determine severity/progression of CKD (staging CKD).

Stage	e-GFR ml/min	Description
1	Equal to or greater than 90	Kidney function normal but some evidence (e.g. proteinuria) of renal disease
2	60–89	Mildly reduced kidney function
3A	45–59	Moderately reduced kidney function
3B	30–44	
4	15–29	Severely reduced kidney function
5	Less than 15	Kidney failure – end stage renal disease

Table 5.3 Recommendations for annual serum creatinine testing.

Annual measurement of serum creatinine and calculation of e-GFR is advised for the following adult patient groups who, because of their condition, are at greater than normal risk of CKD

Those with:

- Diabetes
- Coronary heart disease or history of any other atherosclerosis
- Related disease
- Heart failure
- Hypertension
- Systemic lupus erythematosus
- Rheumatoid arthritis
- Myeloma
- Urine stone disease
- Persistent proteinuria
- Unexplained haematuria
- A long-term prescription of any potentially nephrotoxic drug

range 60–>90 ml/minute). There is thus a potential for over diagnosis of CKD using the MDRD formula alone, that is to say making a diagnosis of early (stage 1 or 2) CKD in those whose kidneys may well be functioning normally. This potential problem prompted research aimed at devising a more accurate formula for estimating GFR based on plasma creatinine concentration. In 2009 a new formula (the CKD-EPI equation) was validated and shown to be more accurate than the MDRD formula[4] in determining eGFR among those with normally functioning kidneys and those with only slight reduction in kidney function. It seems likely that this new CKD-EPI formula will soon be adopted and the MDRD formula abandoned[5].

Effects of increased plasma urea and creatinine concentration

Although it is clear that significant renal disease, whatever the cause, is associated with increased amounts of urea and creatinine in blood, and that actual levels reflect severity, there is no evidence that the clinical signs and symptoms of renal disease are a direct result of either a raised urea or creatinine. However those with a raised plasma urea and creatinine may suffer any of the following major signs and symptoms of renal disease:

- Renal pain, i.e. lower back pain.
- Failure to maintain normal urine flow of 1–2 L/day:
  - anuria, i.e. no urine flow,
  - oliguria <500 ml/day,
  - polyuria >2000 ml/day.
- Raised blood pressure (hypertension).
- Accumulation of fluid in tissues (oedema).
- Presence of blood and/or protein in urine (haematuria/proteinuria).
- Tiredness/fatigue.
- Anaemia.

Uraemic syndrome

This is the constellation of clinical signs and symptoms that arise in those with most advanced renal failure when survival depends on renal replacement therapy (dialysis or transplantation). This degree of renal dysfunction is of course associated with extremely high plasma urea and creatinine concentrations and extremely low GFR (typically <15 ml/minute). It was once supposed that urea was toxic, and responsible for many of the signs and symptoms that constitute uraemic syndrome, hence the name. In fact it has been known for many years that urea is no more than an innocent marker of renal failure. A range of other toxic substances accumulating in blood are in large part responsible for the signs and symptoms of uraemic syndrome, which include:

- Mental confusion, fits and coma.
- Loss of appetite, nausea, vomiting and diarrhoea.
- Itching.
- Breathlessness.
- Electrolyte, water and acid-base disturbances.

Case history 6

Jane Redbridge, a 48 year old housewife, was brought by ambulance to the local accident and emergency department, having collapsed while out shopping. She reported feeling very tired recently, and was concerned that she had been passing black stools, a sign (called melaena) that indicates the presence of blood in the gastrointestinal tract. On examination she appeared clinically anaemic and hypotensive; a provisional diagnosis of gastrointestinal bleed of unknown cause was made. Blood was sampled for full blood count (FBC) and urea and electrolytes (U&E). The following results were obtained:

Sodium   139 mmol/L
Potassium   4.1 mmol/L
Bicarbonate   24 mmol/L
Urea   9.2 mmol/L
Creatinine   65 µmol/L

Questions

(1) Are the urea and creatinine results normal?
(2) Do the urea and creatinine results indicate renal disease?
(3) Do the results support the provisional diagnosis?
(4) Are there other conditions that might be suggested by this pattern of urea and creatinine results?
(5) Would you expect Mrs Redbridge to have a normal eGFR?

Discussion of case history 6

(1) Mrs Redbridge's plasma urea concentration is raised but her creatinine is well within the reference range.

(2) A urea concentration of 9.2 mmol/L is consistent with considerable loss of renal function. Tiredness and anaemia incidentally may also be a feature of CKD. However, a normal creatinine level suggests that Mrs Redbridge's kidneys are functioning normally, and therefore consideration should be given to non-renal causes of raised urea.

(3) Yes. Bleeding into the gut results in a marked increase in protein absorption as the blood is 'digested' by gut enzymes. Such a high protein intake increases urea production. If urea production exceeds urinary excretion, urea accumulates in blood. Creatinine is produced by contracting muscle cells and blood levels are unaffected by increased protein intake. The combination of raised urea and normal creatinine supports the provisional diagnosis.

(4) Whilst a raised plasma creatinine concentration nearly always indicates renal disease, there are several non-renal causes including gastrointestinal bleeding for a marginally raised plasma urea concentration. Chronic starvation, dehydration and a very high protein diet may result in a similar pattern of urea and creatinine levels exhibited by Mrs Redbridge.

(5) If, as seems likely from laboratory results, Mrs Redbridge has normally functioning kidneys, then her e-GFR would be normal.

Case history 7

Brian Trumpton is 68 years old and was diagnosed with Type 2 diabetes 15 years ago. Additionally he has a history of hypertension, which is currently being treated with drugs. At his most recent six month check up, his GP sampled blood for a range of tests including HbA1c and U&E. The next day the GP received the following results:

HbA1c   89 mmol/mol
Sodium   139 mmol/L
Potassium   4.8 mmol/L
Urea   7.2 mmol/L
Creatinine   103 mmol/L
(e-GFR   66 ml/min/1.73 m²)

Questions

(1) Why is it important that diabetic patients have plasma urea and creatinine measured at routine check ups?
(2) Do plasma urea and creatinine results indicate any loss of kidney function?
(3) What, if anything, is revealed by the e-GFR result?
(4) The GP decided on the basis of these results that it would be worth testing Mr Trumpton's urine for the presence of protein. It was positive (2+). Why did the doctor decide to test urine for protein? What is the significance of the result?
(5) What is the significance of the HbA1c result?

Discussion of case history 7

(1) Long standing diabetes is associated with risk of diabetic nephropathy, a CKD. The risk is particularly high for those whose blood glucose is not well controlled. Diabetes is one of the most common causes of CKD and the most common cause of end stage renal disease; a third of all patients requiring regular dialysis or kidney transplant are diabetic. Regular plasma urea and creatinine measurements are necessary to detect diabetic nephropathy. Early detection and medical intervention can halt or at least slow progression of the disease.

(2) Both plasma urea and creatinine are within the reference range and indicate no loss of kidney function.

(3) e-GFR is normally >90 ml/minute, so that a result of 66 ml/minute indicates reduced GFR and therefore reduced renal function. The result indicates possible early (stage 2) CKD (see Table 5.3). The MDRD calculation used to estimate GFR is less than reliable for e-GFR in the range 60–90 ml/minute so that a diagnosis of CKD should not be made without other evidence of kidney disease when eGFR is within this range.

(4) A normally functioning glomerulus is virtually impermeable to protein so that urine normally contains no detectable protein. In deciding to test Mr Trumpton's urine for the presence of protein, the doctor was looking for supportive evidence of CKD that was suggested by the slightly reduced e-GFR. The test proved positive allowing the doctor to confirm that Mr Trumpton is suffering mild CKD (stage 2) secondary to diabetes; hypertension may have been a contributory factor.

(5) The HbA1c result indicates poor blood glucose control (see Chapter 3). To limit the rate of progression of kidney disease it is important that attempts are made to improve this aspect of Mr Turnbull's care. It is also important that hypertension is treated effectively. In this case CKD was detected at a very early stage before plasma creatinine and urea concentration was raised. Although potentially devastating, early recognition and treatment can preserve kidney function and significantly reduce the risk of Mr Turnbull progressing to end stage renal failure at some time in the future.

References

1. NHS (2010) Kidney disease: key facts and figures September 2010 (available at: www.kidneycare.nhs.uk accessed October 2011).
2. Levey, A., Bosch, J., Lewis, J. et al. (1999) A more accurate method to estimate glomerular filtration rate from serum creatinine: a new prediction equation. Modification of diet in renal disease (MDRD) study group, *Ann Intern Med*, 130: 461–70.
3. NICE clinical guideline 073 (2008 reviewed 2011) Chronic kidney disease early identification and management of chronic kidney disease in adults in primary care and secondary care, National Institute for Health and Clinical Excellence (NICE).

4. Levey, A., Stevens, L., Schmid, C. et al. (2009) A new equation to estimate glomerular filtration rate, *Ann Intern Med*, 150: 604–12.
5. Florkowski, C. and Chew-Harris, J. (2011) Methods of estimating GFR – different equations including CKD-EPI, *Clin Biochem Rev*, 32: 75–9.

Further reading

Allsopp, K. (2011) Caring for patients with kidney failure, *Emergency Nurse*, 18: 12–18.

Graves, J. (2008) Diagnosis and management of chronic kidney disease, *Mayo Clinic Proceedings*, 83: 1064–9.

Griffith, K. and Kaira, P. (2010) 10 steps before you refer for chronic kidney disease, *Br J Cardiol*, 17: 81–5.

Martin, R.K. (2010) Acute kidney injury: advances in definition pathophysiology and diagnosis, *AACN Advanced Critical Care*, 21: 35 –356.

Neyhart, C., McCoy, L. and Rodegast, B. (2010) A new nursing model for the care of patients with chronic kidney disease: the UNC Kidney Center Nephrology Nursing Initiative, *Nephrol Nursing Journal*, 37: 121–30.

Piccoli, G., Conijin, A., Attini, R. et al. (2011) Pregnancy in chronic kidney disease: need for a common language, *J Nephrology*, 24: 282–99.

CHAPTER 6

PLASMA/SERUM CALCIUM AND PHOSPHATE

Key learning topics

- Distribution and function of calcium and phosphate in the body
- Regulation of plasma calcium/phosphate concentrations
- The distinction between total and ionised plasma calcium and the concept of 'adjusted' or 'corrected' total plasma calcium
- Principle causes of increased and reduced plasma calcium
- Principle causes of increased and reduced plasma phosphate
- Clinical effects of abnormality in plasma calcium and phosphate concentrations

---

Most of the calcium and phosphate in the body is present in bone, but a small and vital fraction of each is present in blood. The two tests which are the focus of this chapter, measurement of plasma/serum concentration of calcium and phosphate, are often requested together with two other blood tests considered in Chapter 11: albumin and alkaline phosphatase. The four tests, together known as a bone profile, are used in the first line investigation of patients who are suspected of suffering metabolic bone disease. The origins of bone disease often lie in distant organs (parathyroid glands, kidneys and gastrointestinal tract) that are involved in the regulation of plasma calcium and phosphate concentration. Measurement of calcium and phosphate is thus often appropriate in investigation of patients suffering disease of these organs. Three other broad groups of patients in whom plasma calcium is often measured are those suffering malignant disease, the critically ill and preterm babies.

Point of care testing in intensive care units often includes the measurement of plasma calcium. In these circumstances nursing staff may be responsible for the analytical process.

Understanding Laboratory Investigations: A Guide for Nurses, Midwives and Healthcare Professionals, Third Edition. Chris Higgins.
© 2013 John Wiley & Sons, Ltd. Published 2013 by John Wiley & Sons, Ltd.

Normal physiology

Dietary source of calcium (Ca) and phosphorus (P)

A normal western diet contains around 1000 mg Ca/day. Recommended minimum intake for adults is 700 mg/day. The most common source is milk and dairy products; alternative sources include green leafy vegetables, soybean and nuts. Flour and some breakfast cereals are fortified with calcium, and in some areas tap water is a significant source of calcium. Less than half of ingested calcium is normally absorbed from the gastrointestinal tract (small intestine) the rest is excreted in faeces. The actual amount that is absorbed is under hormonal control and so is adjusted to suit requirements at the time.

Most foods contain some phosphorus and a normal diet contains around 1000 mg/day, predominantly from meat and dairy foods.

Body distribution of calcium and phosphate

The adult body contains around 1 kg of Ca and 600 g of P, the latter combined with oxygen and present as phosphate (PO_4). Almost all (99%) of this calcium and 85% of phosphate is contained in bone as hydroxyapatite crystals, which has the chemical formula $Ca_{10}(PO_4)_6OH_2$. Together with the protein collagen, hydroxyapatite crystals are the major structural components of bone and teeth; calcium and phosphate together comprise 65% of bone weight. A small amount (<1%) of the calcium in bone is exchangeable with calcium in blood, this allows movement of calcium into bone when blood concentration is high and in the reverse direction when blood calcium is low.

Just 350 mg (8.7 mmol) of calcium circulates in blood plasma at a concentration of around 2.5 mmol/L. Half of this is bound to the protein albumin and is physiologically inert, the rest circulates as 'free' or ionised calcium (Ca^{++}); it is only this fraction that is physiologically active and therefore of clinical significance. Finally, there is a very tiny but physiologically vital fraction of total body calcium that resides in all cells. The concentration of calcium in cells is of the order of nanomol/L, one thousandth of the concentration in blood plasma.

The 15% of phosphate which is not present in bone is divided between tissue cells and the extracellular compartment, which includes blood plasma. Around 1% of the body's phosphate is present in blood plasma at a concentration of around 1.0 mmol/L.

Function of calcium and phosphate

Both calcium and phosphate have significant roles other than the one they share as major structural component of bones and teeth. The ionised calcium that circulates in blood plasma is an essential cofactor for the enzymes involved in blood coagulation. It is also a source of the calcium required for many cellular processes, including electrical conductance of nerve impulses, cardiac and skeletal muscle contraction and the signalling between nerve and muscle cells (neuro-muscular transmission). Calcium signalling is an essential part of the process by which many hormones affect target tissue cells. Thus the function of many hormones is dependent on ionised calcium. There are in fact few physiological functions that can proceed in the absence of minute quantities of intracellular ionised calcium.

Phosphate is an integral part of many key biological molecules. These include the nucleic acids DNA and RNA, phospholipids (structural components of all cell membranes) and many other substances of intermediary cell metabolism, including adenosine triphosphate (ATP), the most significant source of chemical energy for cell metabolism. Inorganic phosphate, that is the phosphate which is not integrated into larger biological molecules, acts as a buffer in blood and urine, and is thus involved in the vital process of maintaining normal blood pH.

The many functions of calcium and phosphate depend on the maintenance of their plasma concentrations within narrow limits. The next section describes the mechanisms that maintain normal plasma calcium concentration. Disturbance of one or more of these mechanisms is often the cause of abnormal plasma calcium and/or phosphate results.

Normal control of plasma calcium and phosphate concentrations

The concentration of calcium in plasma reflects a balance between dietary derived calcium absorbed via the gastrointestinal tract and that lost from the body in urine. In addition, as outlined above, calcium can move between plasma and bone. These routes of calcium movement, and thereby plasma calcium concentration, are under the control of two hormones: parathormone (PTH) and the vitamin D derived hormone, calcitriol. These hormones also have effect on plasma phosphate concentration.

Source, secretion and effect of PTH

PTH is the calcium regulating hormone produced and secreted by the four tiny (rice grain sized) parathyroid glands, sited close to, or embedded in the surface of, the thyroid gland. By virtue of a protein called the calcium sensing receptor (CaSR) located in the membrane of parathyroid cells, the parathyroid glands are able to sense ionised calcium concentration of blood flowing through the gland and respond to changes in concentration. Reduction in concentration of plasma ionised calcium stimulates parathyroid gland production and secretion of PTH (Figure 6.1). The PTH is transported in blood to its two target organs: kidney and bone. The effect of PTH is to release calcium from bone to blood and decrease renal excretion of calcium in urine. The net result is restoration of normal plasma ionised calcium concentration. As plasma ionised calcium concentration rises towards normal, PTH secretion diminishes. PTH also has a plasma phosphate lowering effect through its action on kidney, where it increases urine excretion of phosphate. Overall then the effect of PTH is to raise plasma ionised calcium and lower plasma phosphate.

Source, secretion and effect of calcitriol

Calcitriol (alternative name 1,25 dihydroxycholecalciferol), the other main calcium regulating hormone, is derived from vitamin D and released to blood from the kidneys.

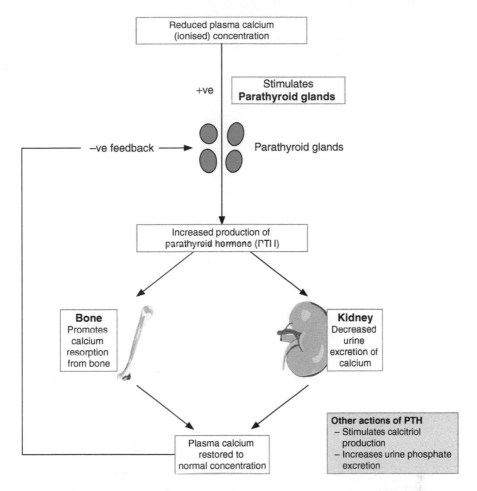

Figure 6.1 Parathyroid hormone (PTH) control of plasma calcium concentration.

Although diet is a source of vitamin D, it is also synthesised in the skin by the action of sunlight on a cholesterol-like substance (7-dehydrocholesterol) present in skin cells. By a two step process vitamin D derived from diet, as well as that synthesised in skin, is converted to calcitriol (Figure 6.2). The first step occurs in the liver and the second in the kidneys. The second step, which results in release of calcitriol to blood from kidney, is under the control of PTH. When plasma calcium is low and therefore PTH levels are high, renal production and secretion of calcitriol is also high. Production and secretion of calcitriol is like that of PTH promoted by reduced plasma ionised calcium and inhibited by rising plasma ionised calcium concentration as well as rising plasma phosphate concentration.

The principle action of calcitriol is on the gastrointestinal tract where it promotes absorption of dietary calcium and phosphate. The net effect is a rise in plasma calcium and phosphate concentrations. By the integrated action of PTH and calcitriol, plasma calcium and phosphate concentrations are maintained within normal limits.

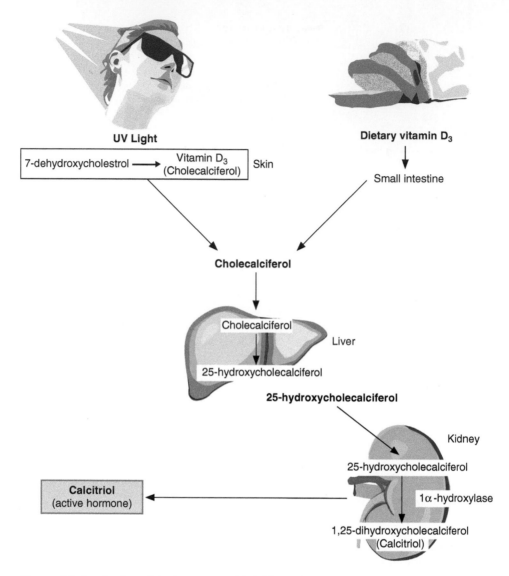

Figure 6.2 Production of the hormone calcitriol from vitamin D.

To summarise, the maintenance of normal plasma calcium and phosphate concentration depends on:

- Normal diet containing adequate calcium, phosphorus and vitamin D.
- Normal gastrointestinal function for dietary absorption of all three.
- Exposure to sunlight for adequate endogenous production of vitamin D.
- Normal parathyroid function: for appropriate secretion of PTH.
- Normal liver and renal function: for conversion of vitamin D to calcitriol.
- Normal renal function: for secretion of calcitriol and appropriate adjustment of calcium and phosphate loss in urine.

- Normal bone metabolism for appropriate movement of calcium (and phosphate) between blood and bone.

The preservation of normal plasma ionised calcium concentration is more important for survival than preserving normal amounts of calcium in bone and, if calcium is in short supply, the body sacrifices bone mineralisation in order to maintain plasma ionised calcium concentration.

Measurement of calcium and phosphate

The concept of 'corrected' or 'adjusted' total calcium

As already discussed, the calcium present in blood plasma comprises two almost equal fractions: half is bound to the protein albumin and the rest is unbound free, ionised calcium (Ca^{++}). Ideally, the physiologically active, clinically important ionised calcium fraction would be measured, but for reasons discussed below it is more convenient and cheaper to measure total plasma calcium (i.e. the calcium bound to albumin plus unbound (free) ionised calcium), and it is total plasma calcium concentration that is routinely measured in the clinical laboratory. The validity of measuring total plasma calcium as a proxy for measuring plasma ionised calcium depends crucially on the concentration of calcium bound to albumin remaining constant in both health and disease, then any change in total plasma calcium concentration can only be due to change in plasma ionised calcium concentration.

In practice, so long as the amount of albumin in plasma (i.e. plasma albumin concentration) is constant then the amount of calcium bound to albumin is constant and total calcium concentration accurately reflects plasma ionised calcium concentration. However, if plasma albumin concentration is abnormal then total plasma calcium is abnormal, providing the false impression that plasma ionised calcium is also abnormal.

To overcome this potential problem it is important to take account of plasma albumin concentration when interpreting plasma total calcium concentration. If plasma albumin is either abnormally high or abnormally low a correction must be made to the total plasma calcium concentration. Various formulae have been devised to make the correction – this is one of the most commonly used:

If plasma albumin is greater than 45 g/L

'corrected' or 'adjusted' total Ca (mmol/L) = measured total Ca (mmol/L) − [0.02 × albumin (g/L) − 45].

If plasma albumin is less than 40 g/L

'corrected' or 'adjusted' total Ca (mmol/L) = measured Ca (mmol/L) + [0.02 × (40 − albumin g/L)].

In essence the 'corrected' or 'adjusted' total calcium is the total calcium value that would be obtained if the plasma albumin concentration were normal.

Although historically not necessarily the case, most laboratories now have a policy of measuring plasma albumin on all samples submitted for total plasma calcium measurement and automatically reporting a 'corrected' or 'adjusted' total calcium result. If this is not the case then a request for plasma albumin must be made with plasma calcium requests if it is thought that plasma albumin *may* be abnormal.

Measurement of plasma ionised calcium

For some patient groups, most notably the critically ill, the formulae used to correct total calcium are invalid[1] and for these patients it is important to measure plasma ionised calcium rather than plasma total calcium. Point of care analysers, including blood gas analysers sited in intensive care units, recovery rooms and emergency departments, usually have the capacity for measurement of plasma ionised calcium. Clinical laboratories may or may not have the capacity to measure plasma ionised calcium but there must be good clinical justification for eschewing request for total plasma calcium estimation in favour of a request for plasma ionised calcium estimation.

Patient preparation

No particular patient preparation is necessary.

Timing of sample

Blood for both calcium and phosphate can be collected at any time of day.

Sample requirements

For laboratory measurement of total plasma calcium

Around 5 ml of venous blood is sufficient for laboratory estimation of calcium and phosphate. Measurement may be made on either plasma or serum recovered from a blood sample. If local policy is to use serum then blood must be collected into a plain collection tube that does not contain anticoagulant. Plasma estimation requires collection into a tube containing the anticoagulant lithium heparin. No other anticoagulant is suitable for calcium and phosphate analysis.

Use of a tourniquet can affect calcium results. Blood for calcium estimation should if possible be collected without the use of a tourniquet. Poor technique during blood collection can cause damage to the membrane of blood cells and resulting haemolysis. Phosphate is present at much higher concentration in the cells of blood than plasma and damage to cells causes release of phosphate to plasma and a falsely raised result. Haemolysed samples are thus unsuitable for phosphate estimation.

For point of care measurement of ionised calcium

Plasma ionised calcium is usually measured at the point of care using the same anticoagulated arterial blood specimen used for blood gas analysis. The same specialised attention to sampling and handling of blood for blood gases is necessary if only ionised calcium estimation is required. The exacting requirements for sample collection and handling is a major reason why ionised calcium measurement is not suited to routine 'high throughput' measurement in the laboratory.

Ionised calcium can be measured on venous as well as arterial blood, provided it is processed in the same way arterial blood is processed for blood gas analysis. Phosphate cannot be measured at the point of care – only laboratory based methods are available.

Interpretation of results

Effect of blood pH on calcium

The proportion of total calcium in blood that is in the ionised 'free' state is affected by the pH of blood. High blood pH (alkalosis) results in less calcium being in the ionised state and low blood pH (acidosis) results in more calcium being in the ionised state. The clinical implication of this effect of blood pH on plasma total calcium is demonstrated in Case history 11, but the general point to be made here is that interpretation of total calcium results, but not plasma ionised calcium results, is a little more complicated if the patient has a condition in which acid-base balance is disturbed.

Approximate reference (normal) ranges

Plasma/serum calcium ('corrected' total)	2.20–2.60 mmol/L
Plasma ionised calcium	1.15–1.30 mmol/L
Plasma/serum phosphate	0.80–1.40 mmol/L

Critical values

Plasma/serum calcium ('corrected' total)	<1.50 mmol/L >3.30 mmol/L
Plasma calcium (ionised)	<0.80 mmol/L >1.60 mmol/L

Terms used in interpretation

Hypercalcaemia   increased amount of calcium in blood, that is plasma/serum calcium ('corrected' total) > 2.60 mmol/L or plasma ionised calcium >1.30 mmol/L.

Hypocalcaemia   decreased amount of calcium in blood, that is plasma/serum calcium ('corrected' total) <2.20 mmol/L or plasma ionised calcium <1.15 mmol/L.

Hyperphosphataemia   increased amount of phosphate in blood, that is plasma/serum phosphate >1.40 mmol/L.

Hypophosphataemia   decreased amount of phosphate in blood, that is plasma/serum phosphate <0.80 mmol/L.

Causes of raised plasma/serum calcium

The two most common causes of hypercalcaemia are malignant disease (cancer) and primary hyperparathyroidism.

Hypercalcaemia and malignant disease

Excessive production by tumour cells of a protein called parathormone-related polypeptide (PTHrP) is thought to be the main cause of the hypercalcaemia that can affect cancer patients[2]. As its name implies, PTHrP is structurally and functionally similar to the calcium regulating hormone parathormone (PTH) produced by the parathyroid glands. The action of PTHrP is like that of PTH to promote calcium movement from bone to blood, with a consequent rise in plasma calcium concentration. However whereas PTH production is controlled by plasma calcium concentration, that is promoted by reduced calcium concentration and inhibited by increased concentration, PTHrP production by tumour cells is under no such control. The inevitable consequence of the uncontrolled PTHrP production by tumour cells is abnormal loss of calcium from bone and increasing blood calcium concentration.

Although hypercalcaemia can occur in all cancer types, it is more common in some than others, so that cancers of the lung, breast, head, throat and oesophagus are more likely to be associated with hypercalcaemia than those of the kidney, bowel and stomach.

Multiple myeloma, a haematological malignancy of the bone marrow is the malignant disease most commonly associated with hypercalcaemia; nearly a half of all myeloma patients are affected. In this case hypercalcaemia is not due primarily to PTHrP, but to the bone destruction (and consequent release of calcium) that results from infiltrating tumour cells.

Generally speaking hypercalcaemia develops late in the evolution of solid tumour cancers, when disease is at an advanced stage and has spread beyond the primary site particularly to bone; it is therefore a poor prognostic sign. Still it is important to detect because treatment is invariably successful in normalising plasma calcium and relief from symptoms of hypercalcaemia can improve the quality of life of cancer patients.

Primary hyperparathyroidism

Persistently raised plasma calcium in the absence of malignant disease is most likely due to primary hyperparathyroidism, the second most common cause of hypercalcaemia among hospitalised patients and the most common cause among the general population. Although this condition can occur at any age and in both sexes, it most commonly affects post-menopausal women. Excessive, uncontrolled secretion of PTH by a benign tumour, called an adenoma, in one of the four parathyroid glands is the cause of the hypercalcaemia in nearly all cases of primary hyperparathyroidism. In a minority of patients increased PTH is a result of an abnormal increase in size (hyperplasia) of all parathyroid glands.

Many cases are discovered by chance when biochemical screening for investigation of apparently unrelated symptoms reveals raised plasma calcium concentration. Non-specific symptoms of hypercalcaemia (e.g. depression, constipation) may have been present for years before diagnosis and some patients (usually those with only very mild hypercalcaemia, in the range 2.60–2.80 mmol/L) are asymptomatic. If left untreated primary hyperparathyroidism can cause bone demineralisation (due to the uncontrolled effect of PTH on bone), deposition of calcium in kidney and consequent renal disease, urinary calcium stones and, in rare cases, hypercalcaemia is of such severity that life is threatened[3]. Surgical removal of the offending adenoma is the only curative treatment.

Rarer causes

The two causes outlined above account for close to 80% of hypercalcaemia cases. Relatively common conditions that are only rarely associated with hypercalcaemia include chronic kidney disease and thyrotoxicosis. Around 10% of patients suffering sarcoidosis, a rare chronic disease predominantly affecting the lungs, are hypercalcaemic because of abnormal increase in calcitriol production and consequent increased absorption of dietary calcium. The same mechanism accounts for the hypercalcaemia that can affect those with tuberculosis (TB) and those who have taken excessive doses of vitamin D. Some drugs, notably thiazide diuretics and lithium, can cause hypercalcaemia. Severe hypercalcaemia is a feature of a life-threatening condition called milk-alkali syndrome[4] caused by excessive use of over the counter medicines (e.g. Rennie tablets) that contain calcium carbonate. The incidence of milk-alkali syndrome (sometimes called calcium-alkali syndrome) has been increasing in recent years and it is now considered a relatively common cause of severe hypercalcaemia. Occasionally no cause can be identified for hypercalcaemia.

The main causes of increased plasma/serum calcium are summarised in Table 6.1

Causes of reduced plasma/serum calcium

Hypocalcaemia is less common than hypercalcaemia. Since the action of calcium regulating hormones, PTH and calcitriol, is to raise plasma calcium, it is to be expected that deficiency or reduced action of either hormone may lead to hypocalcaemia.

Table 6.1 Principal causes of abnormal plasma calcium and phosphate.

Causes of increased plasma calcium (hypercalcaemia)

- Malignancy (common cause)
- Hyperparathyroidism (common cause)
- 'Milk-Alkali' or 'calcium-alkali' syndrome
- Chronic kidney disease
- Thyrotoxicosis
- Sarcoidosis
- Drugs (e.g. lithium, thiazide diuretics)

Causes of decreased plasma calcium (hypocalcaemia)

- Hypoparathyroidism (due to parathyroid/thyroid surgery)
- Hypoparathryoidism (due to autoimmune mediated damage/congenital absence of parathyroid)
- Vitamin D deficiency due to:
  - dietary deficiency
  - lifestyle that reduces skin exposure to sunlight
  - malabsorption due to gastrointestinal/pancreatic disease
- Critical illness
- Chronic kidney disease
- Chronic liver disease
- Neonatal prematurity (immature parathyroid gland)

Causes of increased plasma phosphate (hyperphosphataemia)

- Renal failure (chronic and acute)
- Marked tissue/cell destruction (e.g. rhabdomyolysis, cytotoxic drug)
- Hypoparathyroidism

Causes of decreased plasma phosphate (hypophosphataemia)

- Primary hyperparathyroidism
- Poor nutrition
- Malabsorption due to gastrointestinal disease
- Vitamin D deficiency
- Diabetic ketoacidosis

Hypoparathyroidism – reduced production of PTH

Hypoparathyroidism is rare, most cases being the result of damage to parathyroid glands during surgery. The anatomical intimacy of parathyroid and thyroid render the parathyroid glands and/or their blood supply particularly vulnerable to unintended damage during thyroid surgery. The small size and variable anatomy of parathyroid glands contributes to this vulnerability. The same mechanism accounts for the hypocalcaemia which may develop after surgical removal of parathyroid adenoma, to cure primary hyperparathyroidism.

Around 10% of patients undergoing total thyroidectomy develop temporary hypoparathyroidism. Permanent hypoparathyroidism is much less common, occurring in just 4% of patients[5]. The risk of hypoparathyroidism and consequent hypocalcaemia is reduced by less radical surgery (partial rather than total thyroidectomy), but the post operative management of all patients recovering from thyroid and parathyroid surgery includes careful monitoring of plasma calcium.

Rarer causes of hypoparathyroidism and consequent hypocalcaemia include damage to the parathyroid as a result of autoimmune disease and congenital absence or reduced development of the parathyroid glands.

Reduced production of calcitriol

Hypocalcaemia is a feature of the childhood bone disease rickets and its adult equivalent, osteomalacia. In both cases hypocalcaemia is due to deficiency of vitamin D, the substance from which calcitriol is synthesised. Hypocalcaemia develops because in the absence of adequate calcitriol, normal amounts of dietary calcium and phosphate cannot be absorbed. Deficiency of vitamin D that leads to hypocalcaemia can arise in a number of ways. It may simply be because diet contains insufficient vitamin D or because disease of the gastrointestinal tract (e.g. coeliac, Crohn's disease) or pancreas (chronic pancreatitis) prevents normal amounts of vitamin D being absorbed from food. Lack of exposure to sunshine and consequent reduced synthesis of vitamin D can also cause vitamin D deficiency.

The normal physiological response to reduced plasma calcium, whatever its cause, is increased production of PTH and resulting movement of calcium from bone to blood. If vitamin D deficiency remains uncorrected, PTH secretion remains high. It is the loss of calcium from bone induced by PTH that leads to the bone deforming features of rickets in children and bone demineralisation of osteomalacia in adults.

Hypocalcaemia is a common feature of CKD and a less common feature of some chronic liver disorders and primary biliary cirrhosis. This reflects the key roles that both kidney and liver play in conversion of vitamin D to calcitriol, as well as the specific role that the kidneys play in minimising calcium loss in urine. The hypocalcaemia associated with chronic liver disease is potentiated by vitamin D deficiency, consequent on reduced bile production by the liver (bile acids are required for absorption of vitamin D). Some anticonvulsant drugs, which are metabolised in the liver, reduce vitamin D metabolism in the liver and thereby calcitriol production. Patients taking these drugs are at long-term risk of hypocalcaemia and consequent bone demineralisation.

Hypocalcaemia in the critically ill

Hypocalcaemia is a common feature of critical illness. Up to 85% of patients being cared for in intensive care units develop hypocalcaemia[6]. Only methods that measure ionised calcium should be used to assess calcium status among these patients (already discussed). The conditions most often associated with hypocalcaemia among intensive care patients include: acute kidney injury, alkalosis, sepsis, acute pancreatitis, severe burns and rhabdomyolysis. Massive blood transfusion may cause hypocalcaemia.

Neonatal hypocalcaemia

Hypocalcaemia is not uncommon during the first day or two of life. Foetal bone development requires a relatively high plasma calcium concentration *in utero*. The physiological transition from an intrauterine environment to neonatal independence includes a rapid reduction in plasma calcium during the first 24–48 hours of life. Transient hypocalcaemia during this early period is thought to be an exaggeration of this physiological response due to an insufficient PTH response from immature parathyroid glands (transient hypoparathyroidism). Premature and low birth weight babies being cared for in intensive care are at particular risk of this hypocalcaemic mechanism, as are babies born to diabetic mothers.

Late onset neonatal hypocalcaemia, occurring during the second week after birth is thought be the result of inadequate renal response to PTH due to immature kidneys. Vitamin D deficiency, as a result of maternal deficiency during pregnancy, may also manifest as hypocalcaemia during this early period of life.

The main causes of reduced plasma/serum calcium are summarised in Table 6.1.

Causes of raised plasma/serum phosphate

By regulating the amount of phosphate that is lost from the body in urine, the kidneys have a central role in maintaining normal blood levels. The most common cause of raised plasma/serum phosphate is CKD. It is also a feature of AKI. A failing kidney is unable to excrete excess phosphate as efficiently as normal, so blood concentration rises.

Excessive intake of phosphate is a rare cause of hyperphosphataemia. This may occur in patients who are being fed parenterally. Vitamin D enhances absorption of dietary phosphate so that increased serum phosphate may occur in cases of vitamin D intoxication.

The very high concentration of phosphate within tissue cells as compared with that of extracellular fluid (blood) means that in cases of severe tissue destruction (e.g. rhabdomyolysis) there is an increase in blood levels as phosphate leaks from damaged cells to blood. Any illness or treatment (e.g. cancer chemotherapy) which is associated with marked tissue catabolism can result in raised plasma phosphate.

As already discussed, PTH has an important role in regulating plasma phosphate levels – it increases renal excretion of phosphate. This explains the raised plasma phosphate that is evident in those with PTH deficiency (hypoparathyroidism).

The main causes of increased plasma/serum phosphate are summarised in Table 6.1.

Causes of reduced plasma/serum phosphate

Hypophosphataemia develops as a result of three main mechanisms: reduced phosphate entering the body, increased phosphate losses (in urine) from the body and movement of phosphate from blood plasma into cells.

The presence of phosphate in almost all foodstuffs makes inadequate dietary intake a rare cause of hypophosphataemia, but it can occur if poor nutrition is long standing, for example, in chronic alcoholism and eating disorders (e.g. anorexia nervosa). Inadequate absorption of phosphate may lead to hypophosphataemia in patients with chronic gastrointestinal conditions such as Crohn's disease and coeliac disease; this being part of a wider malabsorption syndrome involving many dietary nutrients. Calcitriol, the hormone derived from vitamin D, is essential for adequate absorption of dietary phosphate so that vitamin D deficiency leads to hypophosphataemia.

One of the actions of PTH is to increase phosphate excretion in urine. It is to be expected then that PTH excess (hyperparathyroidism) is associated with excessive losses of phosphate in urine and consequent hypophosphataemia.

Hypophosphataemia caused by movement of phosphate from blood into tissue cells is a feature of diabetic ketoacidosis and respiratory alkalosis, which is discussed in Chapter 7.

The main causes of reduced plasma/serum phosphate are summarised in Table 6.1.

Consequences of abnormal plasma/serum calcium and phosphate

Many of the clinical consequences of abnormal plasma calcium can be related to the central role that calcium plays in transmission of signal between nerve cells (neural transmission) and between nerve and muscle cells (neuromuscular transmission). The function of central nervous system, skeletal muscle, heart and gastrointestinal tract are particularly dependant on this calcium mediated signalling and any or all of these organ systems may be affected if plasma calcium is abnormal.

Signs, symptoms and consequences of raised calcium

In general, the range and severity of symptoms reflect the degree of hypercalcaemia. So that many patients with mild hypercalcaemia, usually defined as plasma/serum calcium between 2.60 and 3.00 mmol/L are asymptomatic, whilst those with calcium greater than 3.50 mmol/L almost always manifest a range of signs and symptoms, some of which threaten survival.

Common gastrointestinal symptoms include nausea, vomiting and constipation. Central nervous system involvement can result in neuro-psychiatric symptoms including lethargy, depression and confusion; psychosis, seizures and coma may occur. Muscular weakness and fatigue are common. Cardiac involvement includes arrhythmias with characteristic ECG changes. Cardiac arrest can be precipitated by severe hypercalcaemia, so that a plasma total calcium concentration greater than 3.5 mmol/L constitutes a clinical emergency, warranting immediate calcium lowering therapy.

Inability of the kidneys to concentrate urine effectively is a common feature of moderately severe hypercalcaemia, this is manifest as polyuria (increased urine volume) and resulting polydipsia (thirst). Long standing hypercalcaemia, even if it is mild, can lead to deposition of calcium in kidneys and tendency to form renal stones; increasing loss of renal function consequent on either of these can lead in the long term to CKD.

Signs, symptoms and consequences of reduced calcium

Mild hypocalcaemia, roughly defined as total corrected plasma calcium in the range 1.80–2.2 mmol/L, may occur without symptoms, but more severe hypocalcaemia is invariably associated with symptoms of tetany that result from increased neuro-muscular excitability. These include loss of nerve sensation, tingling sensation, painful muscular spasms, twitching and, in severe cases, convulsions and seizures. Laryngeal spasm restricts normal respiration and can be a life-threatening effect of severe hypocalcaemia.

Cardiac arrhythmias with characteristic ECG changes may be a feature. Central nervous system involvement may result in neuropsychiatric symptoms such as anxiety, depression and psychosis among those with long-standing hypocalcaemia. Long-standing hypocalcaemia is associated with higher than normal risk of cataracts and heart failure.

Signs, symptoms and consequences of raised phosphate

There are no symptoms directly attributable to a raised plasma phosphate but by the combined action of several mechanisms, raised phosphate causes a reduction in plasma/serum calcium. For this reason many patients with hyperphosphataemia may be suffering symptoms of hypocalcaemia (outlined already). In the long term, hyperphosphataemia can lead to the precipitation of calcium phosphate in tissues, a pathological process known as calcification. One important aspect of this is that calcification of arteries is involved in the process of atherosclerosis, which leads to coronary heart disease and strokes. It is now suspected that the high risk of a cardiovascular death in patients with CKD is due, at least in part, to the hyperphosphataemia and resulting calcification of arteries that so often occurs in this patient group[7].

Signs, symptoms and consequences of reduced phosphate

Most patients with hypophosphataemia have plasma phosphate in the range 0.5–0.8 mmol/L. Such a mild reduction is not associated with symptoms and is of little clinical significance. However severe hypophosphataemia, usually defined as plasma/serum phosphate <0.3 mmo/L, has important clinical consequence. Symptoms include muscle weakness: this may affect muscles involved in respiration, causing respiratory difficulties. Severe muscle destruction (rhabdomyolysis), consequent on reduced ATP, can occur. Reduced phosphate in erythrocytes can cause increased red cell destruction and resulting anaemia. Central nervous system symptoms include confusion, seizures and rarely coma.

Case history 8

Mrs Riddle, a 42 year old woman, attended her GP surgery on two occasions over a period of a month, complaining of constipation. Physical examination was normal and Mrs Riddle considered herself to be in good health, apart from the constipation. On her second visit when she reported no real resolution of the constipation, blood was taken for a full biochemical profile. The laboratory report included the following results:

Plasma Calcium	2.68 mmol/L
Plasma Albumin	32 g/L
Plasma Phosphate	0.8 mmol/L

Questions

(1) What is Mrs Riddle's 'corrected' plasma calcium?
(2) Which of the following do the results indicate: normocalcaemia, hypocalcaemia or hypercalcaemia?
(3) What is the most likely diagnosis and what is the possible cause of constipation?
(4) What blood test would help to confirm this diagnosis?

Discussion of case history 8

(1) The corrected plasma calcium is 2.84 mmol/L.

(2) Both uncorrected and corrected plasma calcium are greater than 2.60 mmol/L, indicating a raised plasma calcium, that is hypercalcaemia. The severity of the increase as indicated by the laboratory result, 2.68 mmol/L, is masked by a slightly reduced albumin. Only by correcting for this low albumin can the true severity (2.84 mmol/L) be revealed.

(3) Although there are many rare causes of hypercalcaemia, most (80%) are due to either malignant disease (cancer) or primary hyperparathyroidism (excess parathormone, PTH). In most cases of hypercalcaemia due to malignancy, cancer is in an advanced state and already diagnosed. Since Mrs Riddle is relatively young, feels generally fit and well – apart from her complaint of constipation – advanced cancer seems an unlikely cause of her hypercalcaemia. The most likely diagnosis is primary hyperparathyroidism. Constipation is a common symptom of hypercalcaemia. The absence of other symptoms of hyperparathyroidism is not unusual – many patients with the condition are asymptomatic at the time of diagnosis.

(4) The diagnosis of primary hyperparathyroidism depends on demonstrating increased PTH in blood – a request for plasma PTH is indicated.

Case history 9

Ajay, a 12 day old baby boy, was admitted to the special care baby unit because of frequent (up to 6/hour) new-onset focal seizures lasting around 30 seconds. Ajay's mother is Asian. Her pregnancy had been uneventful and Ajay was born at full term by uncomplicated Caesarean section; he was breastfed and had been well since birth apart from seizures for the past three days. Physical examination on admission was unremarkable. Blood was sampled for a range of laboratory tests, including plasma calcium.

Serum total 'corrected' calcium – 1.79 mmol/L

This result prompted doctors to consider the nutritional status of Ajay's mother. On questioning it seemed possible that she might be vitamin D deficient and this was confirmed by blood testing (serum 25-hydoxyvitamin D was 16 nmol/L [normal 20–85 nmol/L]).

Questions

(1) Is Ajay normocalcaemic, hypercalcaemic or hypocalcaemic?
(2) Why did the attending doctor order plasma calcium test?
(3) What lifestyle factors predispose to vitamin D deficiency?
(4) What is the significance of mother's vitamin D deficiency for Ajay's clinical state?
(5) Suggest a final diagnosis and treatment.
(6) Prior to treatment would you expect Ajay to have a normal, reduced or raised level of PTH in his blood?

Discussion of case history 9

(1) Ajay's total 'corrected' plasma calcium is markedly reduced – he is hypocalcaemic.

(2) Seizure in the neonatal period (i.e. the first month of life) has many possible causes, including metabolic disturbances of which the most common are reduced blood glucose (hypoglycaemia), reduced blood calcium (hypocalcaemia) and reduced blood magnesium (hypomagnesaemia). Blood testing for these conditions is routine part of the investigation of babies presenting with unexplained seizure.

(3) The diet is generally quite a poor source of vitamin D because it is only naturally present in oily fish, eggs and liver. Some dairy products and breakfast cereals are fortified with the vitamin. Up to 90% of the vitamin D we need is synthesised in the body by the action of sunlight on skin. Poor diet and limited sun exposure predisposes to vitamin D deficiency as does the use of sun tan lotion. The housebound elderly are at particular risk, as are Asian women living in the UK because they might have limited skin exposure, and dark skin is less efficient at synthesising vitamin D. The body's demand for vitamin D increases during pregnancy and it is now recommended that antenatal care should include a risk assessment for vitamin D deficiency and vitamin D supplementation (10 mg/day) for those pregnant women whose lifestyle and diet indicate high risk.

(4) The vitamin D status of the newborn is determined largely by the vitamin D status of the mother. Since Ajay's mother is vitamin D deficient it seems likely that Ajay too is vitamin D deficient and, because vitamin D is required for adequate absorption of dietary calcium, this has resulted in the hypocalcaemia that is causing the seizures.

(5) Blood testing (serum 25 OH-vitamin D measurement) revealed that Ajay too was deficient of vitamin D, allowing a diagnosis of hypocalcaemic seizures secondary to maternal and infant vitamin D deficiency. Ajay was given calcium gluconate IV, oral calcium and calcitriol (1,25-dihydroxy vitamin D) and the seizures ceased within 24 hours of starting treatment.

(6) The secretion of PTH by the parathyroid glands is controlled by plasma ionised calcium concentration. Reduction in plasma ionised calcium (hypocalcaemia) results in increased PTH secretion. Ajay's PTH was increased, a condition called hyperparathyroidism. Since the hyperparathyroidism in this case is due not to disease of the parathyroid itself but to reduced plasma, ionised calcium it is called secondary hyperparathyroidism rather than primary hyperparathyroidism.

References

1. Byrnes, M., Huynh, K., Helmer, S. et al. (2005) A comparison of corrected serum calcium Levels to ionised calcium levels among critically ill surgical patients, *Am J Surg*, 189: 310–14.
2. Mundy, G. and Edwards, J. (2008) PTH-related peptide (PTHrP) in hypercalcemia, *J Am Soc Nephrol*, 19: 672–5.
3. Van Den Hauwe, K., Oeyen, S., Schrijvers, B. et al. (2009) A 50 year old man with severe hypercalcemia: a case report, *Acta Clin Belg*, 64: 442–6.
4. Swaminathan, K. (2011) A hidden history of heartburn: the Milk-Alkali syndrome, *Indian J Pharmacol*, 43: 78–9.
5. Khan, M. and Waguespack, S. (2011) Medical management of postsurgical hypoparathyroidism, *Endocrin Pract*, 17(suppl 1):18–25.
6. Hastbacka, J. and Pettila, V. (2003) Prevalance and predictive value of ionised hypocalcaemia among critically ill patients, *Acta Anaesthesiologica Scundinavica*, 47: 1264–9.
7. Zheng, C-M., Lu, K-C., Wu, C-C. et al. (2011) Association of serum phosphate and related factors in ESRD-related vascular calcification, *Int J Nephrol*, vol. 2011: article ID: 936613.

Further reading

Hughes, E. (2010) How to care for patients undergoing surgery for primary hyperparathyroidism, *Nursing Times*, 106: 23–6.
Jacobs, T. and Bilezikian, J. (2005) Rare causes of hypercalcemia, *J Clin Endocrin & Metab*, 90: 6316–22.
Mackenzie-Feder, J., Sirrs, S., Anderson, D. et al. (2011) Primary hyperparathyroidism: an overview, *Int J Endocrinol*, vol. 2011: article no 251410.
Peacock, M. (2010) Calcium metabolism in health and disease, *Clin J Am Soc Nephrol*, 5 (Suppl 1): S23–S30.
Shoback, D. (2008) Hypoparathyroidism, *New Eng J Med*, 359: 391–403.

CHAPTER 7

ARTERIAL BLOOD GASES

Key learning topics

- Definition of blood gas parameters
- Principles of oxygen and carbon dioxide exchange in the lungs, and blood transport of these gases around the body
- Defining pH, acid, base and buffer
- Principles of acid-base homeostasis (maintaining normal blood pH)
- Defining the four types of acid-base disturbance
  - respiratory acidosis and respiratory alkalosis
  - metabolic acidosis and metabolic alkalosis
- Causes and consequences of acid-base disturbance
- Causes and consequences of hypoxaemia and hyperoxaemia
- Assessing blood oxygenation (blood gases v pulse oximetry)
- Principles of sampling arterial blood
- Foetal pH monitoring

The use of the term blood gases does not fully describe this test because although it includes measurement of the two significant gases dissolved in blood, oxygen (O_2) and carbon dioxide (CO_2), it also includes measurement of the pH of blood and several other parameters that are calculated from these measurements. In broad terms the test allows assessment of two related physiological functions: the facility of the lungs to simultaneously add oxygen to blood and remove carbon dioxide from blood (the dual process called pulmonary gas exchange); and the ability of the body to maintain the pH of blood within narrow healthy limits (called acid-base balance or acid-base homeostasis). The test is used for monitoring two patient groups in whom either one or both of these physiological functions may be disturbed: the critically/acutely ill and those with chronic respiratory disease. Clinically significant changes in the measured parameters of blood gases can occur over very short periods of time in the critically ill, so that patients may require blood gas measurement every few hours. For this reason blood gas analysers are often sited

Understanding Laboratory Investigations: A Guide for Nurses, Midwives and Healthcare Professionals, Third Edition. Chris Higgins.
© 2013 John Wiley & Sons, Ltd. Published 2013 by John Wiley & Sons, Ltd.

where critically ill patients are being cared for, in intensive care units, emergency departments and recovery rooms. In these circumstances responsibility for blood gas analysis often falls upon nursing staff. It is the only blood test that requires sampling of arterial blood; all other blood tests are performed on venous blood. Strictly speaking then, the test should be, and often is, called arterial blood gases.

Normal physiology

Normal cellular metabolism is associated with continuous production of carbon dioxide (CO_2) and hydrogen ions (H^+), as oxygen (O_2) is consumed. The rates of production and consumption vary according to the level of metabolic activity. Health demands that despite this variation in production and consumption, the blood content of all three be maintained within narrow limits. The mechanism that maintains the three parameters within normal limits is a complex synergy of action involving chemical buffers in blood, the red cells (erythrocytes) that circulate in blood and the function of three organs: lungs, kidney and brain. Blood gases is a test that monitors the ability of the body to maintain these mechanisms. An understanding of test results then depends on a basic knowledge of respiratory physiology and normal acid-base balance. Although interrelated, these two topics are treated separately here for convenience only.

Respiratory physiology

Oxygen is fundamental to life. The cells of all human tissues derive the energy they require to survive and function from the continuous aerobic metabolism of dietary derived nutrients (carbohydrates, fats etc.). This aerobic metabolism requires a constant supply of oxygen and results in continuous production of carbon dioxide, a waste product that must be eliminated from the body. The object of respiration is to supply oxygen, present in inspired air to every tissue cell and eliminate the carbon dioxide these cells produce in expired air. Venous blood returning to the heart from the tissues is low in oxygen and loaded with carbon dioxide (see Figure 7.1). It is mixed in the right side of the heart and pumped to the lungs via the pulmonary artery. In the lungs, carbon dioxide passes from blood in exchange for oxygen. The blood, now with less carbon dioxide but loaded with oxygen, is pumped back to the heart via the pulmonary vein and out, via the aorta through the arterial system, for delivery of oxygen to the tissues.

Basic principles of gases in biological systems: units of measurement and diffusion

The amount of a gas present in systems, including biological systems is defined by the pressure it exerts, traditionally measured as the height in millimetres (mm) of a column of mercury (Hg). For example, the pressure of atmospheric air

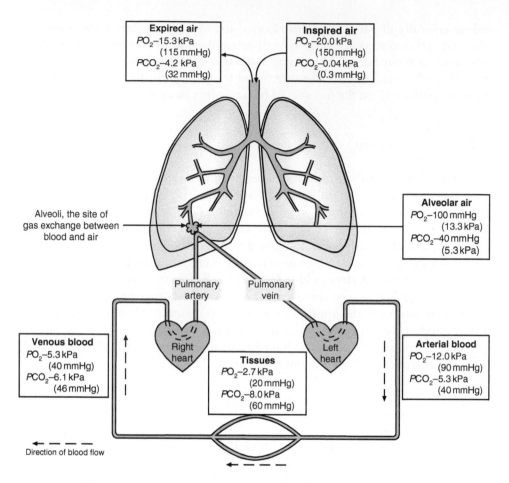

Figure 7.1 Oxygen and carbon dioxide content of air within lungs, systemic blood (venous and arterial) and tissues.

(i.e. barometric pressure) at sea level is 760 mmHg. This means that at sea level, the gases contained in the air we breathe have a combined pressure sufficient to support a column of mercury 760 mm high. In a mixture of gases, as air is, the total pressure is simply the sum of the partial pressures (represented by the symbol P) of each gas. So that since air comprises 21% oxygen, 0.03% carbon dioxide and 78% nitrogen, the partial pressure of oxygen (PO_2) in inspired air at sea level is equal to 21% of total atmospheric pressure (i.e. $21/100 \times 760$) or 150 mmHg and partial pressure of carbon dioxide (PCO_2) = $0.03/100 \times 760$ or 0.2 mmHg.

In clinical laboratories, the Systeme Internationale (SI) unit of pressure, the kilo-Pascal (kPa), has replaced mmHg as the unit of choice when measuring partial pressures of gases. Pressure is defined as force per unit area. The SI unit of force is the Newton (N) and the SI unit of area is the square metre (m^2). Thus the derived SI unit of pressure, the Pascal (named after the seventeenth-century physicist), is defined as 1 Newton per square metre ($1N/m^2$). The kilo-Pascal (kPa) is one thousand Pascals (i.e. $1000N/m^2$). Some physiology texts continue to express the partial pressure of gases in blood in mmHg. To convert mmHg to kPa, simply multiply by 0.133. Figure 7.1 describes the PO_2 and PCO_2 of inspired air, alveolar air (the air deep within the lungs), venous blood, arterial blood and tissues.

The rate of diffusion of a gas across a physiological membrane is determined by the partial pressure of that gas on either side of the membrane. Gas diffuses from high partial pressure to low partial pressure. The greater the difference on either side of the membrane, the faster gas diffuses. The significance of this simple principle will become apparent as the exchange of gases between blood and lungs, and between blood and tissues, is examined more closely.

Gas exchange at the lungs

The site of gas exchange between blood and lungs is the alveolar membrane, the thin lining of the microscopic cul de sacs of lung structure, called alveoli. The millions of alveoli provide a massive alveolar membrane surface area for gas exchange: $80m^2$ in the adult lung. On one side of the membrane is alveolar air. On the other are blood capillaries with diameter so small that red blood cells can only pass through in essentially 'single file'. Gases diffuse across this membrane in an attempt to equalise the partial pressure (amount) of each gas on either side of the membrane. So that oxygen diffuses from alveoli (PO_2 13.3 kPa) to blood (PO_2 5.3 kPa) and carbon dioxide diffuses from the blood (PCO_2 6.1 kPa) to alveoli (PCO_2 5.3 kPa).

Adequate gas exchange between the lungs and blood is dependent on:

- Adequate alveolar ventilation by lungs. This is the mechanical process, due to the elastic recoil of lungs, that ensures movement of air in and out of alveoli.
- Normal numbers of functioning alveoli.
- Sufficient blood flow through the pulmonary capillaries (i.e. adequate perfusion of alveoli).

Transport of oxygen in blood

Oxygen passes across the alveolar membrane into the blood flowing through pulmonary capillaries. Oxygen is poorly soluble in blood and the small amount of oxygen that can be transported simply dissolved in blood (around 3.0 ml of oxygen per litre of blood) is quite inadequate to satisfy the body's demand for oxygen. The oxygen carrying protein, haemoglobin, contained in red blood cells (erythrocytes) provides an additional, far more effective, means of transporting oxygen that increases the oxygen carrying capacity of blood from 3.0 to 200 ml oxygen per litre. In fact only 1–2% of the oxygen transported in blood is dissolved in the blood; this small fraction determines the measured partial pressure of oxygen (PO_2). The remaining 98–99% is transported in erythrocytes bound to haemoglobin.

The product of the reversible binding of oxygen by haemoglobin is called oxyhaemoglobin; the term deoxyhaemoglobin is used to describe haemoglobin that has less oxygen bound to it than is maximally possible. The oxygen delivery function of haemoglobin, that is its ability to 'pick up' oxygen in the lungs and 'release' it in the microvasculature of tissues, is made possible by a reversible conformational change in the quaternary structure (shape) of the haemoglobin molecule that alters its affinity for oxygen. In the deoxy state haemoglobin has low affinity for oxygen and in the oxy state it has high affinity for oxygen. A number of environmental factors in blood determine the haemoglobin state (deoxy or oxy) and thereby relative affinity for oxygen. The most significant of these is the PO_2. Haemoglobin present in blood with relatively high PO_2 (arterial blood) has much greater affinity for oxygen than haemoglobin present in blood with relatively low PO_2 (venous blood). The oxygen dissociation curve (ODC) describes this relationship graphically (Figure 7.2).

The percentage of total haemoglobin saturated with oxygen (i.e. oxygen saturation, SO2) is the measure of haemoglobin affinity in the graph in Figure 7.2. It is clear from the graph that at the high PO_2 that prevails in the blood exposed to alveolar air in the lung (~12 kPa), haemoglobin is almost 100% saturated with oxygen; nearly all of the available oxygen binding sites on the totality of haemoglobin molecules are occupied with oxygen. By contrast in the milieu of the tissues where PO_2 is much lower, haemoglobin affinity for oxygen is also much lower and oxygen is released from haemoglobin to the tissues.

Although arterial PO_2 only reflects a tiny proportion (1–2%) of the oxygen in arterial blood, it is highly significant because it determines the amount of oxygen bound to haemoglobin (the SO_2) and therefore the total amount of oxygen that is contained in arterial blood for delivery to tissues. If PO_2 of arterial blood is reduced then less oxygen can be carried by haemoglobin (i.e. SO_2 is reduced) and less oxygen is available to tissues. Examination of Figure 7.2 reveals that a significant decrease in PO_2 from 16 kPa to 10 kPa has only slight effect on SO_2 and therefore the oxygen content of blood, but there is a sharp fall in SO_2 as PO_2 falls below 10 kPa. The delivery of oxygen to tissues becomes increasingly compromised as PO_2 of arterial blood falls below this level.

For adequate oxygenation of tissues then:

- Blood must contain sufficient haemoglobin.
- That haemoglobin must be >95% saturated with oxygen in arterial blood (SO2 >95%).
- To achieve >95% oxygen saturation, arterial blood PO_2 must be >10 kPa (Figure 7.2).
- Maintenance of arterial PO_2 above 10 kPa is dependent on the factors required for normal gas exchange between lungs and blood (already discussed).

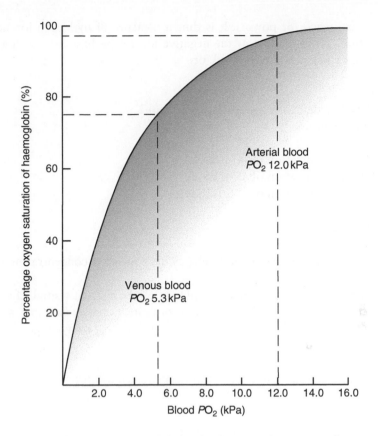

Figure 7.2 Oxygen dissociation curve. Relationship between the amount of oxygen in blood PO$_2$ and the amount of oxygen carried by haemoglobin (% Hb saturation).

Acid-base balance: the maintenance of normal blood pH

Normal cellular metabolism requires that blood pH be maintained within the range 7.35–7.45 despite continuous production of hydrogen ions, which tend to reduce pH. Even slight excursions outside this range have deleterious effects and a pH of less than 6.8 or greater than 7.8 is considered incompatible with life. A brief review of some basic concepts is required for an understanding of acid-base balance in the body.

What is pH?

pH is a logarithmic scale (0–14) of acidity and alkalinity. Pure water has a pH of 7 and by convention neutral (i.e. neither acidic nor alkaline) pH above 7 is alkaline and pH less than 7 is acidic. The term pH is an abbreviation of puissance hydrogen (puissance is French for power). It is thus a measure of hydrogen ion activity or concentration. pH is defined as the negative log to the base 10 (i.e. $\log_{10}$) of the hydrogen ion concentration in mol/L or:

$$pH = -\log_{10}\left[H^+\right]$$ Eqn. 1

where $[H^+]$ = hydrogen ion concentration in mol/L
    From this equation:

pH 7.4 = H^+ concentration of 40 nmol/L
pH 7.0 = H^+ concentration of 100 nmol/L
pH 6.0 = H^+ concentration of 1000 nmol/L

It is evident that:

- The two parameters change inversely; as hydrogen ion concentration increases, pH falls.
- Due to the logarithmic nature of the pH scale, an apparently small change in pH is in fact a large change in hydrogen ion concentration. For example, a reduction of only 0.3 pH unit from 7.4 to 7.1 means a doubling of hydrogen ion concentration from 40 to 80 nmol/L.

Some laboratories report hydrogen ion concentration (units – nmol/L) in preference to pH.

What is an acid and a base?

An acid is a substance that dissociates in solution to *release* hydrogen ions. A base *accepts* hydrogen ions, for example, hydrochloric acid (HCl) dissociates to hydrogen ions and chlorine ions:

$$HCl \rightarrow H^+ + Cl^-$$ Eqn. 2

whereas bicarbonate (HCO_3^-), a base, accepts hydrogen ions to form carbonic acid:

$$HCO_3^- + H^+ \rightarrow H_2CO_3$$ Eqn. 3

A strong acid like hydrochloric acid dissociates easily, yielding many hydrogen ions; it has therefore a very low pH.
    A weak acid by contrast dissociates less easily yielding less hydrogen ions and therefore a relatively higher pH than a strong acid.

What is a buffer?

Chemical buffers are compounds in solution that resist change in pH caused by addition of an acid, by 'mopping up' hydrogen ions resulting from acid dissociation.
    A buffer is the conjugate base of any weak acid. Because of its prime physiological importance for the maintenance of blood pH, the bicarbonate buffer system will be

used as an example (there are several other buffer systems in blood). The buffer in this instance is bicarbonate, the conjugate base of the weak acid, carbonic acid. When a strong acid, for example, hydrochloric acid, is added to a solution of sodium bicarbonate (the buffer), the hydrogen ions from the strongly dissociating hydrochloric acid are incorporated into carbonic acid, a weakly dissociating acid:

$$H^+Cl^- \quad + \quad NaHCO_3 \quad \rightarrow \quad H_2CO_3 \quad + \quad NaCl$$

(Hydrochloric acid)   (Sodium bicarbonate)   (Carbonic acid)
a strong acid   the buffer   a weak acid   Eqn. 4

The important point here is that because the hydrogen ions from hydrochloric acid have been incorporated into a weak acid, which does not dissociate readily, the total number of hydrogen ions in solution and therefore the pH does not change as much as would have occurred in the absence of the buffer. Although a buffer minimises changes in pH due to addition of hydrogen ions, it cannot entirely eliminate them because even weak acids dissociate to some extent. A very useful (if at first sight daunting!) equation defines the pH of all buffer systems in terms of the concentrations of their weak acid and conjugate base, it is called the Henderson-Hasselbach equation. For the bicarbonate buffer system then, this equation is:

$$pH = 6.1 + \log\frac{[HCO_3]}{[H_2CO_3]} \qquad\qquad Eqn.\ 5$$

Where $[HCO_3]$ is the concentration of the conjugate base, bicarbonate and $[H_2CO_3]$ is the concentration of the weak acid, carbonic acid.

This equation reveals that pH is governed by the ratio of the concentration of base (HCO_3^-) to concentration of acid (H_2CO_3).

As hydrogen ions are added to bicarbonate (the buffer), the concentration of bicarbonate falls (as it is converted to carbonic acid) and the concentration of carbonic acid rises (Eqn.3). If acid (hydrogen ions) continues to be added to the system bicarbonate would eventually be consumed (all would be converted to carbonic acid). At this point there would be no buffering capacity and pH would fall sharply with addition of more acid. However if carbonic acid could be continuously removed from the system as it was generated, and bicarbonate continuously replenished, then buffering capacity and therefore pH could be maintained, despite continued addition of hydrogen ions.

As will become clear with more detail of the physiology of acid-base balance that is, in effect, what happens in the body. In essence the lungs ensure removal of carbonic acid (as carbon dioxide) and the kidneys ensure continuous regeneration of bicarbonate. The role of the lungs in maintenance of normal blood pH thus depends on a singular characteristic of the bicarbonate buffering system, the conversion of carbonic acid to carbon dioxide and water. The following equation outlines the relationship of all elements of the bicarbonate buffering system as it operates in the body:

$$H^+ \quad + HCO_3^- \leftrightarrow H_2CO_3 \leftrightarrow H_2O + \quad CO_2$$

Hydrogen ions   Bicarbonate   Carbonic acid   Water   Carbon dioxide

It is important to note that the reactions are reversible. Direction is dependent on the relative concentration of each element. For example, a rise in carbon dioxide forces reaction to the left with increased production of carbonic acid and ultimately hydrogen ions. This explains the acidic potential of carbon dioxide and brings us to the important contribution that the lungs play in preserving normal blood pH.

Lungs and maintenance of normal blood pH

The main contribution of the lungs to the maintenance of a normal pH is regulation of the amount of carbon dioxide in blood. The actual amount of carbon dioxide in blood reflects a balance between that produced by cellular metabolism and that eliminated by the lungs in expired air, during respiration. Respiratory chemoreceptors in the brain detect changes in carbon dioxide content of blood, increasing respiration if carbon dioxide is high and reducing respiratory rate if low. Thus respiratory rate is the main determinant of carbon dioxide excretion by the lungs and therefore the amount of carbon dioxide in blood.

The sequence of events from CO_2 production in the tissues to elimination in expired air is described in Figure 7.3.

Carbon dioxide diffuses out of tissue cells to surrounding capillary blood. A small proportion dissolves in blood plasma and is transported to the lungs unchanged. But most diffuses into red cells, where an enzyme called carbonic anhydrase facilitates its combination with water to form carbonic acid. The acid dissociates, with production of hydrogen ions and bicarbonate. Hydrogen ions combine with deoxygenated haemoglobin (haemoglobin is acting as a buffer here) preventing a dangerous fall in cellular pH, and bicarbonate diffuses along a concentration gradient from red cell to plasma. Thus most of the carbon dioxide produced in the tissues is transported to the lungs as bicarbonate in blood plasma. A small proportion of the carbon dioxide that diffuses into red cells is transported bound to haemoglobin.

At the alveoli in the lungs the process is reversed (Figure 7.3b). Hydrogen ions are displaced from haemoglobin as it takes up oxygen from inspired air. The hydrogen ions are now buffered by bicarbonate which diffuses from plasma back into red cell, and carbonic acid is formed. As the concentration of this rises it is converted to water and carbon dioxide. Finally carbon dioxide diffuses down a concentration gradient from red cell to alveoli for excretion in expired air.

Kidneys and maintenance of normal blood pH

Normal cellular metabolism results in continuous production of hydrogen ions. We have seen that by combining with these hydrogen ions, buffers in blood minimise their effect on pH. However buffering does not remove hydrogen ions from the body and maintenance of normal blood pH depends ultimately on the ability of the body to eliminate hydrogen ions. At the same time, it is important to continuously replenish the bicarbonate used in buffering. These two tasks: elimination of hydrogen ions and regeneration of bicarbonate are accomplished by the kidneys; specifically the renal tubule cells. These cells are rich in the enzyme carbonic anhydrase,

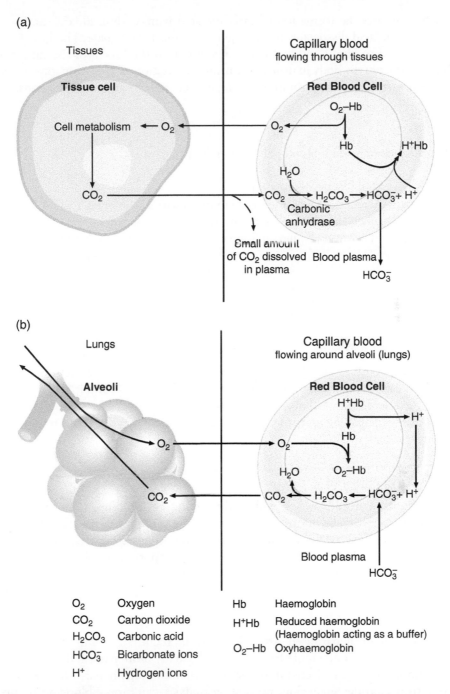

Figure 7.3 (a) Delivery of oxygen (O_2) to tissues and first step in the elimination of carbon dioxide (CO_2); (b) at the lung alveoli bicarbonate is converted back to carbon dioxide (CO_2), which is eliminated by the lungs in expired air.

which facilitates the formation of carbonic acid from carbon dioxide and water. The carbonic acid dissociates to hydrogen ions and bicarbonate. The bicarbonate is reabsorbed to blood and hydrogen ions pass into the lumen of the tubule and eliminated from the body in urine. This urine elimination of hydrogen ions depends on the presence in urine of buffers, principally phosphate and ammonia ions.

Summary

Maintenance of normal blood pH is dependent then on:

- Adequate blood buffering capacity.
- Normally functioning respiratory chemoreceptors in the brain.
- Normally functioning lungs (elimination of carbon dioxide).
- Normally functioning kidneys (elimination of hydrogen ions and regeneration of bicarbonate).

Measurement of blood gases

Patient preparation

Patients who require blood gas analysis may be receiving oxygen therapy or artificial ventilation. Changes in these therapies will affect results and it is preferable to allow the effects of any change to stabilise for 30 minutes before sampling blood. The patient should be warned that arterial sampling may be more painful than venepuncture.

Timing of sampling

Apart from advice already provided, the timing of sampling is not important. Laboratories need to be informed by phone before sampling to ensure that analysis is performed immediately the sample arrives. Blood gases are frequently ordered more than once daily on the same patient; it is important to record the time of blood sampling on the accompanying request card.

Sample requirements

Around 2 ml of heparinised arterial blood is required. An arterial puncture (Table 7.1) is potentially more hazardous and usually more painful than venepuncture. Blood must be collected into a syringe that contains heparin to prevent the blood from clotting. Small clots, preventing analysis, can form if blood is not mixed adequately with the heparin. The metabolic activity of blood cells continues after blood sampling with consumption of oxygen and production of carbon dioxide. For this reason blood for blood gases should be analysed immediately they are sampled. If there is to be any delay (more than 10 minutes), the syringe must be

Table 7.1 A protocol for collection of arterial blood sample.

Arterial blood is routinely sampled from the radial artery in the wrist, the femoral artery in the groin or the brachial artery in the arm.

The syringe must be loaded with 0.5–1.0 ml lithium or sodium heparin solution (1000 units/ml) to prevent blood from clotting in the syringe. Sterile, pre-heparinised syringe packs specifically for arterial blood collection are usually used.

The procedure is more painful than venepuncture so local anaesthetic is sometimes used to dull the arterial puncture site prior to sampling.

Aseptic technique including gloved hands is required to prevent cross-infection.

- Locate the injection site by feeling for pulsating artery.
- Prepare the site by cleaning first with alcohol and then iodine antiseptic solution. Allow to dry.
- Inject local anesthetic to the site (optional).
- Hold the blood gas syringe with needle attached between forefinger and thumb (like holding a dart) and with other hand relocate the artery.
- Warn patient before inserting the needle bevel side uppermost into the skin at an angle of around 45 degrees (90 degrees in the case of a femoral stab) just behind the finger locating the artery.
- Advance the needle in the direction of the artery.
- When the artery is punctured, blood will automatically flow into the syringe due to arterial pressure (a useful signal that an artery rather than a vein has been punctured).
- When sufficient blood has been collected withdraw the needle and immediately place a sterile gauze over the injection site. Firm finger pressure must be applied for minimum of five minutes.
- Discard needle to sharps disposable box, eject any air from the syringe and cap the syringe.
- Invert the syringe several times to ensure adequate mixing of blood and heparin solution.
- Immerse syringe in iced water and arrange immediate transport to laboratory.

packed in iced water to inhibit blood cell metabolism. Any air present in the syringe after blood collection will equilibrate with blood giving falsely raised blood PO_2 if patient's PO_2 is less than that of ambient air or falsely reduced blood PO_2, if patient's PO_2 is more than that of ambient air. It is important to expel all air from the syringe immediately blood has been sampled.

Arterial blood may be sampled from an indwelling arterial line[2]. Capillary blood obtained from a finger prick, earlobe or heel stab may be used if arterial blood collection poses a problem, for example in neonates. The same principles apply; blood sample must be heparinised, contain no air bubbles and be analysed without delay.

Analysis

Blood is injected directly from the syringe into the blood gas analyser. Inside the analyser three separate electrodes measure pH, PCO_2 and PO_2. From these measurements the machine calculates several other parameters, the most frequently used in practice are bicarbonate concentration (HCO_3) and base excess (BE).

The measured and calculated results are printed by the machine within a minute or so after injection of the sample. Most modern blood gas analysers also have the capacity to measure oxygen saturation (SO_2); in older blood gas analysers SO_2 is calculated rather than measured.

Interpretation of blood gas results

[Note: By convention the partial pressure (P) of gases in blood is most often (although not universally) written with a suffix ('a' or 'v') to denote either arterial or venous blood. The standard sample for blood gases is arterial blood so partial pressures of oxygen and carbon dioxide are expressed thus: PaO_2, $PaCO_2$. This convention, which also applies to oxygen saturation (SO_2) (arterial blood SO_2 is expressed: SaO_2), will be adopted for the remainder of the chapter.]

Reference ranges – adults

pH	7.35–7.45
(Hydrogen ion (H^+) concentration 35–45 nmol/L)	
$PaCO_2$	4.7–6.0 kPa (or 35–45 mmHg)
Bicarbonate	22–28 mmol/L
Base Excess	−2 – +2 mmol/L
PaO_2	10.6–13.3 kPa (or 80–100 mmHg)
SaO_2	95–99%

Reference range – neonates (age 36–60 hours)[1]

pH	7.31–7.47
$PaCO_2$	3.8–6.5 kPa (28–49 mmHg)
PaO_2	4.3–8.1 kPa (32–61 mmHg)
Bicarbonate	15–25 mmol/L

Critical values – adults

pH	<7.2 or >7.6
$PaCO_2$	<2.7 kPa or >9.3 kPa
Bicarbonate	<10 mmol/L or >40 mmon/L
PaO_2	<5.3 kPa
SaO_2	<60%

Terms used in blood gas interpretation

Acidosis/acidaemia – pH <7.35 or H^+ concentration >45 nmol/L
Alkalosis/alkalaemia – pH >7.45 or H^+ concentration <35 nmol/L

Hypercapnia (increased amount of carbon dioxide dissolved in arterial blood) – $PaCO_2$ >6.0 kPa

Hypocapnia (decreased amount of carbon dioxide dissolved in arterial blood) – $PaCO_2$ <4.7 kPa

Hypoxaemia (reduced amount of oxygen dissolved in arterial blood) – PaO_2 <10.6 kPa, SaO_2 <95%

Anaemic hypoxaemia (reduced amount of oxygen in blood due to reduced haemoglobin) – PaO_2 and SaO_2 within normal reference range

Hypoxia – reduced oxygen tension in tissues, tissues poorly oxygenated. This may be due to hypoxaemia but can also be due to reduced blood supply. It is important to emphasise that hypoxia can occur even if blood is well oxygenated (i.e. PaO_2, SaO_2 and Hb within their respective normal reference range).

Clinical disturbances of acid-base balance

Most disturbances of acid-base balance can be attributed to one of three broad causes:

- Disease or damage to organs (kidney, lungs, brain) whose normal function is necessary for acid-base homeostasis.
- Disease which causes abnormally increased production of metabolic acids such that homeostatic buffering mechanisms are overwhelmed.
- Medical intervention (e.g. artificial ventilation, some drugs).

To understand how blood gas results (pH, $PaCO_2$ and bicarbonate) can be used to identify the cause and monitor disturbances of acid-base balance we must return to the Henderson-Hasselbach equation

$$pH = 6.1 + \log\frac{\left[HCO_3^-\right]}{\left[H_2CO_3\right]} \hspace{3cm} \text{Eqn. 6}$$

Bicarbonate (HCO_3^-) is calculated during blood gas measurement but carbonic acid (H_2CO_3) is not. However there is a relationship between carbonic acid concentration and $PaCO_2$, a measured parameter of blood gases, which allows restatement of the Henderson-Hasselbach equation in terms of the three measured parameters of blood gas analysis, pH, $PaCO_2$ and bicarbonate:

$$pH = 6.1 + \log\frac{\left[HCO_3^-\right]}{PaCO_2 \times 0.23} \hspace{3cm} \text{Eqn. 7}$$

Removing all constants from this equation we can state that

$$pH \propto \frac{\left[HCO_3^-\right]}{PaCO_2} \hspace{3cm} \text{Eqn. 8}$$

This simple relationship, crucial for an understanding of all that follows concerning acid-base disturbances, states that blood pH is proportional to the ratio of bicarbonate concentration to $PaCO_2$. It allows the following deductions:

- pH remains normal so long as the ratio $[HCO_3]:PaCO_2$ remains normal.
- pH increases (i.e. alkalosis occurs) if *either* $[HCO_3]$ increases *or* $PaCO_2$ decreases.
- pH decreases (i.e. acidosis occurs) if *either* $[HCO_3]$ decreases *or* $PaCO_2$ increases.
- If *both* $PaCO_2$ *and* $[HCO_3]$ are increased by relatively the same amount, the ratio and therefore the pH are normal.
- If both $PaCO_2$ *and* $[HCO_3]$ are decreased by relatively the same amount, the ratio and therefore the pH are normal.

Classification of acid-base disturbances

All acid-base disturbances are classified to one of four groups depending on whether the primary abnormality is in $PaCO_2$ or bicarbonate concentration. Primary disturbance of $PaCO_2$ is referred to as a respiratory disturbance (reflecting the role that the respiratory system plays in regulating $PaCO_2$) and primary disturbance of bicarbonate is called metabolic:

- If the primary disturbance is raised $PaCO_2$ (which causes acidosis – already discussed) the condition is called *respiratory acidosis*.
- If the primary disturbance is reduced $PaCO_2$ (which causes alkalosis – already dicussed) the condition is called *respiratory alkalosis*.
- If the primary disturbance is reduced bicarbonate (which results in acidosis – already discussed) the condition is called *metabolic acidosis*.
- If the primary disturbance is raised bicarbonate (which results in alkalosis – already discussed) the condition is called *metabolic alkalosis*.

Causes of the four acid-base disorders

Respiratory acidosis (i.e. primary increase in $PaCO_2$, reduced pH)
Respiratory acidosis is characterised by increased $PaCO_2$ due to inadequate ventilation (hypoventilation) and consequent reduced elimination of CO_2 in expired air and accumulation in blood. Respiratory disease such as bronchopneumonia, asthma, chronic obstructive pulmonary disease (emphysema, chronic bronchitis) may all be associated with hypoventilation sufficient to cause respiratory acidosis. Some drugs (e.g. morphine and barbiturates) and head injury can cause respiratory acidosis by depressing or damaging the respiratory centre in the brain that regulates respiration. Damage or trauma to chest wall and the musculature involved in the mechanics of respiration may reduce ventilation rate. This explains the respiratory acidosis that can complicate the course of diseases such as poliomyelitis, Guillain-Barre syndrome and recovery from severe chest trauma. Respiratory acidosis can be classified as acute (i.e. rapid onset, for example,

during an acute asthmatic attack) or chronic, for example, in chronic obstructive pulmonary disease, between acute exacerbations. $PaCO_2$ greater than 7.0 kPa defines respiratory failure (type 2).

Respiratory alkalosis (reduced $PaCO_2$, increased pH)

By contrast respiratory alkalosis is characterised by *reduced* $PaCO_2$ due to excessive ventilation and resulting excessive elimination of CO_2 from blood. Reduced oxygen in blood (hypoxaemia) can stimulate increased ventilation sufficiently to cause respiratory alkalosis. Conditions in which this mechanism might operate to cause respiratory alkalosis include severe anaemia, pulmonary embolism and adult respiratory distress syndrome. Stress related hyperventilation sufficient to cause respiratory alkalosis is often a feature of anxiety attacks and response to severe pain. One of the less welcome properties of salicylate (aspirin) is its stimulatory effect on respiratory centre. This effect accounts for the respiratory alkalosis that occurs following salicylate overdose. Finally, excessive rate of artificial ventilation can cause respiratory alkalosis.

Metabolic acidosis (reduced bicarbonate, reduced pH)

Reduced bicarbonate is always a feature of metabolic acidosis. This occurs for one of two reasons: increased consumption of bicarbonate in buffering an abnormal acid load or increased loss of bicarbonate from the body. Diabetic ketoacidosis and lactic acidosis are two pathological conditions characterised by overproduction of metabolic acids with consequent exhaustion of bicarbonate. In the first case, abnormally high blood concentrations of keto-acids (β-hydroxybutyric acid and acetoacetic acid) reflect the severe metabolic derangements that result from insulin deficiency.

All cells produce excess lactic acid if they are deficient of oxygen, so increased lactic acid production and resulting metabolic acidosis occurs in any condition in which oxygen delivery to the tissues is severely compromised, a common feature of critical illness and among those who have suffered major trauma. Examples include: cardiac arrest; any condition associated with hypovolaemic shock (e.g. massive fluid loss) and severe anaemia. The liver plays a major role in removing the small amount of lactic acid that is produced during normal cell metabolism, so that lactic acidosis can be a feature of liver failure.

Abnormal loss of bicarbonate from the body can occur during severe diarrhoea. If unchecked this can lead to metabolic acidosis. Failure to regenerate bicarbonate and excrete hydrogen ions explains the metabolic acidosis that occurs in renal failure.

Metabolic alkalosis (increased bicarbonate, increased pH)

Bicarbonate is always raised in metabolic alkalosis. Rarely, excessive IV administration of bicarbonate or ingestion of bicarbonate in over the counter antacid preparations can cause metabolic alkalosis, but this is usually transient. Abnormal loss of hydrogen ions from the body can be the primary problem; bicarbonate, which would otherwise be consumed in buffering these lost hydrogen ions, consequently accumulates in blood. Gastric juice is acidic and gastric aspiration or any disease process in which gastric contents are lost from the body represents a loss of hydrogen ions. The projectile vomiting of gastric juice, for example, explains the metabolic alkalosis that can occur in patients with pyloric stenosis. Severe potassium depletion can cause metabolic alkalosis due to the reciprocal relationship between hydrogen and potassium ions across cell membranes (potassium passes out of cells to ECF in exchange for hydrogen ions in the context of hypokalaemia).

Consequence of acid-base disturbance – compensation

Because of the prime importance of maintaining a normal blood pH, the body will always attempt to return an abnormal pH to normal. This process is called compensation. To understand compensation it is important to recall that pH is governed by the ratio $[HCO_3]:PaCO_2$. So long as the ratio is normal, pH will be normal. Primary respiratory disturbances of acid-base, in which $PaCO_2$ is abnormal, are compensated for by adjustment of the metabolic component bicarbonate (HCO_3). Conversely, a primary disturbance of bicarbonate is compensated for by adjustment of the respiratory component, $PaCO_2$.

Consider the patient with metabolic acidosis whose pH is low because bicarbonate concentration $[HCO_3]$ is low. To compensate for the low $[HCO_3]$, and restore the all-important ratio towards normal, the patient must lower his or her $PaCO_2$. Chemoreceptors respond to rising hydrogen ion concentration (low pH) causing increased ventilation (hyperventilation) and thereby increased elimination of carbon dioxide; the $PaCO_2$ falls and the ratio $[HCO_3]:PaCO_2$ returns towards normal.

Compensation for metabolic alkalosis in which $[HCO_3]$ is high by contrast, involves depression of respiration and thereby retention of carbon dioxide so that the $PaCO_2$ rises to match the increase in $[HCO_3]$. However depression of respiration has the unwelcome side effect of threatening adequate oxygenation of tissues. For this reason respiratory compensation of metabolic alkalosis is limited. Primary disturbances of $PaCO_2$ (respiratory acidosis and alkalosis) are compensated for by renal adjustments that result in changes in bicarbonate concentration. Thus the renal compensation for respiratory acidosis (raised $PaCO_2$) involves increased renal reabsorption of bicarbonate and compensation for respiratory alkalosis (reduced $PaCO_2$) involves reduced bicarbonate reabsorption.

If the compensatory process is sufficient to return the pH to normal, the patient is said to be fully compensated. If the compensatory process is sufficient to return the pH towards normal, but insufficient to actually achieve normality, the patient is said to be partially compensated. The concept of an 'acid-base balance' allows the process of compensation to be conveyed visually (Figure 7.4).

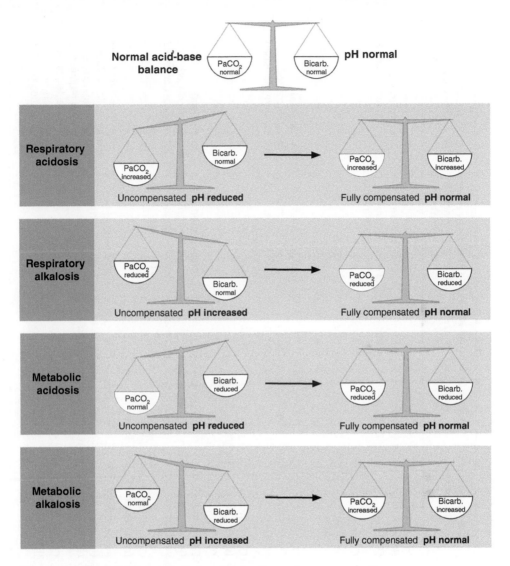

Figure 7.4 The 'acid-base balance': compensation restores normal pH.

It must be remembered that compensation whether partial or complete is not a state of normality; the ratio $[HCO_3]:PaCO_2$ and therefore the pH may be normal, but both $[HCO_3]$ and $PaCO_2$ are abnormal. Only successful treatment of the primary disturbance can return $PaCO_2$ and $[HCO_3]$ to normal. Table 7.2 summarises blood gas results before, during and after compensation of acid-base disorders.

Renal compensation of respiratory disorders is much slower than respiratory compensation of metabolic disorders. In the first case compensation occurs over a period of days or weeks, but in the second evidence of compensation is seen within hours.

Table 7.2 Blood gas results in disturbances of acid-base balance.

Primary disturbance	Some common causes	Compensatory mechanism	Initial blood gas results (uncompensated)	Blood gas results after partial compensation	Blood gas results after full compensation
Respiratory acidosis *i.e. primary increase in* $PaCO_2$	Hypoventilation due to • Pneumonia • Asthma • COPD • Depression of respiratory centre	Increase bicarbonate (kidney and red blood cells) Compensation slow (several days, maybe weeks)	pH decreased $PaCO_2$ increased Bicarbonate normal	pH decreased but closer to normal $PaCO_2$ increased Bicarbonate increased	**pH normal** $PaCO_2$ increased Bicarbonate increased
Respiratory alkalosis *i.e. primary decrease in* $PaCO_2$	Hyperventilation due to • Pain • Anxiety attack • Stimulation of respiratory centre	Decrease bicarbonate (kidney and red blood cells) Compensation slow (several days, maybe weeks)	pH increased $PaCO_2$ decreased Bicarbonate normal	pH decreased but closer to normal $PaCO_2$ decreased Bicarbonate decreased	**pH normal** $PaCO_2$ decreased Bicarbonate decreased
Metabolic acidosis *i.e. primary decrease in* bicarbonate	• Renal failure • Diabetic ketoacidosis • Circulatory failure-shock	Decrease $PaCO_2$ (i.e. increase respiratory ventilation) Compensation rapid (minutes/hours)	pH decreased $PaCO_2$ normal Bicarbonate decreased	pH decreased but closer to normal $PaCO_2$ increased Bicarbonate decreased	**pH normal** $PaCO_2$ decreased Bicarbonate decreased
Metabolic alkalosis *i.e. primary increase in* bicarbonate	• Excessive bicarbonate ingestion • Potassium depletion • Vomiting of gastric acid	Increase $PaCO_2$ (i.e. decrease respiratory ventilation) Compensation rapid (minutes/hours)	pH increased $PaCO_2$ normal Bicarbonate increased	pH increased but closer to normal $PaCO_2$ decreased Bicarbonate increased	Full compensation is rare in metabolic alkalosis because the decreased ventilation required would threaten blood oxygenation. Full compensation prevented by 'hypoxaemic drive'

Consequences of acid base disturbances – clinical signs and symptoms

Whatever the cause, acid-base disturbances themselves result in signs and symptoms. Raised $PaCO_2$ (hypercapnia) has non-specific effects on the central nervous system which may include confusion, headache and hand tremor. Coma may ensue if levels are particularly high. Reduced $PaCO_2$ results in symptoms of light-headedness or dizziness. Acidosis can cause hyperkalaemia; patients affected may have characteristic symptoms and ECG changes. Alkalosis decreases plasma concentration of ionised calcium; this causes symptoms of tetany, which include painful muscle cramps and spasm, pins and needles and paraesthesia. As we have seen potassium depletion is an important cause of metabolic alkalosis, but alkalosis can itself cause hypokalaemia so that symptoms and signs of hypokalaemia often accompany alkalosis, whatever the cause. Compensation for metabolic acidosis involves deep and rapid respiration to eliminate CO_2.

Mixed acid-base disturbances

Thus far it has been assumed that any particular patient with a disturbance of acid-base balance suffers only one of the four categories of acid-base imbalance discussed. Whilst this may well be the case, patients can present with a mixture of two or even three disturbances, making interpretation of blood gas results more complex. As an example of a mixed disturbance, consider a patient with a chronic obstructive pulmonary disease (COPD) who has a heart attack and suffers cardiac arrest. Before the arrest the patient has partially compensated respiratory acidosis due to long standing COPD. The cardiac arrest causes metabolic acidosis. Results of blood gas analysis within a few hours after the arrest will reflect the combined effect of both respiratory and metabolic acidosis. Having regard to the causes of single acid-base disturbances, it is not difficult to imagine many other clinical situations in which a patient might be suffering more than one type of acid-base disturbance.

Causes and consequences of reduced PaO_2 (hypoxaemia)

Breathing air which has relatively low PO_2 (e.g. atmospheric air at high altitude) will result in a low PaO_2, but clinically the most important causes are those in which gas exchange with blood across the alveolar membrane is compromised due to respiratory disease. Reduced PaO_2 may thus occur in any condition that causes respiratory acidosis. However hypoxaemia can occur in the absence of respiratory acidosis. For example, in some respiratory diseases the hypoxic drive induced by low PaO_2 increases respiration (and therefore CO_2 elimination) sufficient to maintain a normal or even low $PaCO_2$. Respiratory acidosis develops when even the hypoxic drive is insufficient to prevent CO_2 retention.

Finally, inadvertent sampling of venous blood rather than arterial blood causes falsely low results and this explanation should be considered if there is no clinical reason for a low PaO_2.

From Figure 7.2 it can be seen that reduction in PO_2 reduces oxygen saturation of haemoglobin and therefore oxygen delivery to the tissues. Respiratory failure (defined as a PaO_2 of <8 kPa) causes breathlessness confusion, sweating, tachycardia and cyanosis. In patients with accompanying respiratory acidosis the symptoms of hypercapnia may also be present. A distinction is made between type 1 respiratory failure (defined as PaO_2 <8 kPa with normal or reduced $PaCO_2$) and type 2 respiratory failure (defined as PaO_2 <8 kPa with increased $PaCO_2$). This distinction highlights the fact that hypoxaemia can occur with or without adequate ventilation.

Causes and consequnces of increased PaO_2 (hyperoxia)

The only cause of increased PaO_2 is supplemental oxygen therapy. The reference (normal) range for PaO_2 assumes patients are breathing ambient air, which comprises 21% oxygen (i.e. fraction of inspired oxygen, $FiO_2 = 21\%$). Depending on the mode of therapeutic oxygen delivery, FiO_2 can range 25–100%. PaO_2 may be transiently raised in patients receiving oxygen therapy, particularly if FiO_2 is high (>50%).

Oxygen is potentially toxic if delivered at high concentration (FiO_2 >60 for extended periods (>24 hours). Newborn babies are particularly vulnerable to the toxic effects of oxygen. Hyperoxia (PaO_2 >13.3 kPa) in newborns is associated with increasing risk of an eye condition called retinopathy of prematurity (ROP), which can lead to blindness. Additionally, hyperoxia can cause lung and brain damage. Premature babies are at particularly high risk of these and other toxic effects of oxygen therapy, which should be used with caution and carefully monitored in these vulnerable babies; it is recommended that for most pre-term babies requiring supplemental oxygen, dosing should be adjusted so that PaO_2 does not exceed 10.7 kPa and SaO_2 is maintained within the range 89–95%.

Monitoring blood oxygenation by pulse oximetry

Measurement of PaO_2 (partial pressure of oxygen in arterial blood) and SaO_2 (oxygen saturation of arterial blood) during blood gas analysis provides the most accurate assessment of a patient's blood oxygenation status. An alternative non-invasive method of continuously monitoring blood oxygenation is provided by pulse oximetry, which has become ubiquitous in most areas of clinical care and so is familiar to all nurses. The pulse oximeter comprises a probe that is attached, usually to the fingertip or earlobe. The probe emits light of two wavelengths directed through the skin and pulsating blood capillaries in the fingertip or earlobe. The amount of light absorbed is detected and this depends on the relative amounts of oxyhaemoglobin and deoxyhaemoglobin in capillary blood. The instrument computes the percentage of oxygen saturation from these measurements and the result is displayed as SpO_2, that is the oxygen saturation in peripheral (capillary) blood.

The validity of pulse oximetry for assessment of oxygenation status depends on SpO_2 being a reliable estimate of the oxygen saturation of arterial blood (SaO_2), the parameter measured during blood gases. Although in healthy individuals and most clinical contexts SpO_2 is more or less equal to SaO_2, there are some situations when that is not the case. It is important to be aware of the limitations of pulse oximetry and clinical situations when there is no alternative to blood gases for accurate assessment of patient blood oxygenation status.

Pulse oximetry is sufficiently accurate in the range 80–100% but underestimates SaO_2 when patients are severely hypoxaemic (SaO_2 <80%). Pulse oximetry depends on adequate peripheral blood flow and may give inaccurate results when this is compromised, for example, in severe hypotension, cardiac arrest or hypovolaemia.

Normally, a small amount (<1%) of the total haemoglobin in blood is carboxyhaemoglobin (COHb) and methaemoglobin (MetHb), both of which are incapable of binding/transporting oxygen. The measuring system in pulse oximeters is unable to distinguish these so-called dysfunctional haemoglobins from normal functioning haemoglobin. This means that pulse oximetry produces inaccurate results in patients who are suffering conditions in which COHb or MetHb levels are abnormally high; these include carbon monoxide poisoning and methaemoglobinaemia. Nail varnish may interfere with measurement if the probe is applied to the fingertip. Finally, shivering (indeed any persisting movement of the probe) can potentially cause inaccurate pulse oximetry results.

Monitoring foetal pH

This is a specialised use of the blood gas analyser in the obstetric/labour ward. Foetal blood sampling/foetal blood pH is a test used to monitor the foetus during childbirth if non-invasive (e.g. cardiotographic) monitoring indicates signs of possible foetal distress. The test result can provide unequivocal evidence of foetal distress and is useful for deciding if immediate birth by caesarean section is indicated.

Foetal distress is characterised by decreased tissue oxygenation (hypoxia) and resulting metabolic acidosis (due to accumulating lactic and pyruvic acid, products of anaerobic glycolysis). Foetal blood pH equal to or greater than 7.25 is considered normal, and reassuring of no foetal distress; only if non-invasive monitoring worsens should a second sample be tested 1 hour later. Foetal blood pH in the range 7.21–7.24 indicates possible acidosis; the test should be repeated 30 minutes later. Finally, foetal blood pH equal to or less than 7.20 is unequivocal evidence of acidosis and a distressed foetus that needs delivering. Blood for this test is sampled from the foetal scalp, using a technique that involves insertion of a tube into the vagina, through the cervix to the foetal head. This tube allows illuminated direct vision of the foetal head, which is cleaned then sprayed with a fluid that provides both local anaesthesia and vasodilation to increase blood flow. A tiny scalpel blade is inserted into the prepared foetal scalp and a small drop of blood (~0.25 ml) is collected anaerobically into a heparinised capillary tube by capillary action.

Case history 10

Recovery during the 24 hours following coronary bypass surgery was uneventful for 68 year old Brian Phelps. For him the major problem was surgical pain that was being treated effectively with increasing doses of morphine. Progress towards hospital discharge was however halted on the second morning after surgery when Brian reported feeling 'weird' and 'definitely not well'. The duty doctor was called but within half an hour Brian had collapsed; he was unresponsive when the doctor arrived and his breathing was slow and shallow (respiratory rate 6/min). Eye examination revealed abnormally constricted pupils with ambient lighting (pin-point pupils), which persuaded the doctor that Brian might be suffering morphine overdose. Oxygen was administered and arterial blood sampled for blood gas analysis 20 minutes later.

pH	7.22
$PaCO_2$	7.6 kPa
Bicarbonate	25 mmol/L
Base excess	1.0 mmol/L
PaO_2	−11.3 kPa
SaO_2	98%

Questions

(1) Brian's arterial blood pH is abnormal. Is he suffering acidosis or alkalosis?
(2) Is Brian's $PaCO_2$ and/or bicarbonate normal?
(3) Is this a metabolic or respiratory acid-base disturbance?
(4) Is this acid-base disturbance uncompensated, partially compensated or fully compensated?
(5) Describe Brian's acid-base status fully and comment on his blood and tissue oxygenation status.
(6) Are the blood gas results consistent with the doctor's provisional diagnosis of morphine overdose?

Discussion of case history 10

(1) The (normal) adult reference range for arterial blood pH is 7.35–7.45. Brian has markedly reduced blood pH, he is suffering severe acidosis.

(2) Brian's $PaCO_2$ is increased but his bicarbonate concentration is well within the reference range (22–28 mmol/L).

(3) The combination of reduced pH and raised $PaCO_2$ indicates a respiratory acidosis. Metabolic acidosis by contrast is characterised by reduced pH and reduced bicarbonate.

(4) Since Brian has an abnormal blood pH, his acid-base disturbance is not fully compensated. The normal compensatory response to respiratory acidosis is increased regeneration of bicarbonate by the kidneys and consequent raised bicarbonate, but this is a relatively slow process occurring over a period of days. Brian currently has a normal bicarbonate so there is no evidence of even partial compensation.

(5) Brian is suffering acute, uncompensated respiratory acidosis. Although blood gas results indicate adequate blood oxygenation (PaO_2 and SaO_2 within the reference range) this is only by virtue of the oxygen therapy he is necessarily receiving. A healthy person given supplemental oxygen for 30 minutes would have a much higher PaO_2. Results (increased $PaCO_2$, (effective) reduced PaO_2) indicate type 2 respiratory failure,

a marked reduction in ventilation and inadequate pulmonary gas exchange. Without oxygen therapy Brian's tissues would be inadequately oxygenated.

(6) Yes, the most dangerous adverse (side) effect of morphine, like many other opioid drugs, operates via its action on the respiratory centre in the brain that normally controls the rate of breathing by sensing $PaCO_2$. Despite rising $PaCO_2$ respiration is depressed in those suffering morphine overdose. Inadequate pulmonary gas exchange with rising $PaCO_2$ and reducing PaO_2 is the inevitable result if respiratory rate falls to six breaths per minute, as was the case for Brian. The opioid antagonist drug naloxone is used to reverse the effects of morphine and normal respiration is rapidly restored.

Case history 11

When Mr Bridges, a 70 year old man with a ten year history of chronic obstructive pulmonary disease (COPD), experienced sudden worsening of his symptoms, his wife called their GP who arranged immediate transfer to hospital. On arrival he was breathless, even while lying still. He was drowsy and confused. Arterial blood was sampled for blood gases. The laboratory reported the following results:

pH	7.28
$PaCO_2$	8.8 kPa
Bicarbonate	35 mmol/L
PaO_2	5.4 kPa

On admission to intensive care, he was mechanically ventilated and given oxygen. After 30 minutes ventilation the patient showed signs of tetany. Results of blood gases at this time were:

pH	7. 59
$PaCO_2$	3.4 kPa
Bicarbonate	33 mmol/L
PaO_2	10.9 kPa

Questions

(1) What was Mr Bridges' acid-base and oxygen status on arrival at hospital?
(2) How does COPD result in such an acid-base disturbance?
(3) Explain the relationship between symptoms and blood gas results.
(4) What is the acid base and oxygen status after mechanical ventilation? Explain the marked change.
(5) What are the symptoms of tetany? Why did Mr Bridges have such symptoms?

Discussion of case history 11

(1) On arrival at hospital Mr Bridges was acidotic (reduced blood pH). Acidosis may be respiratory (due to raised $PaCO_2$) or metabolic (due to reduced bicarbonate). In this case the acidosis is clearly of respiratory origin. Raised bicarbonate indicates some degree of compensation, emphasising the long-standing (chronic)

nature of his condition. However since the pH remains abnormal, compensation is incomplete. A marked reduction in PaO_2, indicates severe hypoxaemia, consistent with respiratory failure; the combination of reduced PaO_2 and increased $PaCO_2$ indicates the respiratory failure is type 2 rather than type 1. At the time of admission then Mr Bridges was suffering severe partially compensated respiratory acidosis and severe hypoxaemia.

(2) COPD is a chronic disease of the lungs in which the normal elasticity of the air sacs (alveoli) is progressively lost. The consequence of the disease process is reduced alveolar area for exchange of oxygen and carbon dioxide between the environment and blood: PaO_2 falls and $PaCO_2$ rises. The accumulation of carbon dioxide in blood results in reduced blood pH (acidosis). To compensate and return pH towards normal, the kidneys regenerate more bicarbonate than usual and bicarbonate concentration increases.

(3) The cardinal symptom of COPD is progressively worsening breathlessness due to hypoxaemia. Eventually, as in the case of Mr Bridges, the PaO_2 drops so low that even at rest the patient is literally gasping for air. Severe hypercapnia may account for the confusion and drowsiness experienced by Mr Bridges.

(4) After 30 minutes of mechanical ventilation, Mr Bridges had a raised pH (alkalosis) which may be respiratory (reduced $PaCO_2$) or metabolic (increased bicarbonate) in origin. Since the bicarbonate level remained unchanged it must be the marked reduction in $PaCO_2$ brought about by mechanical ventilation that caused the alkalosis. As a result of over enthusiastic ventilation then, Mr Bridges suffered respiratory alkalosis. The normal renal compensation for respiratory alkalosis is to decrease blood bicarbonate by renal mechanisms involving increased elimination in urine and decreased regeneration of bicarbonate. But this is a relatively slow process occurring over days rather than minutes so that in this case there was no evidence of compensation. Respiratory alkalosis due to excessive mechanical ventilation can be quickly corrected by reducing the rate of mechanical ventilation.

(5) The symptoms of tetany, which include 'pins and needles' sensation, muscular spasms, and rarely convulsions, are due to a reduction of ionised plasma calcium concentration; ionised calcium is required for normal neuromuscular transmission. Calcium in blood is present in two almost equal fractions: half is bound to the protein albumin and is physiologically inactive, and the other half is 'free' physiologically active, ionised calcium. The proportion of total calcium that is in the ionised state is determined in part by the pH of blood; if the pH of blood is high (i.e. alkalotic) then less calcium than normal is in the ionised physiologically active form and more is present bound to albumin and therefore physiologically inactive. Patients who have a raised blood pH no matter what the cause, often have tetany. The symptoms of tetany disappear as the alkalosis is corrected and blood pH and ionised calcium returns to normal.

References

1. Cousineau, J., Anctil, S. et al. (2005) Neonate capillary blood gas reference values, *Clinical Biochemistry*, 38: 905–7.
2. Woodrow, P. (2009) Arterial catheters: promoting safe practice, *Nursing Standard*, 24: 35–40.

Further reading

Crawford, A. (2004) An audit of the patient's experience of arterial blood gas testing, *Br J Nursing*, 13: 529–32.

Deuber, C. and Terhaar, M. (2011) Hyperoxia in very preterm infants: a systematic review of the literature, *J Perinat Neonatal Nurs*, 25: 268–74.

Hennessey, I., Japp, A. (2007) *Arterial Blood Gases Made Easy*, Churchill-Livingstone.

Jones, B. (2010) Basic interpretation of metabolic acidosis, *Crit Care Nurse*, 30: 63–9.

Sassoon, C. and Arruda, J. (eds.) (2001) Acid base physiology and disorders: a special issue, *Respiratory Care* 46: 328–403.

Valdez-Lowe, C., Ghareeb, S. and Artinian, N. (2009) Pulse oximetry in adults, *AJN*, 109: 52–9.

Woodrow, P. (2010) Essential principles: blood gas analysis, *Nurs Critical Care*, 15: 152–6.

CHAPTER 8

PLASMA/SERUM CHOLESTEROL AND TRIGLYCERIDES

Key learning topics

- Structure and function of cholesterol and triglyceride (TG)
- Blood transport of lipids (including cholesterol and TG)
- Distinction between total cholesterol, LDL-cholesterol and HDL-cholesterol
- Factors to be considered before sampling blood for lipids
- Significance of serum lipids for atherosclerosis
- Serum cholesterol and risk of cardiovascular disease
- Defining those who require cholesterol testing
- Target (healthy) serum cholesterol concentration

The principle use of this blood test is to help assess an individual's overall risk of the cardiovascular diseases that result from atherosclerosis. The most significant of these is coronary heart disease (CHD), which affects an estimated 2.7 million in the UK and currently accounts for close to 88 000 deaths in the UK each year[1]. Despite 50% reduction in annual CHD deaths over the past 20 years, it remains second only to cancer (all types) as the leading cause of death in the UK[1]. There is overwhelming evidence that too much cholesterol and/or triglyceride in the blood increases the risk of CHD and all other atherosclerosis related cardiovascular diseases. The higher the level the greater is this risk. The test is used not only to assess risk but also to monitor the effectiveness of therapy (drugs, most commonly statins, and dietary manipulation) aimed at reducing the amount of cholesterol and triglyceride in blood.

Understanding Laboratory Investigations: A Guide for Nurses, Midwives and Healthcare Professionals, Third Edition. Chris Higgins.
© 2013 John Wiley & Sons, Ltd. Published 2013 by John Wiley & Sons, Ltd.

Normal physiology

What are cholesterol and triglycerides?

Apart from inorganic elements such as sodium, potassium, calcium etc., there are four broad classes of chemical present in the human body and the food we eat. They are: proteins, carbohydrates, nucleic acids and lipids (or fats). Although structurally dissimilar (Figure 8.1), cholesterol and triglycerides are lipids.

They are provided in a normal diet, both being present in meat and dairy products. Eggs are a particularly rich source of cholesterol. In addition to dietary sources, cholesterol and triglyceride are synthesised in the body, principally the liver (both cholesterol and triglyceride) and adipose or fat tissue (triglycerides only).

Function of cholesterol and triglycerides

In common with all lipids, cholesterol and triglycerides are essential components of cell membranes. Their function is however not confined to cell structure. In the liver, cholesterol is converted to bile acids and bile salts, which are excreted from the liver, via the gall bladder, to the intestinal tract in the digestive juice, bile. The presence of bile acids and salts in bile is essential for absorption of dietary fats. Cholesterol is the raw material from which steroid hormones are synthesised; examples include cortisol in the adrenal glands, progesterone in the ovaries and testosterone in the testis. Vitamin D is synthesised in the skin from a cholesterol derived compound.

Triglyceride is the principal fat present in adipose (fat) tissue and as such its main function is energy storage; triglycerides provide an alternative energy source to glucose, during fasting and starvation when glucose is in short supply. During these periods of relative glucose depletion, triglyceride present in adipose cells is broken down to its constituent parts by an enzyme called lipase; the process is called lipolysis. The free fatty acids that result from lipolysis are transported in blood to cells around the body, where they are oxidised (burnt) providing chemical energy. Meanwhile the other product of lipolysis, glycerol, is converted to glucose in the liver.

Blood transport of cholesterol and triglyceride

Like all lipids, cholesterol and triglyceride are insoluble in water. This poses a difficulty for their transport in blood plasma, which is a water-based (aqueous) solution of chemicals. To overcome this difficulty lipids, including cholesterol and triglycerides, are packaged in a water-soluble protein shell called an apoprotein. The total package, lipids plus apoprotein is called a lipoprotein. There are four main types of lipoprotein in blood, each with differing proportions of cholesterol, triglyceride and apoprotein (Figure 8.2). They are defined by their relative density and particle size and are known as:

- Chylomicrons (lowest density, largest particle).
- Very low density lipoproteins (VLDLs).

(a)

Cholesterol structure, like other sterols,
which include steroid hormones, Vitamin D
and bile acids, is based on the six carbon ring.

Six carbon ring

CH_3

CH_3

CH_3

CH_3

CH_3

CH_3

CH_3

HO

Cholesterol $(C_{27}H_{46}O)$

(b)

Triglycerides
are formed by combination of one molecule of glycerol and three fatty acids.

Fatty acid 1

Fatty acid 2

Glycerol

Fatty acid 3

Glycerol

$$CH_2OH$$
$$|$$
$$HO-CH$$
$$|$$
$$CH_2OH$$

Fatty acids

$CH_3-(CH_2)_n-COOH$

General formula for fatty acids (n = number of CH_2
groups which varies)

e.g. $CH_3-(CH_2)_{14}-COOH$

Formula for palmitic acid, a fatty acid with 14 CH
groups

A triglyceride

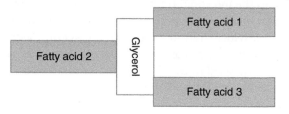

Figure 8.1 (a) Structure of cholesterol; (b) structure of triglycerides.

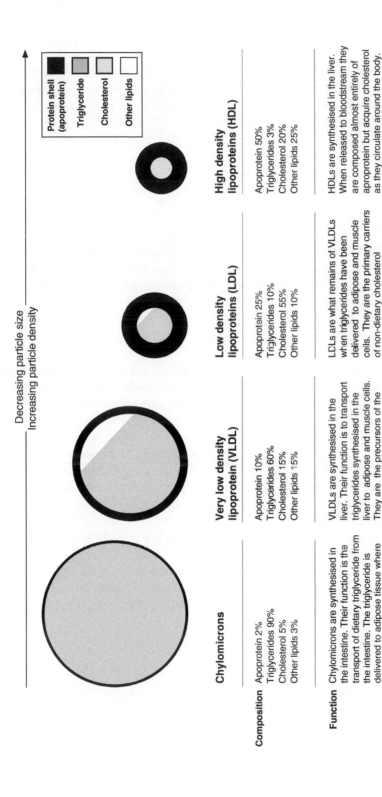

Figure 8.2 Structure, composition and function of lipoproteins.

- Low density lipoproteins (LDLs).
- High density lipoproteins (HDLs).

Around 70% of the cholesterol in blood is present in LDL and most of the remainder is present in HDL. By contrast most of the triglyceride in blood is contained within VLDL. As will become clear, the distinction between LDL-cholesterol and HDL-cholesterol is clinically important.

Laboratory measurement of plasma/serum cholesterol and triglyceride

Patient preparation

The concentration of cholesterol and triglyceride in blood is affected by diet, smoking, alcohol intake, inter-current illness and even changes in posture. It is important that where possible blood is sampled under standard conditions to minimise some of these effects.

- The patients normal diet should be followed in the two to three weeks prior to testing.
- There is a transient and quantitatively unpredictable rise in blood triglyceride level immediately after a meal, making interpretation difficult. For this reason blood for triglyceride estimation must be sampled only after an overnight fast of 12–14 hours. Fasting is not necessary if total cholesterol only is of interest but is necessary if LDL-cholesterol is requested because serum triglyceride is required for calculation of serum LDL-cholesterol concentration (explained further).
- The test should be deferred for three months if the patient has suffered major illness (e.g. myocardial infarction) or major surgery unless blood can be sampled within 12 hours of such an event. The test should be deferred for two to three weeks after minor illness.
- The patient should be well rested and seated for five to ten minutes before blood collection.
- Use of a tourniquet for more than a minute or so before blood collection can cause erroneous results. If possible avoid the use of tourniquet for this test.
- Interpretation of results is not possible if blood is sampled during lipid infusion (e.g. intraplipid).

Sample requirement

Around 5 ml of venous blood is required. The test may be performed on either plasma or serum. If local policy is to use serum then blood must be collected into a plain chemistry tube (i.e. without anticoagulant). If local policy is to use plasma then blood must be collected into a tube containing an anticoagulant (EDTA or heparin) which prevents blood from clotting.

In the laboratory

Three measurements are made in the laboratory:

- Serum or plasma concentration of total cholesterol (i.e. cholesterol contained in LDL, HDL and VLDL).
- Serum or plasma concentration of HDL-cholesterol (i.e. only the cholesterol contained in HDL).
- Serum or plasma concentration of triglycerides (i.e. triglyceride contained in VLDL, LDL and HDL).

The concentration of serum or plasma LDL-cholesterol is technically difficult to measure and in most laboratories is calculated using the results of analysis in the following well validated equation:

LDL-cholesterol = Total cholesterol – HDL-cholesterol – (Triglyceride/2.2)

Interpretation

Reference range – fasting triglycerides
0.45–1.80 mmol/L
Total cholesterol, HDL cholesterol and LDL cholesterol

Unlike most other blood tests the concept of a normal or reference range is not appropriate for cholesterol testing. This is because a large proportion of apparently healthy individuals from which a reference range would normally be constructed have cholesterol levels (total cholesterol, LDL-cholesterol and HDL-cholesterol) that are associated with increased risk of cardiovascular disease. In other words it is 'normal' to have an unhealthy amount of cholesterol in blood. Rather than a reference range, the concept of target values is used to interpret cholesterol results. Target values will be discussed a little later but for now it would be helpful to record some data about serum cholesterol concentration in the UK population.

- The mean plasma/serum total cholesterol for adults (>16 years) is 5.2 mmol/L for men and 5.4 mmol/L for women. The equivalent figures for those aged 45–65 years who have highest levels are: 5.8 mmol/L for men and 6.0 mmol/L for women[2].
- The National Service Framework target for cardiovascular disease prevention is plasma/serum total cholesterol <5.0 mmol/L[3].
- Around 60% of adults have total cholesterol >5.0 mmol/L[2].

Terms used in interpretation

Hyperlipidaemia   raised concentration of lipids in blood, i.e. total cholesterol
>5.0 mmol/L and/or triglyceride >1.8 mmol/L.

Hypercholesterolaemia   raised concentration of total cholesterol, i.e. >5.0 mmol/L.

Hypertriglyceridaemia   raised blood concentration of triglyceride, i.e. >1.80 mmol/L.

Consequences of raised cholesterol or triglyceride cardiovascular disease

As concentration of plasma/serum total cholesterol rises so too does the risk of those cardiovascular diseases that result from the restricted blood flow through arteries diseased by atherosclerosis, and associated thrombotic (blood clotting) consequences. Atherosclerosis may affect any artery, but the most commonly affected are the coronary arteries. The result is coronary heart disease, the most common cardiovascular disease.

Coronary heart disease

Coronary heart disease (CHD) (alternative name ischaemic heart disease) is caused by atherosclerosis in the coronary arteries that supply oxygenated blood to heart muscle (the myocardium). The focal thickening and hardening of the normally elastic walls of coronary arteries that characterises atherosclerosis progressively reduces the internal diameter of the artery, restricting blood flow and therefore oxygen delivery to the cells of which the myocardium is composed. The portion of myocardium affected becomes relatively deficient of oxygen (ischaemic). The first clinical manifestation of this relative oxygen deficit is usually angina pectoris or stable angina, intermittent attacks of chest pain or discomfort precipitated by increased heart rate due to exercise or some other stress. The pain subsides as rest and return of resting heart rate reduces the increased oxygen demand of myocardium.

Atherosclerosis predisposes to the inappropriate activation of the clotting cascade and formation of a blood clot (thrombus) within blood vessels at the site of atherosclerosis. This further occludes or totally occludes blood flow through the artery, effectively starving myocardial cells of the nutrients and oxygen required for survival. The clinical consequence of this is either unstable angina that is chest pain at rest or myocardial infarction (heart attack). The two conditions are referred to as acute coronary syndromes. A diagnosis of unstable angina implies high risk of future myocardial infarction. Myocardial infarction implies tissue necrosis (cell death), that is permanent damage to heart muscle as a result of ischaemia. The damage to the heart may result in sudden death if it causes lethal abnormal rhythms (e.g. ventricular fibrillation).

Stable angina, unstable angina, myocardial infarction and sudden death represent the most common manifestations of CHD in order of severity. They do not necessarily present in this ordered sequence and myocardial infarction or sudden death may be the first indication of coronary disease.

Other cardiovascular disease

Other sites less commonly affected by atherosclerosis include:

- Peripheral arteries that supply oxygenated blood to the limbs.
- Cerebral arteries which supply oxygenated blood to the brain.
- Abdominal aorta, lower half of the main blood vessel (aorta) that delivers oxygenated blood to the body.

Peripheral arterial disease usually affects the legs. Reduced oxygen delivery (consequent on reduced blood flow) to leg causes calf muscle pain on exercise, which is relieved by rest (intermittent claudication). The most severe presentation occurs if a thrombus forms at the site of atherosclerosis, totally occluding blood flow through the affected artery. Without urgent treatment to restore blood flow, resulting acute ischaemia can lead to necrosis, gangrene and necessity for amputation.

Reduced blood flow through cerebral arteries partially occluded by atherosclerosis is a common cause of transient ischaemic attacks (mini-strokes). Occlusion of cerebral arteries by a thrombus formed at the site of atherosclerosis is the most common cause of cerebrovascular accident (stroke), which can result in permanent disability or death.

Atherosclerosis in the abdominal aorta contributes to the weakening of the wall of this large vessel that results in dangerous dilation (aneurysm). This can be asymptomatic or cause abdominal pain. Without surgical repair to the vessel, progressive dilation can lead to catastrophic rupture of the aneurysm, massive haemorrhage and sudden death.

Blood lipids and cardiovascular disease

Atherosclerosis, the underlying pathology of CHD and other cardiovascular disease outlined already, is a complex and as yet not fully understood phenomenon which begins many years before symptoms develop. It is clear however that there are well defined risk factors (Table 8.1) which predispose people to atherosclerosis and subsequent cardiovascular disease. Some, like cholesterol and triglyceride, are modifiable, and some are not.

All risk factors must be taken into account to make the most reliable assessment of an individual's overall risk of CHD.

To understand how the lipids in blood, particularly cholesterol, contribute to CHD and other cardiovascular disease it is necessary to examine in a little more detail what is known about the process of atheroma formation, which leads to atherosclerosis and thrombosis.

Atheroma formation begins with damage to the endothelium that lines the internal surface of arteries, allowing entry of cholesterol-rich LDL particles present in blood. The damage attracts protective cells called macrophages which take up the LDL particles; LDL accumulates in these cells. At this early stage the only evidence of atheroma is a barely visible raised yellowish patch on the internal surface of the

Table 8.1 Major risk factors for coronary heart disease (CHD).

Increasing age

Family history of CHD

Diabetes

  Diabetics have 2–4 times the risk of CHD compared with non-diabetics who in all other respects have a similar risk status

Cigarette smoking*

Hypertension*

Unhealthy bodyweight*

  Defined as body mass index (BMI) >25 [BMI=weight in kg divided by height in m^2]. Obesity (BMI >30) is associated with hypertension, increased total and LDL-cholesterol and reduced HDL-cholesterol

Unhealthy diet*

  High fat diet (i.e. fat more than 30% of total calorific intake)

  High intake of saturated rather than unsaturated fat

  High intake of trans fats (non-natural fats produced by industrial process)

  High cholesterol intake

  Diet devoid of fruit and vegetables, which provide 'protective' antioxidant vitamins

  High salt diet (causes hypertension)

Excess alcohol*

  Although alcohol in moderation (glass of red wine or pint of beer per day) is thought to protect against heart disease, as intake rises above 21 units of alcohol per week so too does risk of CHD; excess alcohol can cause hypertension

Lack of exercise*

  Exercise reduces body weight and increases the amount of 'protective' HDL-cholesterol present in blood

Unhealthy amount of lipids in blood*

  Increased plasma/serum total cholesterol concentration

  Increased plasma/serum LDL-cholesterol concentration

  Reduced plasma/serum HDL-cholesterol concentration

  High ratio of plasma/serum total cholesterol : plasma/serum HDL-cholesterol

*Modifiable risk factors.

artery, known as a fatty streak. Development of the fatty streak to the more ominous and complex fatty plaque that protrudes into the lumen of the artery is thought to involve an inflammatory reaction initiated by the death of the cells engorged with LDL-cholesterol. The normal smooth muscle cells of which arterial walls are composed migrate into the plaque, proliferate and synthesise fibrous proteins like collagen, which renders the growing plaque hard. The atherosclerotic plaque has a lipid rich centre surrounded by a dynamic fibrous cap composed of collagen protein and pro-inflammatory cells. The strength and stability of the cap is of great pathological significance because this determines if thrombosis occurs. A thin and fragile cap may rupture exposing the platelets in blood flowing through the vessel to substances beneath the cap that promote platelet aggregation and activation at the site of the ruptured plaque. This in turn initiates the clotting cascade with formation of a blood clot (thrombus), which may completely occlude blood flow.

In general, stable angina is associated with a stable plaque, whereas acute coronary syndromes (unstable angina and myocardial infarction) are associated with an unstable plaque, plaque rupture and consequent thrombosis.

The growth of atherosclerotic plaques to the point where they can occlude blood flow sufficiently to cause symptoms of cardiovascular disease is very slow, occurring over a period of many years. There is now evidence that by addressing risk factors such as hyperlipidameia it is possible to halt or even reverse plaque progression[4].

Research directed at better understanding of the complexities of atherosclerosis continues, but some aspects are clear:

- Accumulation of cholesterol, specifically LDL-cholesterol is an important requirement for atheroma formation.
- The LDL-cholesterol found in atherosclerotic plaques is derived from the blood.
- The higher the concentration of cholesterol in blood the greater is the risk of CHD and other cardiovascular disease.
- It is specifically LDL-cholesterol that is damaging; the higher the LDL the greater is the risk of CHD.
- By contrast, HDL is protective against CHD because it clears the blood of cholesterol. The lower the HDL-cholesterol the greater is the risk of CHD. A high level of HDL-cholesterol is associated with reduced risk of CHD.
- Reducing the concentration of total cholesterol in a patient with raised levels is effective in reducing overall risk of CHD.
- The link between blood triglyceride and CHD is currently less clear. There is evidence that particularly among those who have an increased LDL-cholesterol or a reduced HDL-cholesterol, a raised blood triglyceride increases yet further the risk of CHD.
- There is little evidence however to suggest that reducing raised triglyceride levels decreases the risk of CHD.

It must be emphasised that blood lipid testing determines risk only; results cannot be used to diagnose or definitively predict CHD for a particular individual. Some have a raised LDL-cholesterol and do not suffer CHD and there is no safe level of cholesterol or triglyceride below which one can be guaranteed not to suffer CHD. The best we can say is that the higher the level of LDL-cholesterol, the greater is the risk of CHD; that risk is increased if triglycerides are also raised, and reduced by a high HDL-cholesterol level. The World Health Organisation (WHO) estimates that if everyone had a serum total cholesterol <3.8 mmol/L then the total number of patients suffering CHD would be reduced by 60%[5]. This gives some notion of the considerable contribution that raised cholesterol makes to overall risk of CHD.

Other effects of raised blood lipids

There are few signs or symptoms to suggest that an individual may have an increased level of cholesterol or triglyceride and the onset of anginal pain or myocardial infarction may be the first indication. Lipid deposits (xanthomata) visible as nodules may form in subcutaneous tissue (most commonly the Achilles tendon) among those with very high levels. Lipid may also accumulate in the cornea. Severe hypertriglyceridaemia is associated with abdominal pain and is a rare cause of acute pancreatitis.

Causes of raised cholesterol and/or triglycerides

Many genetic defects in lipid metabolism have been identified which result in a raised cholesterol, a raised triglyceride or both, so that it is possible to inherit a predisposition to raised blood lipids. This in part explains the observation that CHD runs in families. One of these inherited conditions is extremely common, several are less common and most are extremely rare. All are grouped together in the term primary hyperlipidaemias. A raised cholesterol or triglyceride may arise as a complication of another disease process; this is called secondary hyperlipidaemia. Treatment of the underlying disease often corrects secondary hyperlipidaemia.

Primary hyperlipidaemia

The most common cause of primary hyperlipidaemia is known as 'polygenic' hypercholesterolaemia. As its name implies many genes interact to cause raised cholesterol. The condition results in mild to moderate increase in LDL-cholesterol, the actual level depending to a great extent on diet. Triglyceride levels are usually normal. Much higher levels of LDL-cholesterol, often greater than 9.0 mmol/L, characterise a less common inherited condition known as familial hypercholesterolaemia which affects around 1 in 500 in the UK. This single gene defect is associated with high risk of myocardial infarction in early middle age.

Although rare it is possible to inherit a predisposition to raised triglyceride levels. Familial hypertrigylceridaemia is the most common genetic cause of raised triglyceride. Levels are usually very high (>10 mmol/L). Cholesterol levels are usually normal. Risk of CHD is not greatly increased for this group of patients.

Secondary hyperlipidaemias

The most common cause of secondary hyperlipidaemia is diabetes mellitus. Untreated diabetic patients tend to have a mild increase in LDL-cholesterol and moderate to severe increase in triglyceride. This is at least in part the reason why diabetic patients are at high risk of CHD. Other causes of secondary hyperlipidaemia include hypothyroidism, nephrotic syndrome, cholestatic liver disease and alcohol abuse.

National guidelines (recommendations) for prevention of cardiovascular disease[6,7]

The Joint British Societies guidelines[6] recently endorsed by NICE[7] identify the following groups of people who require careful monitoring of blood cholesterol and cholesterol lowering drug intervention to reduce blood cholesterol because they are all at equally high risk of future cardiovascular disease:

- Those with a history of atherosclerotic cardiovascular disease (e.g. angina, myocardial infarction, stroke etc.).
- Those with diabetes (Types 1 and 2).
- Those with elevated blood pressure (>160 mmHg systolic or >100 mmHg diastolic).
- Those with hypercholesterolaemia (defined as total cholesterol to HDL cholesterol ratio >6).
- Those without any cardiovascular disease but whose quantified risk of developing it during the next ten years is greater than 20%.

[Note: It is recommended that all adults over the age of 40 who have no history of cardiovascular disease be assessed in primary care every five years using the latest Joint British Societies risk charts to quantify their ten year risk of cardiovascular disease. This risk assessment is based on consideration of the following five major risk factors: age, sex, smoking habit, systolic blood pressure and ratio of total to HDL-cholesterol.]

The optimal total cholesterol target for all those in these high risk groups is <4 mmol/L, and that for LDL-cholesterol <2.0 mmol/L. The previous recommended targets contained in the National Service Framework for CHD prevention (total cholesterol <5.0 mmol/L and LDL-cholesterol <3.0 mmol/L) have thus been revised downwards in the light of accumulating evidence that reducing total and LDL-cholesterol yet further has benefit in terms of reducing both morbidity and mortality due to cardiovascular disease.

Case history 12

Michael Oliver, a 41 year old accountant in good health, attended a 'well man' clinic at his GP surgery. A family health history and lifestyle questionnaire revealed a family history of heart disease; his 61 year old father was currently recovering from a heart attack and his grandfather had died of 'heart disease' at the age of 71. His father's recent illness had prompted Michael to quit smoking but he took little exercise. As part of the health screen Michael was weighed, his blood pressure was taken and blood was sampled for blood glucose and lipid screen. Body weight and blood pressure were normal. Clinical examination was unremarkable. The laboratory reported the following blood results:

Blood glucose   5.6 mmol/L
Plasma total cholesterol 5.9 mmol/L
Plasma LDL-cholesterol   4.3 mmol/L
Plasma HDL-cholesterol   0.97 mmol/L
Plasma triglyceride   1.0 mmol/L

Question

In view of his father's illness Michael was most concerned about his own risk of heart disease. Consider the advice that might be given.

Discussion of case history 12

To advise Michael it is necessary to consider all risk factors for CHD. The recommended method for making this risk assessment is the new Joint British Societies risk assessment charts, which take account of age, sex, systolic blood pressure, smoking habit and ratio of total cholesterol to HDL-cholesterol. In Michael's case the cholesterol ratio (5.9/0.97) is 6.1 which places him in a high risk group irrespective of the results of global risk assessment. This indicates that Michael would benefit from reducing his total and LDL-cholesterol. The recommended targets are total cholesterol <4.0 mmol/L and LDL-cholesterol <2.0 mmol/L. This might be achievable by lifestyle changes (e.g. dietary changes, increased exercise) but if this fails a cholesterol lowering drug, most commonly a statin, might be advised. However before embarking on this course it is important to confirm the hyperlipidaemia on two further occasions, because of the biological variability of serum cholesterol. Due consideration should also be given to the possibility that raised cholesterol is due to some underlying disease.

References

1. Scarborough, P., Bhanagar, P., Wickramasinghe, K. et al. (2010) *Coronary heart disease statistics 2010 edition*, British Heart Foundation.
2. Becares, L. and Mindell, J. (2009) Blood analytes. In: *Health Survey for England 2008 Vol 1: Physical Activity and Fitness*, NHS Health and Social Care Information Centre.
3. Dept of Health (2000) National service framework for coronary heart disease, modern standards & service models, Product No: 16602 DOH.
4. Okazaki, S., Yokoyama, T. et al. (2004) Early statin treatment in patients with acute coronary syndrome: demonstration of the beneficial effect on atherosclerotic lesions by serial volumetric intravascular ultrasound analysis during half a year after coronary event: the ESTABLISH study, *Circulation*, 110: 1061–8.
5. Ara, R., Tumur, A., Pandor, A. et al. (2008) Ezetimibe for the treatment of hypercholesterolaemia: a systematic review and economic evaluation, *Heath Technology Assessment* Vol. 12 (21).
6. Joint British Societies (2005) Joint British Societies guidelines on prevention of cardiovascular disease in clinical practice, *Heart* 91 (v): v1–v52.
7. National Institute for Health and Clinical Excellence NICE (2010) Lipid modification: cardiovascular risk assessment and the modification of blood lipids for primary and secondary prevention of cardiovascular disease, NICE clinical guideline 67, NHS.

Further reading

Cooney, M., Cooney, H., Dudina, A. et al. (2011) Total cardiovascular disease risk assessment: a review, *Current Opinions in Cardiology*, 26: 429–37.

Lindsay, G. and Gaw, A. (eds.) (2003) *Coronary Heart Disease Prevention: A Handbook for the Healthcare Team*, 2nd edn, Churchill Livingstone.

Nabel, E. and Braunwald, E. (2012) a tale of coronary artery disease and myocardial infarction, *New Eng J Med*, 366: 54–63.

CHAPTER 9

CARDIAC MARKERS – TROPONIN, CREATINE KINASE (MB) AND BRAIN NATRIURETIC PEPTIDE (BNP)

Key learning topics

- Structure and physiological function of troponin, CK(MB) and BNP
- Blood collection for troponin, CK(MB) and BNP testing
- Myocardial infarction/acute coronary syndrome (ACS)
- Troponin and CK(MB) testing in assessment of patients with chest pain
- Heart failure
- BNP testing in assessment of patients with suspected heart failure

---

Chest pain and breathlessness are two common reasons for adults to seek medical help either in primary care or at the hospital emergency department. This chapter is concerned with how laboratory testing can help in the diagnosis of patients presenting with either of these two symptoms. The three tests for consideration here are: the serum or plasma concentration of cardiac troponins (cTnT and cTnI); the serum or plasma concentration of creatine kinase CK(MB); and the plasma concentration of brain natriuretic peptide (BNP). Although functionally and structurally unrelated all three substances are normally present in cardiac tissue cells and released to blood in abnormal amounts if those cells are damaged or diseased: they are thus blood markers of heart (cardiac) disease and referred to collectively as cardiac markers.

The principle use of the first two tests, troponins and CK(MB) is to help identify those patients whose chest pain is due to myocardial infarction, the acute and life threatening manifestation of coronary heart disease (CHD) commonly known as a 'heart attack'. Every year in the UK around 125 000 people suffer myocardial infarction[1]. The damage to the heart may be sufficient to cause immediate lethal arrhythmia, cardiac arrest and sudden death; around 20% die before medical help

Understanding Laboratory Investigations: A Guide for Nurses, Midwives and Healthcare Professionals, Third Edition. Chris Higgins.
© 2013 John Wiley & Sons, Ltd. Published 2013 by John Wiley & Sons, Ltd.

arrives. For the rest early diagnosis and treatment is usually life-saving; around 90% of those who get to hospital alive now survive myocardial infarction.

The principle use of the third test, serum BNP, is to help identify those patients who are suffering heart failure, the most frequent early symptom of which is breathlessness after only minimal exertion. This is a common, progressively debilitating chronic disease that can result from the damage caused to the heart during myocardial infarction; chronic hypertension is another major cause. Heart failure affects an estimated 900 000 in the UK[2]. This is a disease of advancing years and the vast majority of those affected are aged more than 65 years at the time of diagnosis. Prevalence is highest in the very elderly (>84 years); around one in ten in this age group have heart failure[3].

Normal physiology

Troponin

There are three main muscle types in the human body: smooth muscle, present in the wall of those hollow organs whose function depends on muscle wall contraction (gastrointestinal tract, uterus, blood vessels etc.); skeletal muscle; and cardiac muscle (the myocardium) which makes up the bulk of the heart wall.

Troponin (Tn) is a protein constituent of cardiac and skeletal muscle cells where it functions as a structural component of the contractile assembly (myofibrils) that enables muscle contraction. It is composed of three sub-units: troponin C (TnC), troponin I (TnI) and troponin T(TnT). The whole troponin complex is located on the actin filament of the myofibril. The interaction between actin and myosin filaments that facilitates muscle contraction is initiated by calcium ions binding to troponin C. TnI binding of actin inhibits contraction. By these two opposing effects, one initiating contraction of myofibrils the other inhibiting the process, troponin plays a major role in regulating contraction of both skeletal and cardiac muscle.

There are tissue specific isoforms of troponins C, I and T. This means that it is possible to distinguish cardiac muscle troponin (cTn) from skeletal muscle troponin. Normally all the troponin in the body is contained within skeletal and cardiac muscle cells; it is virtually undetectable in blood. However if muscle cells are damaged, their contents, including troponin, are released to the bloodstream and plasma concentration rises. If only cardiac muscle is damaged, only troponin composed of the cardiac isoforms of troponin sub-units C, I and T (i.e. cTnC, cTnI, and cTnT) will appear in blood. There are two troponin tests currently used for assessment of patients with chest pain. Some laboratories measure serum or plasma concentration of cTnT; others measure serum or plasma concentration of cTnI. Of many potential candidates, the troponins cTnT and cTnI have emerged as the cardiac markers of choice for diagnosis and exclusion of myocardial infarction because of their superior specificity and sensitivity for cardiac muscle (myocardial) damage.

Creatine kinase (MB) CK(MB)

Creatine kinase (alternative name, creatine phosphokinase CPK) is an enzyme that catalyses the transfer of phosphate from creatine phosphate to adenosine diphosphate. The products of the reaction are creatine and the energy rich compound, adenosine triphosphate (ATP).

$$\text{Creatine phosphate} + \text{Adenosine diphosphate} \longrightarrow \text{Creatine} + \text{Adenosine triphosphate}$$

CK is present in many types of tissue cells, but three sorts of tissue contain most of the body's CK. They are: cardiac muscle (myocardium), skeletal muscle and the brain.

CK is composed of two protein subunits, M and B, allowing three functionally identical, but structurally different, isoenzymes: CK(MM), CK(BB) and CK(MB). CK isoenzymes are tissue specific. Most of the CK(BB) is found in the brain; most of the CK(MM) is in skeletal muscle and most of the CK(MB) is in cardiac muscle cells. Thus CK(MB) is a fraction of total CK which is confined to the cells of which heart muscle are composed. Normally blood plasma contains very little CK(MB) but following damage to heart muscle, blood plasma concentration rises. CK(MB) is considered the best alternative cardiac marker, if troponin is not available.

Brain natriuretic peptide (BNP)

Peptide is the generic name for all substances that comprise a simple chain of a small number of amino acids (usually less than 50). Brain natriuretic peptide was first isolated from the brain of pigs, hence the name, but in humans most is actually synthesised in the heart, specifically in the muscle cells (myocytes) that comprise the muscular wall (myocardium) of the two ventricles of the heart. A closely related peptide, atrial natriuretic peptide (ANP) is synthesised in the myocytes that comprise the wall (myocardium) of the two atria of the heart. All natriuretic peptides (there are two other types, not synthesised in the heart) are hormones that are involved in the regulation of the amount of sodium and water in blood and thereby blood volume, blood pressure and ultimately cardiac function. The mode of action and physiological effect of these hormones is complex but an important aspect is that via action on the renin-angiotensin system, they promote the excretion of sodium in urine (natriuresis) and it is this action that is reflected in their collective name.

The physiological impetus for BNP synthesis and secretion to blood is ventricular stretching and distension that occurs when the heart is working harder than normal (e.g. during vigorous exercise). The ventricular myocytes do not actually secrete BNP in response to ventricular stretching but a larger peptide (a pro-hormone) called proBNP, which is composed of 108 amino acids. This is split during secretion, and the derived two substances are both present in blood. The first is the physiologically active hormone BNP, composed of 32 amino acids and the second is a physiologically inactive peptide called N-terminal pro-brain natriuretic peptide (NTproBNP) comprising 76 amino acids. Some laboratories measure BNP concentration and some measure NTproBNP concentrations. The two assays are equally valid for clinical purposes, but because BNP and NTproBNP are metabolised at different rates, each assay has its own, quite different reference (normal) range.

Laboratory measurement of troponins (cTnT cTnI) and CK(MB)

Patient preparation

No particular patient preparation is necessary.

Timing of blood collection

Most hospitals have a protocol for timing of blood sampling for troponin and CK(MB) among patients presenting with chest pain. Commonly blood is sampled on admission and again 6–12 hours later. Further testing at 24 hours may be necessary. Interpretation of test results depends crucially on knowing when the blood was sampled in relation to the time of onset of symptoms of chest pain. For these reasons it is important to record on the accompanying request card both the time blood is sampled and the time of onset of symptoms (if known) or time of admission.

Amount and type of sample

Around 5 ml of blood is sufficient for cardiac markers. The assays are performed on either plasma or serum. If local policy is to use plasma then blood must be collected into a tube containing the anticoagulant lithium heparin. If local policy is to use serum then blood must be collected into a plain glass tube, without any additive. Haemolysed samples are unsuitable for troponin testing – repeat blood sampling is necessary if haemolysis is present.

Interpretation of results

Reference ranges

It would be inappropriate to provide definitive reference ranges for these two tests because of variable and continually evolving laboratory methodology. An important aspect of this, so far as troponin is concerned, is development of assays that are increasingly sensitive in detecting troponin. Interpretation of patient results should always be made using reference ranges provided by the laboratory that performed the test(s). Suffice to say there is normally very little (often undetectable quantities) of any of these cardiac markers in blood.

The now recommended unit of measurement for TnI and T is nanograms/litre (ng/L) but some laboratories continue to use other units (ng/ml or mg/L). To convert results expressed as either ng/ml or mg/L to the recommended ng/L, simply multiply the result by 1000.

Causes of raised serum or plasma concentration of cTnT, cTnI and CK(MB)

Cardiac muscle cell death (myocardial necrosis) is the only cause for an increase in serum or plasma concentration of cTnT and cTnI. It is also the principle but not the sole cause for an increase in plasma or serum concentration of CK(MB). The most common cause of myocardial necrosis is myocardial infarction.

Myocardial infarction/coronary heart disease

All cells require a continuous supply of oxygen rich blood for survival. Ischaemia is the term used to describe deficient blood supply to an area of tissue, and infarction is the term for the death of tissue that results if ischaemia is sufficiently severe or prolonged. Myocardial infarction is thus the death of an area of heart muscle tissue due to ischaemia. Almost invariably in cases of myocardial infarction, ischaemia is the result of CHD.

The atherosclerotic plaque is the pathological lesion that defines CHD. This is a focal accumulation of lipid and cellular material beneath a fibrous cap on the internal surface of a coronary artery. During a long sub-clinical period of many years the plaque may grow to the point where it reduces blood flow sufficiently to cause symptoms of reduced oxygen delivery to an area of heart muscle. The main symptom is ischaemic chest pain, which is often experienced as discomfort rather than as a sharp or stabbing pain. Tightness, pressure, constriction and strangling are common descriptors of ischaemic chest pain. It is usually diffusely located across the chest and may radiate to neck, throat, jaw, shoulders or arm.

The least severe and most common manifestation of CHD is the ischaemic chest pain associated with stable angina. A patient with stable angina experiences chest pain or discomfort only during periods of increased oxygen demand, for example, during exertion or other stress (e.g. emotional stress) that causes heart rate to increase. Symptoms disappear as the heart's demand for oxygen is reduced by rest. The reduced oxygen delivery to heart muscle cells that causes ischaemic pain in those with stable angina is not sufficient to cause cell death. There is therefore no increase in the serum or plasma concentration of either of the two cardiac markers among patients whose chest pain is the result of stable angina.

The first manifestation of CHD may not be stable angina but the more serious acute coronary syndrome (ACS). This is not a single entity but a spectrum of disease of increasing severity that includes myocardial infarction. The pathological feature that defines ACS is plaque instability. For reasons that remain poorly understood, the fibrous cap that protects the underlying lipid and cellular contents of an atherosclerotic plaque from the blood flowing through an affected artery, may be thin, fragile and prone to disruption (rupture). It is the patients whose plaques have these vulnerable characteristics that are most at risk of the life threatening consequences of CHD. Plaque rupture exposes the platelets in blood to the pro-coagulant environment of the plaque contents. A single thrombus may form at the site of the exposed plaque, partially or totally occluding blood flow. Alternatively debris from the plaque along with fragments of thrombi may embolise to smaller vessels where they may occlude blood flow at a site remote from the plaque. It is in the context of these variable effects of plaque disruption that ACS is evident.

The mildest clinical presentation of ACS is unstable angina. This is the same ischaemic chest pain or discomfort as that experienced by patients suffering stable angina. However in the case of unstable angina, symptoms are experienced at rest or on minimal exertion, and are generally of longer duration and greater intensity. A definitive feature of unstable angina and one that distinguishes it from the more serious presentation of ACS, myocardial infarction, is the absence of myocardial necrosis. As with stable angina, the ischaemia associated with unstable angina is not sufficient to cause cell death, so that cardiac markers remain within normal limits. However unstable angina is clinical evidence of an unstable plaque and therefore high risk of myocardial infarction in the immediate future or later. Around 15% of patients with unstable angina suffer myocardial infarction during the seven days following diagnosis.

Myocardial infarction and cardiac markers

If the ischaema induced by thrombus or other occlusion of an artery is severe and prolonged, the myocardial cells that are supplied by the vessel simply die. This is myocardial infarction. The volume of myocardium affected varies greatly from <1 to >25 g depending on the site of occlusion, and this is reflected in the variable electrocardiographic (ECG) changes and mortality associated with myocardial infarction. In all cases there is an increase in the plasma concentration of cardiac markers, indeed an increase in the plasma concentration of troponin (either cTnT or cTnI) or CK(MB) is an essential criteria for diagnosis of myocardial infarction [4] (Table 9.1). The magnitude of the increase reflects the amount of tissue destroyed and therefore severity of the infarct.

Crushing ischaemic chest pain, usually lasting no less than 20 minutes marks the onset of severe myocardial infarction in the majority of cases. Additional symptoms include breathlessness, light-headedness, sweating, nausea and vomiting. Extensive tissue ischaemia is reflected in the early characteristic electrocardiograph (ECG) change (ST elevation) that gives this severe presentation its name: ST elevation myocardial infarction (STEMI). Myocardial necrosis is not immediate and begins only after a finite period ($\approx$10–15 minutes) of ischaemia. Necrosis of all the tissue at risk occurs gradually over the following four to six hours or longer, providing a window of therapeutic opportunity to limit the damage with thrombolytic/reperfusion therapy that restores blood flow.

The rise in plasma concentration of cTnI, cTnT and CK(MB) following myocardial infarction is a transitory phenomenon, related to the time of infarction and typically begins between three and six hours after onset of symptoms, although may be earlier in particular cases (Figure 9.1). Peak levels occur at about 12–24 hours after onset of symptoms. CK(MB) concentration returns to normal within

Table 9.1 Definition of myocardial infarction[4].

The following criteria satisfy the diagnosis of acute, evolving or recent MI:

Detection of rise and/or fall of a blood cardiac marker (preferably troponin), with at least one value above the 99th percentile of the upper reference limit. This evidence of myocardial necrosis must be accompanied by evidence of ischaemia; that is, at least one of the following:
- Symptoms of ischaemia (see text)
- ECG changes indicative of new ischaemia [ST segment elevation/depression or left bundle branch block (LBBB)]
- Development of Q waves on ECG
- Imaging evidence of new loss of viable myocardium or regional wall motion abnormality

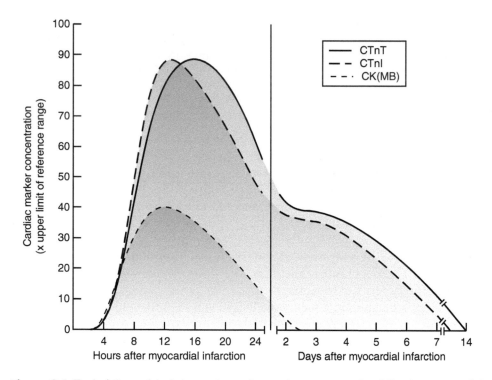

Figure 9.1 Typical time related change in cardiac marker concentration following myocardial infarction.

two or thress days but both cTnI and cTnT remain raised for much longer, up to two weeks in some cases.

Myocardial infarction can usually be excluded as the cause of chest pain if plasma or serum concentration of CK(MB), cTnT or cTnI remains within normal limits during the 12 hours following onset of symptoms. There may still be clinical doubt, in which case repeat testing at 24 hours is indicated. If this confirms previous normal results, myocardial infarction is definitively excluded. However this does not exclude the possibility that chest pain is of cardiac origin, because cardiac markers remain within normal limits in patients with stable and unstable angina.

Other causes of myocardial necrosis

Although the ischaemia associated with myocardial infarction is by far and away the most common cause of myocardial necrosis it is not the only cause, so that cardiac markers may be raised in conditions other than myocardial infarction[5].

These conditions include myocarditis (inflammatory infection of heart muscle), pericarditis (inflammation of the membrane that covers the heart), pulmonary embolism, renal failure, trauma to the heart and sepsis. In general these conditions are associated with only slight increase in cardiac markers compared with the increase associated with myocardial infarction.

Laboratory measurement of BNP

Patient preparation

No particular patient preparation is necessary.

Timing of blood collection

Blood can be sampled at any time of the day.

Amount and type of blood sample

Around 5 ml of blood is sufficient. The collection bottle depends on the exact nature of laboratory measurement; as outlined already, some laboratories measure plasma BNP concentration and some measure serum NTproBNP concentration. Plasma BNP estimation requires that blood be collected into a bottle containing the anticoagulant EDTA, whereas serum NTproBNP estimation requires that blood is collected into a plain tube, containing no anticoagulant.

Interpretation of results

Adult reference range (approximate)

Plasma BNP	10–150 pg/ml
Serum NT-proBNP	80–250 pg/ml

Females have higher values than males, and in both genders concentration increases significantly with age. So that males less than 60 years of age normally have values at the lower end of these two ranges, and females greater than 80 years of age normally have values at the high end of these two ranges.

Use of BNP, NT-pro BNP in heart failure

Both BNP and NT-proBNP are raised in a range of cardiac and non-cardiac conditions (e.g. myocardial infarction, myocarditis, renal failure, pulmonary hypertension) but the tests currently only have clinical application in the diagnosis of heart failure.

The pathogenesis of heart failure is complex but the condition is essentially a chronically progressive disorder in which the heart becomes increasingly less able to pump blood fast enough to meet the demands of the body. There are a number of possible causes, but previous myocardial infarction and chronic hypertension are two common causes that account for the vast majority of cases. The reduced oxygen delivery to tissues that results from reduced blood flow accounts for some of the signs and symptoms of heart failure, including low exercise tolerance, dizziness and fatigue. The condition is associated with compensatory mechanisms that help in the short term, but ultimately increase the workload of the heart and thereby exacerbate the condition. Retention of fluid to increase blood volume is one such compensatory response. This leads to peripheral odema and pulmonary congestion both of which have symptomatic effect in the form of painful swollen ankles (ankle oedema) and increasing breathlessness after only mild exertion. The condition is progressively debilitating, and eventually breathlessness and fatigue is experienced, even when resting.

Compensatory mechanisms associated with heart failure also include remodelling of the structure of the heart; it becomes larger (a condition called cardiomegaly). Ventricles of the heart are distended and the associated stretch in ventricle walls results in increased production and secretion of pro-BNP from the cells (myocytes) of which they are composed. Increase in plasma BNP and serum NT-proBNP concentration is the inevitable consequence; as heart failure worsens levels rise inexorably.

Since there are other conditions that cause an increase in BNP and NT-proBNP, the tests cannot be used to reliably diagnose heart failure. The most reliable routinely available diagnostic tool is echocardiography a non-invasive imaging technique that involves production of a real time image of the working heart by ultrasound scan. The now established clinical value of BNP and NTproBNP, which is based on the well validated observation that virtually all patients with symptomatic heart failure have raised BNP/ NT-proBNP, is to *exclude* a diagnosis of heart failure. The finding of a normal BNP/NTproBNP in a patient with symptoms (breathlessness, fatigue etc.) suggestive of heart failure makes a diagnosis of heart failure extremely unlikely and therefore excludes the necessity for echocardiography. Two recent clinical guidelines[6,7] endorse this use of the two tests and provide identical detail for interpretation of test results (Table 9.2). The NICE guidelines[7] state that BNP/NTproBNP should be a first line test in the diagnostic process for patients with suspected heart failure and no history of myocardial infarction. Only those with raised BNP (>100 pg/ml) or raised NTproBNP (>400 pg/ml) need be submitted for echocardiography. Those with particularly high levels (BNP > 400 pg/ml, NTproBNP > 2000 pg/ml) have a poorer prognosis and should be referred for echocardiography urgently (within two weeks).

Since BNP/NTproBNP concentration correlates with severity of heart failure, it follows that the tests might be useful for monitoring response to treatment. A diagnostic role for BNP/NTproBNP is now well established but it is currently less certain if either test can serve reliably as a routine monitoring tool in heart failure. This however remains the object of continuing research interest[8].

Table 9.2 Natriuretic Peptides (BNP/NTproBNP) in the first line investigation of patients with suspected heart failure[7].

	Heart failure excluded	**Uncertain diagnosis**	**Heart failure likely**
BNP (pg/ml)	<100	100–400	>400
NT-proBNP (pg/ml)	<400	400–2000	>2000

Unless there is a history of myocardial infarction, only those in the 'uncertain diagnosis' and 'heart failure likely' categories need be submitted for echocardiography. Those in the 'heart failure likely' category should be submitted for echocardiography urgently (within 2 weeks).

Patients with a history of myocardial infarction and symptoms suggestive of heart failure should receive urgent echocardiography, irrespective of BNP/NTproBNP result.

Case history 13

Henry Jarvis, a 58 year old retired teacher with a history of myocardial infarction three years previously, developed chest pains while working in the garden. Within an hour he arrived by ambulance at his local hospital emergency department. Clinical history and examination suggested a provisional diagnosis of myocardial infarction but ECG trace was normal, save evidence of previous infarct. He was admitted to coronary care. Blood was collected for measurement of cardiac markers according to local protocol, on admission (sample 1); at 9 hours post admission (sample 2); and again at 24 hours post admission (sample 3).

Sample 1 serum cTnT   12 ng/L
          serum CK(MB)   3.9 mg/L
Sample 2 serum cTnI   45 ng/L
          serum CK(MB)   3.8 mg/L
Sample 3 serum cTnI   32 ng/L
          serum CK(MB)   4.1 mg/L
Laboratory upper limit of the reference range
          cTnT   15 ng/L
          CK(MB)   5.0 mg/L

Questions

(1) Would you expect the results of sample 1 to show elevated cTnT and CK(MB) if Mr Jarvis had suffered a myocardial infarction?
(2) What do the serum cTnT results indicate?
(3) What do the serum CK(MB) results indicate?
(4) Did Mr Jarvis suffer myocardial infarction?

Discussion of case history 13

(1) Not necessarily. There is a delay between the onset of chest pain and a rise in the concentration of cardiac markers. The increase in cTnT and CK(MB) starts on average between four and six hours after onset of pain and Mr Jarvis's blood was sampled just an hour after onset of symptoms. Normal cardiac markers on admission cannot be used to exclude a diagnosis of myocardial infarction.

(2) The serum cTnT results at 9 hours and 24 hours were marginally raised. The combination of raised cTnT and typical clinical symptoms of ischaemic disease suggest a diagnosis of myocardial infarction. The magnitude of the increase in cTnT was small, indicating only minimal tissue loss. The results are consistent with a diagnosis of myocardial infarction.

(3) The serum CK(MB) remains normal throughout the period of 24 hours following the onset of chest pain. These results do not indicate myocardial infarction.

(4) Yes, on the basis of the cTnT results Mr Jarvis suffered a myocardial infarction. These results demonstrate the superior sensitivity of cTnT for detecting myocardial necrosis. In this case, the amount of tissue destroyed during infarction was not sufficient to cause an increase in CK(MB). The ischaemia that caused the minimal loss of tissue, was not sufficiently extensive to cause any of the ECG changes normally associated with evolving myocardial infarction.

Case history 14

Helen Blackmore is a retired teacher now aged 78 with a three year history of hypertension. She was diagnosed with Type 2 diabetes seven years ago. At her most recent GP visit she complains of being 'really tired all the time' and has noticed becoming unusually breathless when walking. This sense of breathlessness has increased gradually over several months and she now really struggles to complete her usual ten minute walk with her dog. After physical examination including auscultation of her lungs and heart, Helen's GP suspects she might be suffering heart failure and takes blood for a range of tests including serum NTproBNP estimation.

Two days later the local laboratory reports the following result:

Serum NTproBNP – 545 pg/ml

Questions

(1) What are essential features of the case history that suggest possible heart failure. Is the result normal?
(2) Is it possible to make or exclude a diagnosis of heart failure on the basis of this result?
(3) Can you suggest another test that might help to identify the cause of Helen's breathlessness and fatigue?

Discussion of case history 14

(1) The symptoms Helen reports – progressive breathlessness and fatigue – are very common presenting symptoms among patients who are later diagnosed with heart failure. Of course they are by no means specific for heart failure; many other medical conditions are commonly associated with breathlessness and fatigue. Her advancing years and medical history provide additional support for the suspicion. Heart failure is a disease predominantly of the elderly and both hypertension and diabetes increase the risk of heart failure.

The result is abnormally high and consistent with a diagnosis of heart failure.

(2) No, the result is only consistent with a diagnosis of heart failure, there are a number of other conditions that can give rise to increased serum NTproBNP. A normal result makes a diagnosis of heart failure extremely unlikely.

(3) The result along with clinical finding is highly suggestive of heart failure and the next step to definitively make the diagnosis is referral to the local hospital for echocardiography. If Helen's serum NTproBNP result was normal this referral would, almost certainly, not have been appropriate.

References

1. Scarborough, P., Bhanagar, P., Wickramasinghe, K. et al. (2010) *Coronary heart disease statistics*, 2010 edition, British Heart Foundation.
2. Peterson, S., Rayner, M., and Wolstenholme, J. (2002) *Coronary heart disease statistics: heart failure supplement*, British Heart Foundation.
3. Majeed, A., Williams, J., deLusignan, S. and Chan, T. (2005) Management of heart failure in primary care after implementation of the national service framework for coronary heart disease: a cross-sectional study, *Public Health*, 119: 105–11.
4. Thygesen, K., Alpert, J. and White, H. et al. (2007) Joint ESC/ACA/AHA/WHF task force for the redefinition of myocardial infarction, *Eur Heart J*, 28: 2525–38.
5. Tanindi, A. and Cemri, M. (2011) Troponin in conditions other than acute coronary syndromes, *Vascular Health Risk Management*, 7: 597–603.
6. Dickstein, K., Cohen-Solal, A., Filipatos, G. et al. (2008) Guidelines for the diagnosis and treatment of acute and chronic heart failure, *Eur Heart J*, 29: 2388–442.
7. National Institute for Health and Clinical Excellence (2010) NICE clinical guideline 108 chronic heart failure, NICE.
8. Porapakkham, P., Porapakkam, P., Zimmet, H. et al. (2010) B-type natriuretic peptide-guided heart failure therapy, *Arch Int Med*, 170: 507–14.

Further reading

Babuin, L. and Jaffe, A. (2005) Troponin: The biomarker of choice for detection of cardiac injury, *CMAJ*, 173: 1191–202.

Fox, K. (2004) Management of acute coronary syndrome: an update, *Heart*, 90: 698–706.

French, J. and White, H. (2004) Implications of the new definition of myocardial infarction, *Heart*, 90: 99–106.

Grange, J. (2005) The role of nurses in management of heart failure, *Heart*, 91 Suppl 2: ii 39–42; discussion ii 43–8.

Mair, J. (2008) Biochemistry of B-type natriuretic peptide – where are we now?, *Clin Chem Lab Med*, 46:1507–14.

Nabel, E. and Braunwald, E. (2012) A tale of coronary artery disease and myocardial infarction, *New Eng J Med*, 366: 54–63.

Sutherland, K. (2010) *Bridging the Quality Gap: Heart Failure*, The Health Foundation.

CHAPTER 10

TESTS OF THYROID FUNCTION – THYROXINE (T4), TRIIODOTHYRONINE (T3) AND THYROID STIMULATING HORMONE (TSH)

Key learning topics

- Structure and function of the thyroid hormones: T4 and T3
- Control of thyroid hormone production – role of the pituitary hormone, TSH
- Causes and consequences of overactive thyroid gland (hyperthyroidism)
- Causes and consequences of underactive thyroid gland (hypothyroidism)
- How measurement of blood concentration of T4, T3 and TSH aids in diagnosis of thyroid disorders
- Thyroid testing and pregnancy

The focus of this chapter is endocrinology, that branch of medical science which is concerned with organs or parts of organs responsible for production and secretion of hormones. These hormones or 'biochemical messengers' are transported in blood to distant target organs where they exert their various and specific effects. The thyroid gland is an endocrine organ responsible for production and secretion of the thyroid hormones, thyroxine (T4) and triiodothyronine (T3). Of all endocrine disorders, those involving the thyroid are the most common. Thyroid disease affects around 3–5% of the adult population[1] and there is evidence that incidence is increasing[2], so that thyroid hormones are by far and away the most frequently measured hormones in clinical laboratories. In this chapter we consider how the laboratory contributes to diagnosis and monitoring of thyroid disorders.

Understanding Laboratory Investigations: A Guide for Nurses, Midwives and Healthcare Professionals, Third Edition. Chris Higgins.
© 2013 John Wiley & Sons, Ltd. Published 2013 by John Wiley & Sons, Ltd.

Normal anatomy and physiology

Thyroid gland

The thyroid gland (Figure 10.1), weighing around 20 g, is butterfly shaped and situated in the neck. The two lobes of the thyroid sit on either side of the trachea, just below the larynx and are connected by a bridge of tissue, the thyroid isthmus. Thyroid enlargement (goitre), a feature of many thyroid disorders may be visible as a swelling of the neck, or at least palpable on physical examination.

The gland is composed of two types of hormone producing cell, the bulk of the cells are so called follicle cells that produce the two thyroid hormones, T4 and T3. Interspersed between these cells are the parafollicular cells or C-cells that synthesis calcitonin, a hormone not considered here that is involved in calcium metabolism.

Function of thyroid hormones, T3 and T4

Thyroid hormones are delivered via the bloodstream to every part of the body and with few exceptions have an effect on the cells of all tissue types. Although T3 is the more potent of the two hormones, both increase the speed of many cellular metabolic reactions. For example, mobilisation and breakdown of body fat is increased in the presence of thyroid hormone, as is the speed of many reactions involved in the metabolism

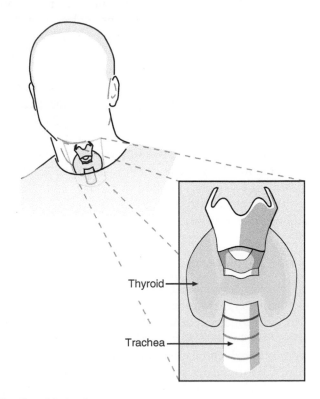

Figure 10.1 The thyroid gland.

of carbohydrates and proteins. This overall stimulatory effect on the body's metabolism determines that thyroid hormones are essential for normal growth and development, including sexual maturation. Specific effects of thyroid hormones are evident in relation to the heart and central nervous system. Cardiac output is influenced by the concentration of thyroid hormones in blood. Mental development from birth is dependent on adequate amounts of thyroid hormone: a deficiency at this time can lead not only to impaired growth but also to severe and irreversible mental retardation.

Thyroid hormone production

Dietary derived iodine is essential to thyroid hormone production and around 95% of the body's iodine is concentrated in the thyroid. This element is present in sufficient amounts in a normal diet and absorbed to blood from the small intestine in the form of iodide. By an energy consuming process, iodide is removed from blood and 'trapped' in thyroid follicular cells, where it is required for production of T4 and T3. In the thyroid follicular cells iodide is oxidised to iodine and hormone synthesis begins with addition of iodine to the amino acid tyrosine, a process called iodination (Figure 10.2). Both the oxidising process and iodination are facilitated by the action of a key enzyme, thyroidal peroxidase (TPO).

Iodination results in monoiodotyrosine and diiodotyrosine. Two molecules of diiodotyrosine combine to form T4, which contains four iodine atoms; and one molecule of monoiodotyrosine combines with one molecule of diiodotyrosine to form T3, which contains three iodine atoms. Both T4 and T3 are released into the bloodstream from follicular cells, although 80% of circulating T3 is formed not in the thyroid but by enzymatic deiodination (removal of one molecule of iodine) of T4 in peripheral tissue, notably the liver and kidney. Two forms of T3 are formed in this way: physiologically active T3 and physiologically inactive reverse T3 (rT3); rT3 is a stereoisomer (structural mirror) of T3. More than 99% of both T4 and T3 that circulates in blood is bound to specific proteins, predominantly thyroxine binding globulin (TBG). In this protein bound form the hormones are inactive but serve as a reservoir or store of thyroid hormones. Less than 0.05% of total T3 and T4 in blood is present in a free (i.e. unbound to protein) and therefore physiologically active form. The nomenclature FT3 and FT4 is used to specifically identify these free thyroid hormone fractions.

Control of thyroid hormone production

The maintenance of thyroid hormone blood concentration within normal limits is essential for good health so that production and secretion from the thyroid gland is finely controlled. This control depends on the pituitary gland, a pea sized organ located at the base of the brain (Figure 10.3). Among several hormones produced by this tiny gland is thyroid-stimulating hormone (TSH), also called thyrotropin. As its name implies, TSH stimulates production and secretion of thyroid hormones from the thyroid gland. The secretion of TSH is in turn controlled by thyrotrophin releasing hormone (TRH) secreted by the hypothalamus in the brain. Release of

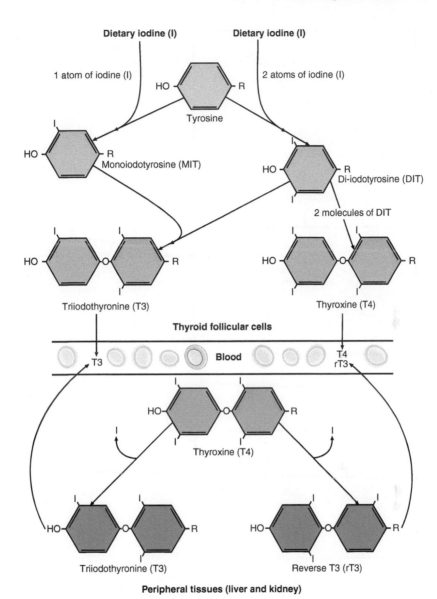

Figure 10.2 Formation of thyroid hormones T4, T3 and reverse (r)T3.
Note: R = CH₂. CHNH₂. COOH

both TSH and TRH are controlled by the plasma concentration of circulating free thyroid hormone (FT4 and FT3). As thyroid hormone concentration falls, TRH and TSH secretion increases, stimulating the thyroid to secrete more thyroid hormone. Conversely as thyroid hormone concentration rises, TRH and TSH secretion decreases and consequently thyroid hormone production and secretion decrease. This continuous process of negative feedback maintains the amount of thyroid hormone in blood within normal limits.

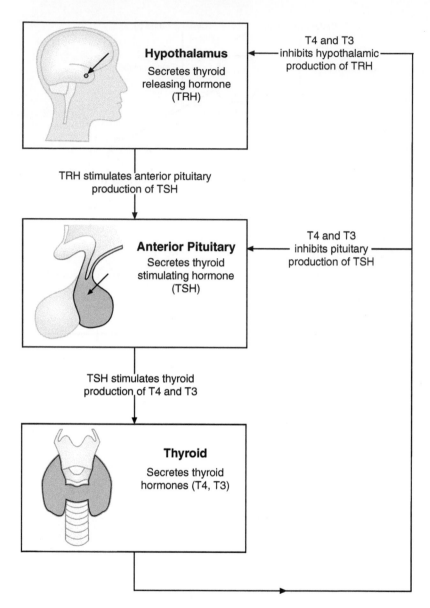

Figure 10.3 Control of thyroid hormone production (by negative feedback).

Normal concentration of thyroid hormones in blood is dependent on:

- An adequate amount of dietary iodine for manufacture of thyroid hormones.
- A normally functioning thyroid gland.
- Adequate production of TSH and therefore normally functioning pituitary gland.
- Adequate production of TRH and therefore normally functioning hypothalamus.

Laboratory assessment of thyroid function

Patient preparation

No particular patient preparation is necessary.

Sample requirements

Around 5 ml of venous blood is required. The tests may be performed on blood plasma or blood serum; if local policy is to use plasma, then blood must be collected into a tube containing an anticoagulant (usually heparin) but if local policy is to use serum, blood must be collected into a plain tube (i.e. without any additive).

Request card information

Since drugs and pre-existing non-thyroid disease can affect interpretation it is important to record drug and brief clinical history. In addition to its role in the diagnosis of thyroid disorders, the test may also be used to monitor the effectiveness of therapy among those already diagnosed; it is important that the reason for requesting the test and dosage of any prescribed thyroxine replacement or antithyroid drugs are recorded.

In the laboratory

Two tests are used in the first line investigation of patients suspected of suffering thyroid disease:

- Thyroid stimulating hormone (TSH). The TSH test measures concentration in blood serum or plasma of the pituitary hormone TSH.
- Free thyroxine (FT4). The FT4 test measures the concentration in blood plasma or serum of free thyroxine (the biologically active fraction of total thyroxine that is not bound to protein).

A third test may be useful in particular circumstances:

- Free triiodothyronine (FT3). The FT3 test measures the concentration in blood serum or plasma of free triiodothyronine (the biologically active fraction of total triiodothyronine that is not bound to protein).

Before development of the highly sensitive laboratory methods required to detect the minute (picomole) concentration of free thyroid hormones (FT4 and FT3) present in blood, the only way of assessing thyroid function was to measure the concentration of total (free plus bound) T4 and T3. Although technically less demanding, measurement of total T4 and T3 (TT4, TT3) concentration is a less satisfactory means of assessing thyroid function, not least because results are affected by the plasma concentration of thyroid binding globulin (TBG), which varies in both healthy and disease states. The concentration of TBG has no effect on free hormone concentration, allowing clearer interpretation of results. Most laboratories now only offer the FT4 and FT3 tests but some may still be using the older TT4 and TT3 tests. For completeness these older tests will be included in the list of reference ranges below, but for the rest of the chapter attention will be focused on the now preferred tests, FT4 and FT3.

Interpretation of test results

Approximate reference ranges

TSH   0.3–4.5 mU/L
FT4   9–26 pmol/L
FT3   3.0–9.0 pmol/L
TT4   60–150 nmol/L
TT3   1.1–2.6 nmol/L

Terms used in interpretation

Euthyroid (ism)   normal thyroid activity.
Hyperthyroid (ism)   overactive thyroid gland.
Hypothyroid (ism)   underactive thyroid gland.
Goitre   enlargement of the thyroid gland. Depending on the cause, goitre may be a feature of euthyroidism, hyperthyroidism or hypothyroidism.
Thyrotoxicosis   the clinical syndrome which results from hyperthyroidism, often used as a synonym for hyperthyroidism.
Myxoedema   a clinical syndrome that includes accumulation of fluid (oedema) in skin tissue, which is associated with severe hypothyroidism.

Causes of abnormal thyroid function test results

Over activity of the thyroid gland and associated increased production of thyroid hormones is called hyperthyroidism. In most instances this is due to disease of the thyroid gland itself, in which case the condition is known as primary hyperthyroidism. Very rarely hyperthyroidism occurs because a normally functioning thyroid gland is being over stimulated by inappropriately increased secretion of TSH from a diseased pituitary gland; this is known as secondary or central hyperthyroidism.

Similarly, under activity of the thyroid gland and concomitant reduced production of thyroid hormones, called hypothyroidism is most commonly due to disease of the thyroid gland (primary hypothyroidism) but can rarely result from decreased production of TSH by the pituitary gland (secondary or central hypothyroidism).

Primary hyperthyroidism

Graves' disease is the most common cause of primary hyperthyroidism accounting for around 80% of cases. This is an autoimmune disease that is ten times more common among women than men; 0.5–2% of adult women have Graves' disease[1]. Patients often report a family history of the condition; it is possible to inherit a predisposition. The thyroid gland of those suffering Graves' disease is diffusely enlarged (smooth or diffuse goitre) and non-tender. The cause of the increased hormone production is abnormal thyroid stimulating antibodies, produced by the patient's immune system, that act in the same way as TSH and stimulate the thyroid to produce thyroid hormones. Unlike TSH however, the production and action of these autoantibodies is not under negative feedback control, and continues despite rising thyroid hormone levels.

Three other less common conditions, toxic adenoma, toxic multinodular goitre and subacute thyroiditis, account for most of the remaining 20% of primary hyperthyroidism cases. Toxic adenoma is characterised by a single abnormal 'nodule' in the thyroid gland that secretes excessive thyroid hormone autonomously, whereas in toxic multinodular goitre the problem is many hypersecreting nodules. Leakage of thyroid hormone from follicular cells damaged by inflammation is the cause of the hyperthyroidism in those with subacute thyroiditis, a self-limiting, usually painful and debilitating condition that follows viral infection. The hyperthyroid phase is typically followed by a hypothyroid phase before recovery, which may take many months.

Amiodarone, a drug used to treat cardiac arrhythmias, is the most significant of a number of drugs that can cause hyperthyroidism. Whatever the cause, primary hyperthyroidism is characterised by increased concentration of thyroid hormone in blood and it is this feature which accounts for the many signs and symptoms (Table 10.1) that reflect the significance of thyroid hormones for all organ systems.

Since increased thyroid hormone production suppresses pituitary secretion of TSH (Figure 10.3), a reduction in serum or plasma TSH is an important diagnostic

Table 10.1 Major signs and symptoms of hyperthyroidism.

Thyroid hormone excess causes a general speeding of body metabolism and physiological process, resulting in any of the following signs and symptoms:

- Weight loss
- Increased appetite
- Intolerance of heat
- Increased sweating: warm, moist hands
- Increased heart rate (tachycardia)
- Palpitations
- Diarrhoea
- Nervousness/anxiety
- Inability to concentrate
- Fine hand tremor
- 'Staring' prominent eyes (exophthalmos)*
- Disturbance of menstrual cycle

*This is a feature of Graves' disease only.

feature of primary hyperthyroidism. Measurement of TSH is the single most important biochemical test for investigation of those suspected of suffering primary
hyperthyroidism because a diagnosis can almost always be excluded if TSH is
within the reference range.

The blood results that would be expected in primary hyperthyroidism, no matter
what the cause, are:

- Plasma/serum TSH concentration always reduced (undetectable in severe cases).
- Plasma/serum FT4 and FT3 concentrations increased.
- Occasionally FT4 is normal and only FT3 is increased (this is called T3
  thyrotoxicosis).

Secondary (central) hyperthyroidism

Very rarely excessive thyroid hormone production is the result not of a problem
within the thyroid but rather as a result of uncontrolled secretion of TSH due to
disease (over activity) of the pituitary gland. For example, pituitary tumours secrete
abnormally high amounts of TSH. In these rare cases, the thyroid is responding
normally to abnormal increased stimulation. Typical blood results in secondary
hyperthyroidism are:

- Plasma/serum TSH concentration raised.
- Serum FT4 and FT3 concentration raised.

Subclinical (mild) primary hyperthyroidism

Sometimes patient testing reveals reduced plasma concentration of TSH, indicating primary hyperthyroidism, in association with a normal (usually high normal)
plasma concentration of FT4 and FT3, indicating euthyroidism. This pattern indicates that TSH production is partially suppressed by overactive thyroid, but there
remains sufficient TSH to maintain thyroid hormone concentration within the
reference range. It is not usually associated with symptoms because thyroid hormone concentration is not increased, so it is called subclinical hyperthyroidism.
However it is not normal and represents a stage between normality and overt
hyperthyroidism. Patients with sub-clinical hyperthyroidism are at greater than
normal risk of developing overt hyperthyroidism, usually Graves' disease in the
long term, and should be offered thyroid testing every 6–12 months. In addition
there is evidence that sub-clinical hyperthyroidism increases the risk of atrial fibrillation (an abnormal heart rhythm) in the elderly and reduced bone density (osteo-
porosis) in postmenopausal women[3]. Blood results to be expected in sub-clinical
hyperthyroidism are:

- Plasma/serum TSH reduced.
- Plasma/serum FT4 and FT3 normal (often high normal).

Primary hypothyroidism

Like primary hyperthyroidism, primary hypothyroidism is ten times more common in women than men and, overall, primary hypothyroidism affects an estimated 1–2% of the UK population[1]. Incidence increases with age; close to 10% of elderly women are likely affected by hypothyroidism. Most cases of hypothyroidism are the result of slowly progressive autoimmune mediated destruction of thyroid tissue. There are two main forms: atrophic autoimmune thyroiditis and goitrous autoimmune thyroiditis (alternative name Hashimoto's thyroiditis). In the first the thyroid is shrunken in size (atrophic) and function, and in the second the thyroid is enlarged (goitrous) – but still 'shrunken' in function. In both cases destructive autoantibodies are detectable in the patient's serum and the same infiltration of the thyroid by inflammatory cells is evident; they are probably different stages of the same disease, with atrophy of the gland being the final stage.

The other major cause of primary hypothyroidism is two commonly employed treatment regimes for primary hyperthyroidism: thyroid surgery and irradiation of the thyroid gland. The aim of both treatments is destruction of thyroid tissue and an inevitable consequence of this destruction is increased long-term risk of primary hypothyroidism. Together, autoimmune destruction and treatment of hyperthyroidism account for more than 90% of all cases of primary hyperthyroidism.

Some drugs, notably lithium (Chapter 14) can cause hypothyroidism. Around 1 in 3500–4000 babies are born with a deficiency of thyroid hormone. All babies are screened at birth for this condition, which is called congenital hypothyroidism and considered further in Chapter 23. In some parts of the world a diet severely deficient of iodine and consequent reduced thyroid hormone production is a major cause of hypothyroidism.

Whatever the cause, primary hypothyroidism is associated with reduced thyroid hormone production and it is this hormone deficiency that accounts for symptoms in adults (Table 10.2). The normal response of the pituitary to reduced thyroid hormone production is increased production of TSH. An increased concentration of TSH in blood is the most important diagnostic feature of primary hypothyroidism.

Table 10.2 Major signs and symptoms of hypothyroidism.

Thyroid hormone deficiency causes a general slowing of body metabolism and physiological process, resulting in any of the following signs and symptoms:

- Weight gain
- Puffy face particularly below the eyes
- Decreased appetite
- Intolerance of cold
- Dry skin, dry 'lifeless' hair
- Decreased heart rate (bradycardia)
- Constipation
- Depression
- Slowing of metal agility
- Hoarse 'gruff' voice

The blood results that would be expected in primary hypothyroidism whatever the cause are:

- Plasma/serum TSH concentration always increased (usually >10 mU/L).
- Plasma/serum FT4 concentration reduced.

Secondary (central) hypothyroidism

Very rarely hypothyroidism is the result not of thyroid disease but of an inability to adequately stimulate a normal thyroid gland because of a deficiency of TSH. This occurs if there is trauma to or tissue damaging disease of the pituitary gland. Damage to the hypothalamus has the same effect. The blood results that would be expected in secondary hypothyroidism whatever the cause are:

- Plasma/serum TSH concentration reduced.
- Plasma/serum FT4 concentration reduced.

Sub-clinical (mild) hypothyroidism

Relatively frequently patient testing reveals raised serum TSH (indicating primary hypothyroidism) in association with serum FT4 within the reference range (indicating euthyroidism). This pattern indicates that although the thyroid gland is producing enough thyroid hormone to maintain concentration within the reference range, it is not producing sufficient to fully suppress TSH production. Thyroid hormone blood levels are only maintained within the reference range by virtue of the abnormally increased amount of TSH being released from the pituitary. Since thyroid hormone concentration is normal there are usually no symptoms, so the condition is called sub-clinical hypothyroidism. This represents a stage between normality and overt hypothyroidism. Patients with sub-clinical, sometimes called mild hypothyroidism are at long-term risk of developing overt hypothyroidism, especially if TSH is found to be particularly high (>10 mu/L), and should be offered annual thyroid testing.

The effect of non-thyroid illness on TSH, FT4 and FT3

The laboratory diagnosis of hyper and hypothyroidism whether sub-clinical or overt is rarely a problem in otherwise well patients, but interpretation of thyroid function test results is often more difficult in patients who are suffering acute illness. The term euthyroid sick syndrome or non-thyroidal illness syndrome is applied to those patients whose thyroid function tests (TSH, FT4 and FT3) are transiently abnormal due to acute illness. By definition the thyroids of these patients are working normally, the cause of the abnormal thyroid blood tests results is the acute illness. Euthyroid sick syndrome may reflect a protective adaptive response to acute illness or perhaps a maladaptive result of acute illness that impairs recovery from the illness. Either way, the practical clinical problem is that there is often difficulty in knowing if abnormal blood tests results are due to euthyroid sick syndrome or thyroid disease.

Table 10.3 Summary of typical changes to thyroid function test results in thyroid and non-thyroid disease.

THYROID DISEASE	FT4	FT3	TSH
Primary hyperthyroidism Common cause: Graves' disease Less common causes: • Toxic adenoma • Toxic multinodular goitre • Thyroiditis	Increased (at high end of normal range in sub-clinical disease)	Increased	Marked decrease (may be undetectable)
Primary hypothyroidism Common causes: • Hashimoto's disease • Treatment of hyperthyroidism Less common causes: • Congenital hypothyroidism • Iodine deficiency (common in some parts of the world)	Decreased (at low end of normal range in sub-clinical disease)	Decreased (occasionally normal)	Marked increase
NON-THYROID DISEASE			
Secondary hyperthyroidism (rare) Cause: over-activity of pituitary gland or hypothalamus	Increased	Increased	Increased
Secondary hypothyroidism (rare) Cause: under-activity (damage) to pituitary gland or hypothalamus	Decreased	Decreased	Decreased
Euthyroid sick syndrome (common) May be a feature of any acute, severe illness, e.g. cancer, advanced liver disease, renal failure, major trauma or surgery, extensive burns, starvation	Usually normal but may be decreased	Decreased	Usually normal but may be decreased or increased

The range of acute illnesses that might be associated with euthyroid sick syndrome is wide and includes: acute infectious disease (especially sepsis), myocardial infarction, malignancy, severe trauma (e.g. surgery), indeed any acute illness may be affected in this way. Those being cared for in intensive care units are a patient group at particularly high risk; close to 50% of such patients have euthyroid sick syndrome[4].

Abnormal results of all three tests may be found in those with severe acute illness; the most consistent finding is reduced FT3. FT4 may be normal or reduced. TSH is usually normal but this too may be reduced and, rarely, raised.

The confounding effect of acute illness makes laboratory diagnosis of thyroid disease particularly difficult. Repeat testing after resolution of the acute illness may be the only way of making or excluding a laboratory diagnosis of hypothyroidism or hyperthyroidism.

A summary of the abnormal changes in thyroid function tests for both thyroid and non-thyroid disease is contained in Table 10.3.

Monitoring treatment of thyroid disease

The blood tests described above for the identification of patients suffering thyroid disorders are also useful in monitoring the effectiveness of therapy among those already diagnosed.

Treatment of hyperthyroidism

There are three possible treatment regimes for those with hyperthyroidism. Most patients are treated initially with anti-thyroid drugs. In the UK, carbimazole, a drug that inhibits the key enzyme TPO required for normal thyroid hormone production, is most often prescribed. Typically a daily dose of carbimazole for 12–18 months effects a cure for around half of patients. For those in whom drug therapy is either contraindicated or unsuccessful, an alternative is radioactive iodine treatment. Like all ingested iodine, radioactive iodine is concentrated in the thyroid gland. Here the radioactivity destroys thyroid tissue. Surgical removal of thyroid tissue (partial thyroidectomy) offers a third treatment option.

The object of therapy is to reduce thyroid hormone levels to normal (biochemical euthyroidism) and thereby remove symptoms; that is achieve a state of clinical euthyroidism. All therapies carry a high risk of 'over-treatment', rendering patients hypothyroid so that monitoring of blood hormone levels during and after treatment is an essential part of the care of patients being treated for hyperthyroidism. The dose of anti-thyroid drug is adjusted in the first instance in the light of serum FT4 results; the serum TSH often remains suppressed for a month or two after treatment begins but will eventually return to normal. Since there is a long-term risk of hypothyroidism developing or recurrence of hyperthyroidism in those treated for hyperthyroidism, continued blood testing of thyroid function (FT4 and TSH) at least every 12 months is necessary for all patients.

Treatment of primary hypothyroidism

The only treatment for primary hypothyroidism is thyroid hormone replacement therapy, usually in the form of thyroxine tablets to be taken daily, for life. The object is to increase thyroid hormone levels (T4 and T3) to normal; this will reduce the abnormal high level of TSH secretion to normal and remove symptoms. The dosage required to achieve this state of biochemical and clinical euthyroidism varies and can only be assessed by gradually increasing the dose at four to six week intervals in the light of serum TSH results; the primary target being to achieve a serum TSH that is within the reference range. Too low a dose and symptoms of hypothyroidism persist; too high a dose and T4 and T3 levels rise above normal, TSH levels drop below normal and the patient develops symptoms of hyperthyroidism. Once a maintenance dose has been achieved, which results in both biochemical and clinical euthyroidism, the dose usually remains the same for life and blood levels (TSH and FT4) need only be checked annually.

Thyroid testing in pregnancy

Over the past decade or two it has become apparent that maternal hypothyroidism is common during pregnancy. In most cases this is asymptomatic (sub-clinical hypothyroidism). But whether symptomatic or not, hypothyroidism during pregnancy is associated with higher than normal risk of several adverse outcomes, including: miscarriage, preeclampsia, premature birth, postpartum haemorrhage and foetal and neonatal distress. The greater part of foetal brain development occurs in the first trimester and this development is dependent on adequate amount of thyroid hormone in maternal blood. Even very mild maternal deficiency of thyroid hormone (i.e. hypothyroidisim) at the time of conception and through the first trimester threatens cognitive development in the long term, with risk of reduced intelligence quotient (IQ) in childhood.

Given that undiagnosed sub-clinical hypothyroidism is relatively common in women of child bearing age and that it has adverse effect for both mother and baby but is easily treated (with replacement thyroxine), some experts suggest that all pregnant women should have blood tested for TSH/FT4 early in pregnancy.

At the present time justification for this universal screening policy remains controversial and it has yet to be adopted. However current recommendations[5,6] are that all of the following groups of pregnant women, considered at particularly high risk of thyroid disease, be offered TSH/FT4 testing at the time of first antenatal booking:

- Those with a family or personal history of thyroid disease.
- Those with goitre or other signs and symptoms suggestive of thyroid disease.
- Those with a history of any autoimmune disease, e.g. Type 1 diabetes.
- Those who have had a previous miscarriage or previous pre-term delivery.

Postpartum thyroiditis is quite a common inflammatory disease of the thyroid that affects around 5% of women in the months following birth. It is classically characterised by an initial phase of hyperthyroidism, one to three months after birth, followed by a phase of hypothyroidism during subsequent months. Quite frequently, the condition is not recognised until the second hypothyroid phase, but any sign or symptom of hypothyroidism, including depression, arising up to a year after giving birth should raise suspicion of postpartum thyroiditis and prompt TSH/FT4 testing. Although the condition eventually resolves, women with a history of postpartum thyroiditis have a greater than normal risk of developing permanent primary hypothyroidsim later in life and should therefore be offered annual TSH testing.

Case history 15

Mrs Hollingsworth, a 35 year old PE teacher, has visited her current GP only for antenatal visits during two uneventful pregnancies in her twenties and for annual 'well woman' checks over the previous five years. She now goes to see her GP because for a period of several months she has been feeling 'constantly tired and washed out' despite increasingly less activity at work and sleeping more than usual. She tells the doctor that she thinks she might be anaemic because of several heavy periods over the past few months. The doctor feels that this normally lively lady appears unusually depressed. On questioning she admits feeling depressed but attributes this to tiredness and hopes that some 'iron tablets' will put things right. She also reports being frustrated at recent increase in body weight despite eating less than normal; she feels she has lost her appetite for food. The weight gain is confirmed by comparing her current weight with measurements made at previous well woman clinics. Although there are no clinical signs of anaemia, the doctor agrees to take blood to test for anaemia but also takes a further sample for thyroid function tests.

The full blood count results are entirely normal, excluding anaemia as a cause for the tiredness.

The thyroid function test results are:

FT4   8.0 pmol/L
TSH   26 mIU/L

Questions

(1) What symptoms suggested that thyroid function tests were appropriate?
(2) Are the thyroid function results normal?
(3) What do the results suggest?

Discussion of case history 15

(1) As the GP suspected from clinical examination, Mrs Hollingsworth was not anaemic. Tiredness, depression, excessive menstrual blood flow (menorrhagia) and weight gain without increased food intake can all result from a deficiency of thyroid hormone, that is hypothyroidism. The condition is particularly common in middle-aged women. The extent and severity of symptoms among patients with hypothyroidism vary greatly so that the absence of more clinical features of hypothyroidism does not exclude the diagnosis.

(2) No, FT4 is reduced and TSH is increased.

(3) The results suggest a diagnosis of primary hypothyroidism (Table 10.3). Mrs Hollingsworth's thyroid is producing insufficient thyroid hormone despite increased secretion of TSH by the pituitary gland and would benefit from thyroid replacement therapy if repeat testing confirms these abnormal results.

References

1. Vanderpump, M. (2011) The epidemiology of thyroid disease, *British Medical Bulletin*, 99: 39–51.
2. Leese, G., Flynn, R., Jung, R. et al. (2008) Increasing prevalence and incidence of thyroid disease in Tayside, Scotland: the thyroid epidemiology audit and research study (TEARS), *Clinical Endocrinology*, 68: 311–16.
3. Wilson, G. and Curry, R. (2005) Subclinical thyroid disease, *Am Fam Physician*, 72: 1517–24.
4. Pilkat, K., Langgartner, J., Buettner, R. et al. (2007) Frequency and outcome of patients with non-thyroidal illness syndrome in a medical intensive care unit, *Metabolism*, 56: 239–44.

5. Guidelines Development Group (2006) UK guidelines for the use of thyroid function tests, available at: http://www.british-thyroid-association.org/Guidelines/.
6. Ablovich, M., Amino, N., Barbour, L. et al. (2007) Management of thyroid dysfunction during pregnancy and postpartum: and endocrine society clinical practice guideline, *J Clin Endocrinol Metab*, 92: S1–S47.

Further reading

Carson, M. (2009) Assessment and management of patients with hypothyroidism, *Nursing Standard*, 23(18): 48–56.

Jones, D., May, K. and Geraci, S. (2010) Subclinical thyroid disease, *American J Medicine*, 123: 502–4.

Kapustin, J. (2010) Hypothyroidism: an evidence based approach to a complex disorder, *Nurse Practitioner*, 35(8): 44–53.

Lazarus, J. (2011) Thyroid function in pregnancy, *British Med Bulletin*, 97: 137–48.

Lechan, R. (2008) The dilemma of the non-thyroidal illness syndrome, *Acta Biomed*, 79: 165–71.

Todd, C. (2009) Management of thyroid disorders in primary care: challenges and controversies, *Postgrad Med J.* 85: 655–9.

CHAPTER 11

LIVER FUNCTION TESTS: ALANINE TRANSFERASE (ALT), GAMMA GLUTAMYL TRANSFERASE (GGT), ALKALINE PHOSPHATASE (AP), BILIRUBIN AND ALBUMIN

Key learning topics

- Liver and biliary tract: anatomy, physiology and function
- Bilirubin metabolism and excretion
- Albumin – a marker of liver synthesis
- Liver enzymes (ALT, GGT and AP): markers of liver injury
- Laboratory test results in liver and biliary tract disease
- Adult jaundice
- Neonatal jaundice

This chapter is concerned with the measurement of the concentration of five substances in blood plasma/serum. Although structurally and functionally distinct they are treated together here because they are routinely measured together in a profile commonly known as liver function tests (LFTs). The principle use of the profile is identification of patients who are suffering liver or biliary tract disease. Depending on the exact nature of liver disease, one or more of these tests may be normal but it is unlikely that all would be normal in any patient suffering significant liver or biliary tract disease. Thus, the combination of five LFTs has more power to detect liver or biliary tract disease than each individual test. None of the five tests are specific for a particular liver or biliary tract disease, or indeed specific for liver/biliary tract disease generally, so that there are other diseases, not involving the liver or biliary tract, in which one or more of these tests might be abnormal.

Understanding Laboratory Investigations: A Guide for Nurses, Midwives and Healthcare Professionals, Third Edition. Chris Higgins.
© 2013 John Wiley & Sons, Ltd. Published 2013 by John Wiley & Sons, Ltd.

Normal anatomy and physiology

The liver

The liver, the largest internal body organ weighing around 2 kg, is located in the right upper quadrant of the abdomen, protected for the most part by the lower rib cage. (Figure 11.1a) The narrower left lobe extends from the rib cage over the stomach. It is red-brown in colour due to its copious blood supply: the organ receives around 30% of total cardiac output every minute from two sources, the portal vein and hepatic artery. The products of ingested food are transported to the liver directly from the gastrointestinal tract in blood via the portal vein and oxygenated blood is supplied via the hepatic artery. Blood leaves the liver by way of the hepatic vein, draining to the inferior vena cava for return to the heart (Figure 11.1b).

The complexities of liver function can be broadly summarised under three interconnected headings:

- Metabolic function.
- Synthetic function.
- Excretory function.

Hepatocytes, the cells the bulk of the liver is composed of, play a central role in the metabolism of ingested carbohydrates, proteins and fats. That is why these products of digestion are transported first to the liver, via the portal vein. Glucose derived from ingested carbohydrates can be stored until required, in hepatocytes, as glycogen. Between meals when glucose is in short supply, these glycogen stores are mobilised. During starvation, when even glycogen stores are depleted, hepatocytes are able to convert amino acids derived from ingested and body proteins to glucose. By these effects on carbohydrate metabolism, the liver plays a central role in regulating blood glucose concentration.

Dietary derived amino acids are synthesised into proteins in the liver; these include many of the proteins, like albumin, that are present in blood plasma. The vital process of blood clotting depends on the liver synthesis of the specific plasma proteins (clotting factors) of the clotting cascade. Urea, a waste product of amino acid metabolism is synthesised in the liver before transport in blood to the kidneys, where it is excreted in urine. The liver plays a major role in the metabolism of ingested fats (lipids) by synthesising the lipoproteins necessary for transport of these fats, including cholesterol and triglycerides, around the body in blood. Synthesis of bile acids from cholesterol in the liver provides a further example of the way liver affects lipid metabolism and leads nicely to the excretory role of the liver.

Production of bile – the biliary tract

The liver is the source of bile, an alkaline watery yellow/green fluid that contains the bile acids produced from cholesterol. These bile acids have to be conveyed in bile to the intestine where they are required for absorption of dietary lipids. Bile

(a)

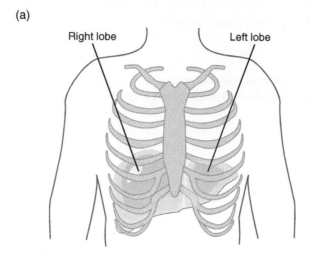

(b)

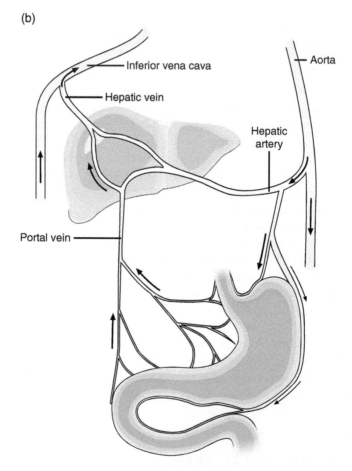

Figure 11.1 (a) Location of the liver, (b) hepatic circulation.

also provides the route for excretion of drugs and other waste products of metabolism that are not excreted from the body by kidneys in urine. The production of bile thus fulfils the excretory role of the liver.

Bile is produced within and secreted from hepatocytes to microscopic tube like structures called bile canaliculi that coalesce within the liver to form larger bile ducts. These in turn join to form the larger hepatic bile ducts that conduct bile from the liver. Left and right hepatic bile ducts join outside the liver forming the common hepatic bile duct, and this is connected via the common bile duct to the duodenum of the intestinal tract. The pancreatic duct that conveys pancreatic digestive juice from the pancreas joins the common bile duct a few centimetres from the duodenum, so that bile and pancreatic juice enter the intestinal tract through the same opening in the duodenum. Bile production by the liver is continuous, amounting to around 500 ml/day. Between meals, when its digestive property is not required, the passage of bile (and pancreatic juice) to the duodenum is blocked by closure of a sphincter (sphincter of Oddi) sited at the junction of common bile duct and duodenum. When this sphincter is closed bile is stored in the gall bladder, which is connected to the common bile duct via the cystic duct. When food is ingested the sphincter opens and bile passes from the gall bladder via cystic duct and common bile duct, to the lumen of duodenum. The biliary tract is the totality of structure that conveys bile from hepatocytes to the intestine and includes bile ducts (cananliculi) within the liver, hepatic bile ducts, gall bladder, common bile duct and sphincter of Oddi.

Although bile acids represent a major constituent of bile, it is by no means the only one; bile is a chemically complex fluid containing of course water but also electrolytes and many waste products of metabolism destined for excretion in faeces. Among them is bilirubin, a waste product of haemoglobin catabolism.

Bilirubin

Many patients suffering liver or biliary tract disease have a yellow discoloration of the skin and mucous membranes, first evident in the sclerae (whites) of the eye. This clinical sign, known as jaundice (derived from the French word for yellow, jaune) which, as will become clear, is not confined to those suffering liver or biliary tract disease, is due to an abnormally high concentration in the blood of the potentially toxic yellow pigment, bilirubin.

Most of the 250–300 mg bilirubin normally produced each day is derived from the breakdown (catabolism) of haemoglobin, the oxygen carrying protein contained in red blood cells (Figure 11.2). At the end of their normal 120 day life span, red blood cells are removed from circulating blood to the spleen and other parts of the reticuloendothelial (RE) system. In macrophage cells within the RE system, haemoglobin released from dead red cells is split into its constituent parts: haem and globin. The haem portion is converted to bilirubin, which is then tightly bound to albumin for transport in blood from RE-macrophages to the liver and eventual excretion in bile. Before entry to liver cells bilirubin is released from albumin.

Bilirubin is water insoluble and must be made water soluble for excretion in bile. This is achieved within hepatocytes by conjugation (joining) of bilirubin to a

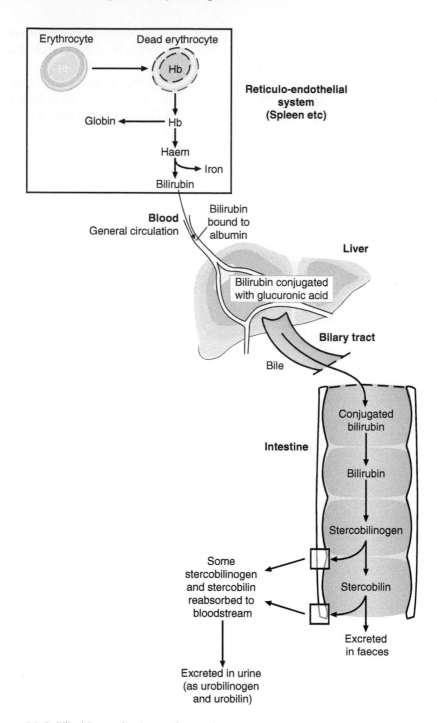

Figure 11.2 Bilirubin production and excretion.

substance called glucuronic acid. The resulting so called conjugated bilirubin is secreted from the hepatocyte to bile canaliculi and onwards in bile, out of the liver via the biliary tract to the duodenum. The action of bacteria normally present within the gut deconjugates bilirubin (that is releases bilirubin from glucuronic acid) and converts bilirubin to stercobilinogen and then stercobilin. Almost all of these final products of bilirubin metabolism are excreted from the body in faeces (stercobilin is an orange-brown pigment responsible for the brown colour of faeces). However a little stercobilinogen and stercobilin is reabsorbed to blood during passage through the gut. Most of this is recycled by the liver and re-excreted into the gut, but some is excreted in urine as urobilinogen/urobilin (urobilinogen/urobilin are the names given to stercobilinogen/stercobilin when they are not in the intestine or faeces).

The bilirubin that is normally present in blood plasma/serum and measured in the laboratory is comprised of two fractions: unconjugated bilirubin and conjugated bilirubin. In health by far the biggest proportion is unconjugated bilirubin; this is the bilirubin that is being transported (bound to albumin) in blood to the liver for excretion. Conjugated bilirubin is, as outlined already, the form in which bilirubin is excreted from the liver in bile to the intestine. Now, although nearly all conjugated bilirubin is normally excreted via bile and gastrointestinal tract in faeces, a very small proportion returns to blood, from hepatocytes, bile canaliculi or intestine. The bilirubin test routinely performed in the laboratory measures total bilirubin concentration (i.e. the sum of unconjugated bilirubin – normally around 80–90% of total bilirubin and conjugated bilirubin normally 10–20% of total bilirubin). The distinction between unconjugated and conjugated bilirubin is important in the differential diagnosis of the jaundiced patient because depending on its cause, jaundice can result from either predominant increase in unconjugated bilirubin or predominant increase in conjugated bilirubin. Most laboratories have the capacity to measure not only total bilirubin concentration but also conjugated bilirubin concentration, in the relatively rare circumstance that this extra testing is diagnostically necessary.

Albumin

Blood plasma contains a mixture of many proteins each with its own function. These include proteins required to fight infection (immunoglobulins or antibodies), enzymes, blood clotting factors, specific transport proteins and many more. Albumin is the single most abundant protein in plasma comprising as it does around 40–60% of total plasma protein; it is the most frequently measured plasma protein in clinical laboratories.

Like many other proteins present in plasma, albumin is synthesised from amino acids in the liver. It has two main functions. The first of these is as a transport protein. Many water insoluble substances can only be transported in blood plasma when bound to specific proteins. Albumin is one of these proteins and is, as we have already seen, required for transport of unconjugated bilirubin. Around half the calcium present in blood plasma is bound to albumin, as are free fatty acids and many drugs.

The other important function of albumin is maintenance of blood plasma volume. As the single most abundant protein in plasma, albumin is a major contributor to colloid osmotic pressure or plasma oncotic pressure. This pressure opposes the tendency of fluid to escape from capillary blood vessels into the surrounding interstitial space due to blood pressure within vessels. Oedema (which may be visible as swelling) is the term used to describe an abnormal accumulation of fluid in the interstitial space and this occurs if albumin concentration of plasma and therefore plasma oncotic pressure fall below normal.

Solution of albumin may be administered therapeutically via an intravenous line to patients who have suffered major trauma, burns or clinical shock, to restore plasma volume.

Gamma glutamyl transpeptidase (GGT), alanine transferase (ALT) and alkaline phosphatase (AP)

GGT, ALT and AP are all enzymes. They are present in the cells of the liver and biliary tract where they function as catalysts of specific metabolic reactions that are required for cell function and survival. The enzymes have no function in blood plasma and the small amount that is normally present (compared with that in cells) is due to normal cell turnover. As cells naturally die they release their contents to blood plasma. The cell injury or death (necrosis) associated with liver or biliary tract disease results in increased amounts of these intracellular enzymes being released to blood plasma. These enzyme measuring tests then are not strictly speaking measuring liver function, they are merely convenient blood markers of liver/biliary tract cell injury/death.

If the source of these enzymes were only the cells of liver or biliary tract tissue, then raised levels would always indicate liver or biliary tract disease. In fact, although GGT, ALT and AP are frequently referred to as 'liver enzymes', they are also present in other tissues, and damage or disease of these non-liver, non-biliary tract tissues may also be associated with a rise in serum concentration of either GGT, ALT or AP. The most significant non-liver non-biliary tract source of GGT is the pancreas. ALT is present predominantly in the hepatocytes of the liver but also, albeit at far lower concentration, in kidney tissue, heart muscle (myocardium) and skeletal muscle. AP is present not only in the liver cells of the bile canaliculi, but also in bone cells, intestinal tissue cells and placental tissue cells.

Laboratory measurement of liver function tests (LFTs)

Patient preparation

No particular patient preparation is necessary.

Timing of sample

Blood for LFTs may be sampled at any time. It is however important that there is not undue delay (more than a few hours) in transporting specimens to the laboratory for separation of serum (or plasma) from cells.

Sample requirement

Around 5 ml of venous blood is required for LFTs. Blood should be collected into a plain tube without additives if local policy is to use serum for analysis, and into a tube containing the anticoagulant lithium heparin if local policy is to use plasma. A falsely raised albumin level occurs if a tourniquet is left in position for a more than a minute or two before sampling blood. If possible the use of a tourniquet should be avoided. Bilirubin is slowly destroyed by both artificial and sun light, leading to falsely low results. To reduce this effect samples should be protected as far as possible from exposure to light both before and during transport to the laboratory.

Neonatal measurement of bilirubin only

For reasons still to be discussed new born babies (particularly those born prematurely) frequently need monitoring of serum bilirubin concentration. In these cases only bilirubin need be measured, reducing the sample requirement to 0.5 ml or less. Capillary blood obtained by a heel stab (Chapter 2) is usually used in these circumstances. Particular care is required to avoid haemolysis during blood collection as such samples are unsuitable for bilirubin estimation. A special dark plastic container (to protect bilirubin from exposure to light) is often used for collection of blood samples for neonatal bilirubin measurement.

Interpretation of results

Approximate reference ranges

Plasma/serum bilirubin (total)	<21 µmol/L
Plasma/serum albumin	35–50 g/L

Plasma/serum ALT, GGT and AP. Methods used to measure enzyme levels vary between laboratories; each method has its own reference range. It would be misleading therefore to quote even approximate reference ranges for these enzyme tests. Always use local laboratory reference range when interpreting results. The unit of measurement for all enzyme assays is the international unit (IU) and results are expressed in terms of number of IUs per litre of plasma/serum (i.e. IU/L).

Bone is a source of AP, and during periods of bone growth (childhood and adolescence) the amount of AP in plasma/serum is markedly increased compared with that which prevails in adulthood. Each laboratory publishes AP reference ranges that refer to specific age ranges. It is vitally important the age of the patient be taken into account when interpreting AP results. The presence of AP in placental tissue determines that AP is higher during pregnancy.

Causes of raised bilirubin – jaundice

The concentration of bilirubin in serum reflects the balance between the amount produced by the normal process of red cell destruction and that removed from the blood by the liver and excreted in bile. An abnormally raised serum bilirubin occurs in three broad pathological situations:

- Diseases in which the rate of bilirubin production exceeds the normal rate of liver processing and excretion. Bilirubin consequently accumulates in blood. These are the haemolytic anaemias, which are characterised by increased red cell destruction and therefore increased catabolism of haemoglobin and consequent increased bilirubin production. Liver and biliary tract are functionally normally, so that haemolytic anaemias serve to remind that jaundice can occur in patients without liver or biliary tract disease. The jaundice that occurs in these conditions (called haemolytic jaundice) is the result of increase in unconjugated (rather than conjugated) bilirubin.
- Diseases in which rate of bilirubin production is normal but the rate at which the liver can process a normal bilirubin load is compromised by disease. These are diseases solely of the liver and the resulting jaundice (called hepatocellular jaundice) is the result of predominant increase in conjugated (rather than unconjugated) bilirubin.
- Diseases in which the rate of production of bilirubin is normal, the rate at which liver cells process bilirubin is normal but the rate of excretion is reduced due to disease of the biliary tract (either within the liver or at some other point in the biliary tract between the liver and the duodenum). The disorders in this group are characterised by cholestasis, which means reduction in bile flow. The resulting jaundice (called cholestatic or obstructive jaundice) is caused by a predominant increase in conjugated (rather than unconjugated) bilirubin.

Generally speaking haemolytic jaundice is associated with only a slight increase in bilirubin; concentration rarely rises above 70 μmol/L. An important exception is haemolytic disease of the newborn (discussed further). Since the liver is functionally normal in this condition, all other LFTs are normal.

Higher serum bilirubin concentration is seen in liver disease in which there is injury to liver cells. For example, acute inflammation of the liver (acute hepatitis), which is usually the result of viral infection (Table 11.1) or alcohol abuse (acute alcoholic hepatitis), causes peak concentrations (up to 300 μmol/L) at around the tenth day after symptoms develop. During the four to eight week recovery period, bilirubin gradually returns to normal. In some cases inflammation does not resolve and becomes chronic and progressively destructive. The term chronic active hepatitis is used to describe such cases, and bilirubin, though not as high as during acute hepatitis, may remain raised. Cirrhosis, that is irreversible liver damage, most often the result of prolonged alcohol abuse or unresolved viral hepatitis (there are many rarer causes), may be associated with a near normal serum bilirubin

Table 11.1 Viral causes of hepatitis and therefore abnormal liver function tests.

	Hepatitis A virus (HAV)	Hepatitis B virus (HBV)	Hepatitis C virus (HCV)	Hepatitis D virus (HDV)	Hepatitis E virus (HVE)
Relative significance as a cause of hepatitis in the UK	Most common cause of viral hepatitis; accounts for around 40% of all cases	Common cause of viral hepatitis: accounts for around 35% of all cases	Less common cause of viral hepatitis: accounts for around 15% of all cases	Infection only occurs in association with HBV infection. Never the sole cause of viral hepatitis	Rare. Cases are almost always the result of travel to areas of the world, e.g. Far East, where the virus is endemic
Mode of transmission/ risk factors	Faecal-oral route. Close contact with infected individual. Eating uncooked contaminated food/water	Inoculation/contact with infected blood/body fluids. Can be sexually transmitted. Those at risk include health workers, sex workers and injecting drug abusers	As for HBV Blood transfusion or receipt of blood product prior to 1993 (when testing was introduced) is a major risk factor for chronic infection	As for HEV	Faecal-oral route. Eating uncooked contaminated food/ water in areas of the world where the virus is endemic (not the UK)
Symptoms of acute infection	Infection does not always result in symptoms, particularly during childhood. When they do occur symptoms begin with a 'flu-like' illness with fever and generalised aches and pains. This is followed a few days later by symptoms that may include: nausea, vomiting, abdominal pain, and fatigue that can be extreme. Generally, HAV infection is associated with milder symptoms and HCV infection is quite often asymptomatic. For the great majority, symptoms gradually resolve over a period of six to eight weeks. Rarely, acute viral hepatitis can quickly evolve to liver failure.				
Long-term consequences of acute infection: progression to chronic liver disease or liver cancer	No long-term consequences	Around 5–10% of acutely infected patients progress to chronic liver disease (chronic active hepatitis/cirrhosis) and a small minority of these subsequently develop liver cancer	Progression common Around 70% of HCV infected patients eventually develop chronic liver disease and some of these subsequently progress to liver cancer, usually decades after infection	Risk of chronic disease among HBV infected persons is greatly increased if they are also infected with HDV	No long term consequences

concentration in the early stages but rises as the disease progresses, often over many years, to liver failure. Secondary spread (metastases) of primary cancers to the liver is often associated with raised bilirubin; jaundice is a poor prognostic sign in patients with such secondary cancer spread.

Obstruction of bile flow and consequent failure to excrete conjugated bilirubin is the cause of the raised serum bilirubin that can complicate gallstone disease if gallstones become lodged in the cystic duct or common bile duct. A similar mechanism accounts for the very high bilirubin that can occur in cancers of the biliary tract and cancer of the head of pancreas. In these cases it is the malignant growth that obstructs bile flow.

Several inherited defects of bilirubin metabolism result in raised bilirubin but all are rare, except Gilbert's syndrome. This is an entirely benign condition affecting around 5% of the population and often discovered quite by chance during routine blood testing. The only abnormality is a slight increase in serum (unconjugated) bilirubin, often, though not necessarily, precipitated by inter-current illness. Total serum bilirubin rarely exceeds 50–70 μmol/L in those with Gilbert's syndrome and all other liver function tests are normal. The finding of a slightly raised serum bilirubin in association with no other signs, symptoms or laboratory evidence of liver disease is not uncommon, and in the vast majority of cases is due to the quite harmless Gilbert's syndrome.

Neonatal jaundice

All babies, by comparison with adults, have a raised bilirubin at birth, and concentration rises sufficiently during the first week of life to cause jaundice in around 60% of full term babies and 80% of preterm babies. In the vast majority of cases this is due to so called 'physiological' jaundice. Two factors contribute to physiological jaundice. Firstly, the days after birth are associated with increased red cell destruction and therefore increased unconjugated bilirubin production. In addition liver metabolism is not fully mature at this time so that newborn babies are unable to conjugate bilirubin at a sufficient rate for excretion to balance production. Physiological jaundice is transitory with serum bilirubin (predominantly unconjugated bilirubin) concentration peaking usually no higher than 200–250 μmol/L on the third or fourth day of life before falling to a level at which jaundice is no longer evident over the next few days. Jaundice persisting beyond the first 10–14 days of life, or jaundice associated with bilirubin levels in excess of 250 μmol/L, cannot be regarded as physiologic or 'normal'. The most common reason for persistence of neonatal jaundice is breast milk feeding. Up to a third of exclusively breast fed babies develop some degree of jaundice that can persist for up to 12 weeks after birth, before spontaneous resolution[3].

Less benign causes of persistent jaundice in newborn babies include haemolytic disease of the newborn (HDN), which is discussed in Chapter 20, congenital hypothyroidism, which is discussed in Chapter 23, neonatal hepatitis, biliary atresia and very rare inherited defects of bilirubin metabolism.

Causes of abnormal plasma/serum albumin concentration

Since albumin is synthesised in the liver, it might be expected that liver disease is always associated with reduced synthesis and abnormally low serum levels. This however is not the case. Serum albumin is reduced only in chronic liver disease (e.g. cirrhosis) and liver failure but usually remains normal if damage is acute and self-limiting (e.g. acute hepatitis). Albumin may also be reduced in conditions other than liver disease. Inadequate supply of dietary amino-acids required for albumin synthesis is the cause of the low albumin associated with severe malnutrition and malabsorption. Abnormal loss of albumin from the body may also result in low levels. For example, the abnormal loss of albumin in urine accounts for the low serum albumin in diseases of the kidney (particularly marked in nephrotic syndrome). Albumin is frequently low in patients who have suffered extensive burns due to the loss of albumin through skin.

The level of hydration although not affecting the total amount of albumin in the body, does affect the concentration of albumin. In dehydrated patients serum albumin concentration is raised and in overhydrated patients serum albumin concentration is reduced.

Causes of abnormal enzyme results

Alanine transferase (ALT)

Highest ALT results (in extreme cases up to 50 or even 100 times the upper limit of normal) are seen in any disease associated with acute and massive liver cell necrosis (death). In acute viral hepatitis, for example, liver cell necrosis causes ALT to rise to a peak during the first few days following development of first symptoms, usually before jaundice develops. As the disease resolves over the following six to eight weeks, ALT gradually falls back to normal. A similar picture follows the liver cell necrosis that results from hypoxia due to acute circulatory failure (clinical shock) and that which results from ingestion of liver toxins (e.g. overdose of paracetamol in which ALT levels may be in excess of 100 times the upper limit of normal). A moderately raised ALT (up to ten times the upper limit of normal) that persists for more than one month suggests the development of chronic liver disease. Chronic hepatitis, cirrhosis and malignant disease of the liver are frequently associated with such moderate rises. ALT is usually normal or only slightly increased in diseases associated with reduced bile flow.

An isolated mild increase in ALT (up to 5 times the upper limit of normal) with all other liver function tests normal is a quite common finding. Causes of this pattern include chronic hepatitis C infection and drug induced hepatic damage, but the most common cause is non-alcoholic fatty liver disease (NAFLD).

NALFD is a condition characterised by the abnormal accumulation of fat in the liver that, like Type 2 diabetes, results from obesity and associated metabolic syndrome (the two conditions Type 2 diabetes and NALFD co-exist in some patients). Just as the obesity epidemic has given rise to a massive increase in the diabetic population, it has also given rise to ever increasing incidence of this obesity associated liver disease, that can in a minority of affected patients progress, like chronic viral hepatitis and chronic alcoholic hepatitis, to cirrhosis, liver cancer or liver failure. NALFD is now the most common cause of persistently raised liver enzymes, indeed the most common liver disease affecting an estimated 30% of those living in developed countries like the UK[1]. Because it is clinically silent (symptomless) in the early stages and only detected if liver function blood tests are performed, or liver biopsy examined, the vast majority of those with NALFD remain undiagnosed and are quite unaware of their condition.

Gamma glutamyl transpeptidase (GGT)

GGT is usually raised (up to five times the upper limit of normal) in all types of liver and biliary tract disease (acute and chronic hepatitis, cirrhosis, obstructive jaundice etc.) The test can help to identify those with disease of the liver or biliary tract disease but is not very useful in narrowing down the nature of that disease. Measurement of GGT has however been found to be useful in the management of patients who are at risk of liver disease due to alcohol abuse. Unlike the other two liver enzymes, GGT production is induced by alcohol, so that if patients are drinking excessive alcohol, GGT is often raised, even if there is no liver damage; the level returns to normal on withdrawal of alcohol. Persistently raised GGT in a patient with a history of alcohol abuse suggests that the patient continues to drink alcohol or that some damage to the liver has occurred (alcoholic hepatitis or cirrhosis). This use of the test does not however provide full proof because GGT remains within normal limits in an estimated 30% of patients who continuously abuse alcohol, and of course alcohol use and abuse is by no means the only cause of increased GGT. Indeed raised GGT is a feature of NAFLD, which is defined by the absence of alcohol abuse.

Some drugs, including the anticonvulsants phenytoin, phenobarbitone, tricyclic antidepressants and paracetamol, also induce GGT production. For patients taking these and other drugs, a slight increase in GGT can be expected and does not necessarily imply any liver damage. Disease of the pancreas (e.g. acute pancreatitis) usually results in an increased GGT and a slight increase in GGT is often noted in diabetic patients.

Alkaline phosphatase (AP)

AP levels may be raised in liver disease, biliary tract disease and some diseases of the bone. So far as liver and biliary tract diseases are concerned, highest levels are seen in diseases that obstruct the flow of bile, after it has left the liver (e.g. gall stones in the common bile duct and carcinoma of the head of the pancreas). AP is also usually raised in cirrhosis and liver cancers (including liver metastases). Levels are generally only slightly raised in acute hepatitis and may be normal.

AP is present in high concentration in the osteoblastic cells of bone. The function of these cells is formation and constant remodelling of bone. Any condition associated with increased osteoblastic activity results in increased levels of AP in blood. The increase in osteoblastic activity associated with growth spurts in childhood, as new bone is formed, accounts for the increased levels of plasma AP throughout childhood. Some diseases of the bone are associated with abnormally increased osteoblastic activity. Among these is Paget's disease, a painful and bone deforming condition usually diagnosed in middle age, and osteomalacia (called rickets in children) caused usually by vitamin D deficiency. Paget's disease is characterised by particularly high levels of plasma AP. A raised AP is often seen during the healing process following bone fracture, as new bone is formed. Finally AP is raised in patients who have tumours of the bone (either primary or secondary). Primary tumours often metastasise first to the bone. An isolated raised AP in a cancer patient is a poor prognostic sign as it may indicate tumour spread beyond the primary site.

Drugs and liver function tests

Liver damage can be caused by a wide spectrum of drugs, including some antibiotics (especially those used in the treatment of TB), paracetamol, aspirin, some antidepressants, cytotoxic drugs etc. It has been estimated that 10% of cases of jaundice among hospital patients are the result of drug therapy. Other drugs induce (or promote) synthesis of liver enzymes, and thereby cause increased plasma levels without causing jaundice or indeed liver damage. A full drug history is essential for interpretation of liver function test results in particular cases. The main causes of abnormal Bilirubin, Albumin, ALT, GGT and AP are summarised in Table 11.2.

Table 11.2 Causes of abnormal Bilirubin, Albumin, ALT, GGT and AP.

Most common causes of abnormal bilirubin and albumin result	
Increased plasma/serum bilirubin	**Reduced plasma/serum albumin**
Failure of liver cells to conjugate or excrete conjugated bilirubin: ● Acute/chronic hepatitis ● Cirrhosis ● Primary biliary cirrhosis ● Heart failure ● Primary liver cancer ● Liver metastases (cancer spread to liver from other site) ● Toxic liver damage (drugs, e.g.paracetamol)	Failure to synthesise normal amount of albumin: ● Any chronic liver disease, e.g. cirrhosis, chronic hepatitis ● Severe malnutrition ● Disease associated with malabsorption of digested food, e.g. Crohn's or coeliac disease
Failure to excrete bilirubin due to post-hepatic obstruction of bile flow: ● Gall stone obstructing common bile duct ● Carcinoma head of pancreas	Abnormal loss of albumin in urine: ● Nephrotic syndrome Movement of albumin from plasma to interstitial space: ● Any severe acute illness or tissue damage (e.g. common finding post-operatively)
Increased production of bilirubin due to increased rate of red cell destruction: ● Haemolytic anaemia ● Physiological jaundice (neonates only) ● Haemolytic disease of newborn (HDN)	Serum/Plasma albumin affected by state of hydration: increased in those who are dehydrated and reduced in those who are overhydrated.
Inherited defect of bilirubin metabolism: ● Gilbert's disease	

(Continued)

Table 11.2 *(Cont'd)*

Most common causes of abnormal liver enzyme results		
Increased plasma/ serum ALT	Increased plasma/ serum AP	Increased plasma/ serum GGT
Marked increase – 10 to 100 times the upper limit of normal may occur in any condition associated with acute severe liver cell death: • Acute viral hepatitis • Acute toxic hepatitis (e.g. paracetamol overdose, alcohol abuse) • Acute liver failure (irrespective of cause) Moderate increase – up to 10 times the upper limit of normal (non-acute liver diseases): • NAFLD • Cirrhosis • Chronic hepatitis • Primary liver cancer • Secondary spread of cancer to the liver • infectious mononucleosis (glandular fever) Mild increase – up to five times the upper limit of normal may occur in disease not affecting the liver: • Severe tissue damage (e.g. trauma, surgery) • Severe myocardial infarction • Disorders involving muscle cell destruction (e.g. rhabdomyolysis, severe exercise)	Marked increase – up to five times the upper limit of normal seen in liver and biliary tract diseases that cause obstruction to bile flow: • Gallstones • Primary biliary cirrhosis • Pancreatic cancer • Liver cancer (both primary and secondary) Moderately raised levels - up to three times the upper limit of normal may be a feature of any acute or chronically active liver disease: • Acute (toxic or viral) hepatitis • Chronic active hepatitis • Cirrhosis • Infectious mononucleosis Increased in bone disease: • Paget's disease • Bone fracture • Bone cancer (both primary and secondary)	Liver and biliary tract disease: • Acute hepatitis (whatever cause) • Gallstones • Liver cancer • Infectious mononucleosis • NAFLD Non-liver disease: • Pancreatitis • Pancreatic cancer • Diabetes (Type 2) (Temporary) Increased synthesis induced by: • Alcohol • Some drugs (e.g. phenytoin, phenobarbitone)

Specific clinical effects of abnormal liver function tests

Bilirubin

A raised serum bilirubin is the cause of jaundice, although this clinical sign is not evident if concentration is below around 50 µmol/L, so it is possible to have a raised bilirubin (in the range 20–50 µmol/L) and not be jaundiced. As serum bilirubin concentration rises in excess of 75–100 µmol/L, jaundice becomes clearly evident to the untrained observer. Although jaundice is a clinical sign of what might be a serious, even life threatening, disease, it does not of itself have harmful consequence except when it occurs in the neonatal period.

Jaundice during the neonatal period is almost always due to a rise in unconjugated bilirubin. The major concern of neonatal jaundice is that if unconjugated bilirubin concentration rises in excess of 350 µmol/L there is increasing risk of a devastating complication of extreme increase in serum bilirubin, called kernicterus. This is the deposition of free (i.e. not bound to albumin) unconjugated bilirubin in the basal ganglia of the brain with neuronal cell death. The permanent brain damage caused by kernicterus can result in cerebral palsy, loss of hearing and sight problems; the condition is potentially fatal. Intensive monitoring of neonatal jaundice with frequent (6–12 hourly) measurement of serum bilirubin concentration and, if necessary, timely induction of treatment with whole body ultraviolet (UV) phototherapy, prevents kernicterus. The rationale for the treatment is that UV light converts bilirubin to a nontoxic product that is rapidly excreted in urine. In exceptional cases in which the rate at which bilirubin is being formed exceeds the rate at which it is being destroyed by phototherapy, an exchange transfusion is indicated. This involves removal of a significant volume of the neonate's blood and simultaneous transfusion of an equal volume of donated blood (which, of course, has normal plasma bilirubin concentration).

Detailed expert recommendations for monitoring and treatment of neonatal jaundice are contained in recently published guidelines from the National Institute of Clinical Excellence (NICE)[3]. These include the following recommendations regarding initiation of phototherapy based on serum bilirubin concentration:

- For full term babies (gestation >38 weeks) aged more than 96 hours, phototherapy need only be initiated if serum bilirubin exceeds 350 µmol/L.
- For full term babies aged less than 96 hours, the recommended triggering bilirubin concentration is progressively lower as age decreases, so that, for example, for babies aged 72 hours the serum bilirubin trigger for initiation of phototherapy is 300 µmol/L; for babies aged 48 hours it is 250 µmol/L; and for babies aged 12 hours, just 150 µmol/L.
- For preterm babies (gestation <38 weeks) aged more than 72 hours it is recommended that the serum bilirubin trigger for initiation of phototherapy be based on gestational age according to the following formula:

$$\text{triggering bilirubin concentration} = (\text{gestational age} \times 10) - 100$$

So, for example, a five day old baby born prematurely at 32 weeks should be given phototherapy if his or her serum bilirubin concentration exceeds $(32 \times 10) - 100$, i.e. 220 µmol/L.

- For preterm babies aged less than 72 hours the recommended triggering bilirubin concentration is defined in a series of tables provided in the guidance that define triggering bilirubin concentration in terms of both gestational age and actual age (in hours). The lower the gestational age and the lower the actual age the lower is the bilirubin concentration that should trigger initiation of phototherapy. For example, these tables dictate that a preterm baby with a gestational age of 35 weeks who is now 24 hours old should be given phototherapy if his bilirubin is greater than 110 µmol/L whereas an extremely preterm baby with gestational age of just 25 weeks who is now also 24 hours old should be given phototherapy if bilirubin is greater than just 70 µmol/L.

These recommendations are based on the general notion that the risk of severe hyperbilirubinemia (i.e. clinically significant jaundice requiring treatment) increases with degree of prematurity and decreases with advancing age (days since birth). Thus clinically evident jaundice at birth or during the first 24 hours of life is cause for much greater concern than the same degree of jaundice first becoming evident a few days later.

Albumin

A reduced plasma albumin concentration is one of several contributory causes of oedema, the abnormal accumulation of fluid within the interstitial fluid, sometimes causing visible swelling (e.g. ankle oedema). Of particular relevance to liver disease is the abdominal swelling that complicates the course of cirrhosis in some patients. This swelling is the result of accumulation of so called ascitic fluid in the peritoneal cavity. This form of oedema, known as ascites is thought in part to be due to low plasma albumin concentration, a feature of cirrhosis.

ALT, GGT, AP

There are no clinical signs or symptoms that can be directly attributable to raised liver enzymes.

Case history 16

Jamie Conrad, a 22 year old heroin addict, attended his GP surgery complaining of a two day history of vomiting, abdominal pain and unusual tiredness. On questioning he revealed that he had felt unwell and feverish for a day or two a fortnight before, but those symptoms had passed. Apart from that, he judged himself to have been in good health until the current symptoms developed. The GP considered hepatitis might be the cause of his symptoms and sampled blood for LFTs. The laboratory reported the following results:

Bilirubin	28 μmol/L
Albumin	42 g/L
ALT	104 U/L (laboratory normal range <20 U/L)
AP	56 U/L (laboratory normal range <150 U/L)
Gamma GT	203 U/L (laboratory normal range <50 U/L)

Questions

(1) What might have persuaded the GP to investigate Jamie for possible hepatitis?
(2) What laboratory results are abnormal?
(3) Are the results consistent with a diagnosis of hepatitis?

Discussion of case history 16

(1) Some viruses that cause hepatitis (notably Hep B virus) can be transmitted by inoculation with infected blood. For this reason injecting drug users like Jamie who may share syringes with those harbouring the virus are at particular risk of hepatitis. The symptoms that Jamie describes are consistent with a diagnosis of early hepatitis.

(2) The bilirubin level is raised though not sufficiently to cause visible jaundice. There is a significant increase (five times the upper limit of normal) in serum AST. Gamma GT is also raised (four times the upper limit of normal).

(3) The results are consistent with early hepatitis. If Jamie does indeed have hepatitis then it can be expected that increase in bilirubin and AST particularly will become more marked over the next week to ten days. Peak bilirubin concentration is usually sufficient to cause jaundice.

Case history 17

Andrew McIntyre is a 23 year old student who attends his GP because over the past three weeks while preparing for his final exams he has been feeling increasingly 'tired and stressed out'. He is worried that in his present state he will not perform well at his examinations in a few weeks time. During the consultation the doctor notes that the whites of Andrew's eyes are tinged very slightly yellow, and thinks he might be jaundiced. Andrew agrees that a few counselling sessions with the practice nurse might help to resolve his obvious anxiety, and the GP suggests that Andrew returns to see him after his college examinations. In the light of possible jaundice, despite no obvious cause revealed during physical examination and history taking, the doctor takes blood for liver function tests. The next day he receives the following results from the laboratory:

Plasma bilirubin	61 µmol/L
Plasma albumin	40 g/L
Plasma ALT	8 IU/L (reference range <25 IU/L)
Plasma gamma GT	24 IU/L (reference range <50 IU/L)
Plasma alkaline phosphatase	40 IU/L (reference range <120 IU/L)

At follow up three weeks later Andrew reports feeling much better now that the exams are over; the relaxation strategies taught by the practice nurse had, he said, proven very helpful. His jaundice had apparently resolved, but to be on the safe side the GP took blood for repeat liver function tests:

Plasma bilirubin	29 µmol/L
Plasma albumin	38 g/L
Plasma ALT	15 IU/L
Plasma gamma GT	21 IU/L
Plasma alkaline phosphatase	46 IU/L

Questions

(1) Do blood test results confirm that the GP was right in his clinical judgement that Andrew was jaundiced?
(2) The GP was concerned that because Andrew was apparently jaundiced he might have some kind of liver disease – is there any evidence from blood results that Andrew has liver disease?
(3) Can you suggest the most likely diagnosis and what blood test(s) might help to confirm the diagnosis?

Discussion of case history 17

(1) Yes, on his first appointment Andrew's serum bilirubin was slightly raised to a level that allows jaundice to be just discernible to the trained medical eye. On the second visit his bilirubin remained raised, but not sufficiently raised to cause jaundice. Jaundice is usually not apparent if serum bilirubin is less than around 50 µmol/L.

(2) No, on both occasions there was no laboratory evidence of liver disease apart from the marginally raised serum bilirubin concentration.

(3) The most likely cause of marginally raised bilirubin, when all other liver function tests are normal, is Gilbert's syndrome, a common condition that affects around 5% of the population. This is an inherited defect in the process of bilirubin conjugation

that occurs in liver cells and is vital for excretion of bilirubin in bile. In those with Gilbert's syndrome this process occurs but at a slightly slower rate than normal. The only effect of the condition is permanent slight increase in serum bilirubin, usually not sufficient to cause jaundice. Sometimes, as in this case, stress (or inter-current illness) can cause serum bilirubin to rise sufficiently high to cause very mild jaundice, but the condition is entirely harmless. Indeed there is growing evidence that the permanent slight increase in serum bilirubin provides some protection against cardiovascular disease for those with Gilbert's syndrome.

One of the features that distinguishes jaundice due to Gilbert's syndrome from jaundice due to liver disease is that in Gilbert's syndrome the increase in total serum bilirubin is due entirely to increase in unconjugated rather than conjugated bilirubin. By contrast the jaundice that occurs in those with liver disease is due to a predominant rise in conjugated bilirubin. The finding of normal serum conjugated bilirubin in this case would have provided confirmatory evidence of Gilbert's syndrome, but this is not usually considered necessary.

The condition, although entirely harmless, is important to identify because it can, if not recognised, cause unnecessary testing for liver disease. It is important that Andrew be made aware that he has Gilbert's syndrome, so that he can pass this information on to medical staff if he becomes unwell at any time in the future.

Although Gilbert's syndrome is – because of its commonness – the most likely diagnosis, the same pattern (increased unconjugated bilirubin in combination with all other liver function tests being normal) is consistent with a diagnosis of haemolytic anaemia. A normal full blood count (FBC) test result, would exclude this diagnosis.

References

1. Smith, B. and Adams, L. (2011) Non-alcoholic fatty liver disease, *Crit Rev Clin Lab Sci*, 48: 97–113.
2. Preer, G. and Philipp, B. (2011) Understanding and managing breast milk jaundice, *Arch Dis Child (Fetal Neonatal ed)*, 96: F461–F466.
3. National Institute for Clinical Excellence (2010) *Neonatal Jaundice – Clinical Guideline*, Royal College of Obstetricians and Gynaecologists.

Further reading

Alex, M. and Gallant, D. (2008) Towards understanding the connection between infant jaundice and infant feeding, *J Pediatr Nurs*, 23: 429–38.
Aragon, G. and Younossi, Z. (2010) When and how to evaluate elevated liver enzymes in apparently healthy patients, *Cleve Clin J Med*, 77: 195–204.
Coates, P. (2011) Liver function tests, *Aust Fam Phys*, 40: 113–15.
Kim, C. and Younossi, Z. (2008) Non alcoholic fatty liver disease: a manifestation of the metabolic syndrome, *Cleve Clin J Med*, 75: 721–8.
Kirk, J. (2008) Neonatal jaundice: a critical review of the role and practice of bilirubin analysis, *Ann Clin Biochem*, 45: 452–62.

Limdi, J. and Hyde, G. (2003) Evaluation of abnormal liver function tests, *Postgrad Med J*, 79: 307–12.

Moore, M. and Nelson-Piercy, C. (2011) Pregnancy and the liver, *Br J Hosp Med*, 72: M170–M173.

Olsen, M. and Jacobsen, I. (2011) Role of the nurse practitioner in the management of patients with chronic hepatitis, *C J Am Acad Nurse Pract*, 8: 410–20.

Watson, R. (2009) Hyperbilirubinemia, *Crit Care Nurs Clin North Amer*, 21: 97–120.

CHAPTER 12

PLASMA/SERUM AMYLASE

> **Key learning topics**
> * Anatomy and physiology of the pancreas
> * Function of pancreatic and salivary amylase
> * Serum amylase in diagnosis of acute pancreatitis
> * Non-pancreatic causes of raised serum amylase

The measurement of amylase in blood plasma or serum is used almost exclusively in the investigation of patients with acute abdominal pain, a very common symptom especially among patients admitted urgently to hospital. Acute abdominal pain is almost invariably a major presenting symptom of common surgical emergencies like acute appendicitis, intestinal obstruction, perforated peptic ulcer and ruptured aortic aneurysm, so that rapid diagnosis, sometimes with the help of blood and urine tests, is important. A small proportion (around 3%) of patients whose principal symptom is acute abdominal pain will be suffering acute pancreatitis, a potentially life-threatening inflammatory disease of the pancreas. The serum amylase test is particularly useful in identifying these patients; a marked increase in serum amylase in a patient with acute abdominal pain is strongly suggestive of acute pancreatitis.

Normal physiology

The pancreas

The pancreas is a soft, pale yellow/tan coloured organ, around 12–15 cm in length and weighing approximately 100 g. Its shape somewhat resembles a tadpole, with a just recognisable 'head', 'body' and 'tail'. The organ lies transversely across the upper abdomen, with the 'head' positioned in the inner curve of the C shape formed by the first loop of the duodenum, the 'body' lying behind the stomach and

Understanding Laboratory Investigations: A Guide for Nurses, Midwives and Healthcare Professionals, Third Edition. Chris Higgins.
© 2013 John Wiley & Sons, Ltd. Published 2013 by John Wiley & Sons, Ltd.

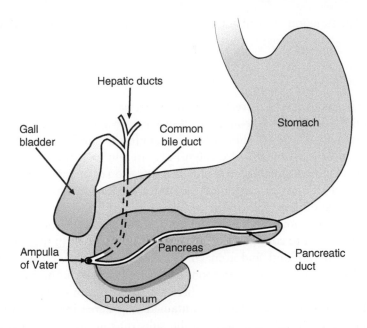

Figure 12.1 Gross anatomy of the pancreas and spatial relationship to nearby organs.

the 'tail' extending from behind the stomach towards the spleen (Figure 12.1). The micro-anatomy of the pancreas reveals two sorts of functionally distinct tissue reflecting the dual (exocrine and endocrine) role of the pancreas. Around 90% of the pancreas comprises so called acinar (exocrine) tissue which is responsible for the production of pancreatic juice, a thin watery fluid required for intestinal digestion of dietary foodstuffs.

Pancreatic acinar cells are arranged like a bunch of grapes around a microscopical central tube or duct; acinar tissue comprises millions of these functional units. The ducts from each unit join, forming progressively larger ducts, which eventually drain all the pancreatic juice from the acinar cells into one large central duct called the duct of Wirsung, running the length of the pancreas. This central duct leaves the head of the pancreas and joins with the bile duct conveying bile from the gall bladder before joining with an opening in the duodenum called the hepato-pancreatic ampulla. Here, pancreatic juice (and bile) drains into the duodenum. Some people (around 20%) have a second pancreatic duct which drains pancreatic juice into the duodenum around 1 cm above the hepato-pancreatic ampulla.

Dispersed throughout the acinar tissue of the pancreas are highly vascularised islands of quite distinct (endocrine) cells that have no ductal connection with the duodenum. These are the islets of Langerhans, which are responsible for production of pancreatic hormones. There are three main cell types within the islets: alpha (α), beta (β) and delta (δ), each producing a specific hormone. β-cells, by far the most numerous, produce insulin; α-cells produce glucagon; and δ-cells produce somatostatin. These pancreatic hormones are released directly into the blood flowing through the islets and have their effect on cellular metabolism throughout the body. The function of insulin and glucagon in regulating blood glucose concentration is discussed in Chapter 3.

Pancreatic juice

The exocrine product of pancreatic acinar tissue, pancreatic juice, is a thin watery alkaline fluid (pH around 8) containing a mixture of many digestive enzymes, and electrolytes, most notably sodium, potassium, chloride and bicarbonate ions. With the exception of bicarbonate, electrolytes are present at similar concentration to that found in blood plasma; bicarbonate concentration of pancreatic juice is around four times higher. The relatively high bicarbonate concentration accounts for the alkaline reaction of pancreatic juice.

Pancreatic juice drains into the duodenum at the rate of 1500–3000 ml per day. Its principle function is to continue the digestion of food process in the small intestine, already begun in the mouth and stomach. The alkaline pH of pancreatic juice ensures that acid chyme (partially digested food) emptying from the stomach into the duodenum is rendered sufficiently alkaline (pH 7–7.5) for optimum pancreatic enzyme activity. The many digestive enzymes contained in pancreatic juice can be broadly divided into three groups according to the substrates in food on which they act: amylase for the digestion of carbohydrates, lipases for the digestion of fats and proteases for the digestion of proteins. Amylase and lipases are secreted in their active form, whereas proteases are secreted as proenzymes, capable of digesting proteins only after they have been activated within the duodenum. For example, trypsin, a protease present in intestine is derived from the inactive pancreatic pro-enzyme, trypsinogen. Pancreatic production and secretion of inactive pro-enzymes rather than their highly reactive product protects the pancreas from enzymic destruction.

The volume and content of pancreatic juice is controlled principally by hormonal pathways. Cholecystokinin (CCK), a gastrointestinal hormone released in response to gastric emptying of food into the duodenum, stimulates acinar cell production of digestive proenzymes. Secretin another gastrointestinal hormone promotes acinar cell production of bicarbonate. Neural pathways also affect pancreatic juice production. The vagal nerve, which is stimulated by the site, smell and thought of food, as well as the presence of food in the mouth, stimulates production of pancreatic juice. Release of pancreatic juice to the duodenum is controlled by a sphincter (the sphincter of Oddi) sited at the hepato-pancreatic ampulla. The sphincter opens when food is present in the duodenum. By a synergy of these and other subtle hormonal and neural mechanisms, the body is able to adjust the volume, content and release of pancreatic juice to suit its digestive requirement at the time.

Once pancreatic juice has performed its digestive function, around 99% of its water and electrolyte content is reabsorbed to the blood from the large intestine.

Amylase

Amylase is just one of several digestive enzymes delivered to the intestine in pancreatic juice. It is also secreted in saliva by three pairs of salivary glands in the mouth.

Salivary and pancreatic amylase function only within the gastrointestinal tract where together, they are responsible for the breakdown of starch, the principal form of dietary carbohydrate. Starch is essentially many glucose molecules joined together. The product of amylase action on starch is a mixture of three sorts of molecule: the disaccharide maltose (2 molecules of glucose joined together); dextrin, a short chain of around eight glucose molecules; and some single molecules of glucose. Any glucose formed by the action of amylase on starch is absorbed to blood by active transport across the cells of the intestinal wall, but maltose and dextrin require further enzymic degradation by the intestinal enzymes, maltase and iso-maltase to single glucose molecules, before absorption can occur.

Like all enzymes, amylase will only work to maximum effect within a narrow pH range; for amylase the optimum pH is 7.1. Digestion of starch begins in the mouth with the action of salivary amylase, during the process of chewing. As soon as food reaches the acidic medium of the stomach (pH 2–3), salivary amylase action ceases In practice, unless food is masticated in the mouth for a prolonged period, salivary amylase contributes little to overall starch digestion and most starch is broken down in the duodenum and jejenum by pancreatic amylase.

Normally a small amount of amylase circulates in blood plasma. Most of this is of pancreatic origin; some is derived from salivary glands. Amylase has no function in blood plasma and is present there only as a result of normal pancreatic and salivary cell turnover. By comparison with most other enzymes, amylase is a small molecule. Indeed it is small enough to pass through the glomeruli of the kidneys, so that it is one of very few plasma enzymes normally found in urine.

Laboratory measurement of serum amylase

Patient preparation

No particular patient preparation is necessary.

Sample requirements

Between 2 and 5 ml of venous blood is required.

The test is performed on either blood serum or blood plasma. If local policy is to use serum then blood must be collected into plain tube containing no anticoagulant. If local policy is to use plasma then blood must be collected into a tube containing an anticoagulant (usually heparin).

Timing of blood sampling and transport

Blood may be collected without reference to time. In many instances the result is required urgently so must be transported to the laboratory without delay. If the request is non-urgent the sample may be stored at room temperature before routine transport to the laboratory.

Interpretation of results

Approximate reference range serum (plasma) amylase: 50– 200 U/L
  [*Note: it is particularly important to use local reference range when interpreting enzyme results.*]

Terms used

Hypoamylasaemia　　serum amylase below normal.
Hyperamylasaemia　　serum amylase above normal.

An abnormally low serum amylase has no known clinical significance apart from limited research that suggests it might be associated with higher than normal risk of cardiovascular disease for diabetic patients. Discussion will be confined to the interpretation of a raised serum amylase.

Causes of raised serum (plasma) amylase

Acute pancreatitis

Acute pancreatitis is a relatively common condition with an annual incidence of 22 per 100 000 population in the UK. Incidence has been increasing gradually over the past two decades, at a rate of 3% per year, with greatest increase among younger adults (11% increase per year for women aged less than 35 years and 5.6% annual increase for men aged 35–45 years).

There are two main causes: gall stones and alcohol abuse. Together these account for around 80% of cases. Excess alcohol consumption among young adults is thought to be responsible for increasing incidence in this age group.

A long list of much less common causes of acute pancreatitis include: trauma to the pancreas; over activity of the parathyroid gland (hyperparathyroidism); viral infections (e.g. mumps virus , Epstein-Barr virus, cytomegalovirus); parasitic worm infection; and marked increase in plasma triglycerides concentration. Very rarely acute pancreatitis occurs as a post-operative complication following upper abdominal surgery. Equally rare are those cases reported to be caused by prescribed drugs (e.g. thiazide diuretics, ACE inhibitors and steroids). Acute pancreatitis is a well documented but rare adverse effect of the invasive diagnostic procedure, endoscopic retrograde cholangiopancreatography (ERCP), occurring in around 4% of patients submitted for ERCP.

Acute pancreatitis is an acute inflammatory disease that is thought to result from the premature activation of proteolytic (protein splitting) enzymes. Activation of these enzymes within pancreas leads to a process of 'autodigestion', in essence self-destruction of the pancreas. Activation of trypsinogen to trypsin within acinar cells is widely proposed as the initiating event, though it remains unclear precisely how alcohol abuse or gall stone disease leads to this initiating event or promotes the autodigestion and inflammation that flows from it. Obstruction to the flow of pancreatic juice by gall stones transiently lodged in the hepato-pancreatic ampulla is significant among those with gallstone related acute pancreatitis.

The cardinal symptom is sudden onset of severe upper abdominal pain, which often radiates to the back. Vomiting and pyrexia is common. The course of acute pancreatitis is variable. In the majority (75–80%) of patients, the inflammation is self-limiting, confined to the pancreas and resolves over a period of a few days to a week with no serious long-term consequences. However, this is not the case for the 20–25% of patients who suffer severe acute pancreatitis. This is a life threatening condition in which the local inflammation leads to systemic inflammatory response syndrome (SIRS) with high risk of sepsis and multiple organ failure. Complications of severe disease include overwhelming infection consequent on massive tissue necrosis (which may not be confined to pancreas), acute respiratory distress syndrome, jaundice, anaemia, hyperglycaemia, hypocalaemia, disseminated intravascular coagulation and haemorrhage. Early (within 12–24 hours) admission to intensive care is necessary and usually lifesaving but, despite intensive care, around 20–30% of patients with severe acute pancreatitis die, usually due to overwhelming infection and associated multiple organ failure.

Damage to acinar cells, the central pathological feature of acute pancreatitis, results in a sudden and massive increase in release of pancreatic enzymes into the blood stream; among these is amylase. This increase in serum amylase has no clinical consequences of itself, that is no signs or symptoms of acute pancreatitis can be attributed to an increase in serum amylase. It does however provide a marker in the blood, of damage to the pancreas. Serum amylase begins to rise 2–12 hours after the onset of symptoms and remains elevated for three to five days. A serum amylase level between three and five times the upper limit of normal (i.e. 800–1000 U/L) in a patient with acute abdominal pain is widely considered to be strongly suggestive of acute pancreatitis. The probability that acute pain is due to pancreatitis increases as amylase level rises above 1000 U/L. A minority of patients with acute pancreatitis do not show such a marked increase so that a serum amylase less than 800 U/L cannot be used to exclude the diagnosis and, rarely, serum amylase may be within normal limits in a patient with acute pancreatitis. It might be assumed that the higher the serum amylase, the more severe the pancreatitis; that is not the case. In fact no prognostic information can be derived from measurement of serum amylase at the time of diagnosis. However failure of amylase to return to normal following an acute attack suggests the presence of a pancreatic pseudocyst (a late complication of acute pancreatitis).

Chronic pancreatitis

Natural repair of the damage caused by inflammation of acute pancreatitis leaves the pancreas of someone who has recovered from acute pancreatitis, functioning normally. By contrast chronic pancreatitis is a chronic inflammation in which damage to the pancreas is slow but irreversibly progressive. The most common cause is long-term alcohol abuse. It may be a feature of haemochromatosis, a disease of iron overload in which excess iron is deposited in the pancreas and other organs. Continuous or at least recurrent abdominal pain is the cardinal symptom of chronic pancreatitis. Long term the condition results in malabsorption of food and consequent weight loss, due to failure of pancreatic enzyme production, and diabetes as a result of islet cell damage. Serum amylase may be slightly raised in the early stages but as acinar cell production of digestive enzymes (including amylase) becomes increasingly compromised, serum amylase falls to normal or even to levels below normal. Since amylase may be raised, normal or reduced, the test serves no useful purpose in the diagnosis of chronic pancreatitis.

Cancer of the pancreas

Apart from acute and chronic pancreatitis, cancer of the pancreas is the only other significant disease of the pancreas. Serum amylase is either marginally raised or normal; the test is not useful for the diagnosis of cancer of the pancreas.

Non pancreatic disease

Serum amylase may be mildly to moderately raised (i.e. rarely greater than 800 U/L) in some non-pancreatic disorders, for example, perforation of peptic ulcer, intestinal obstruction and gall bladder disease (acute cholecystitis). All these conditions are usually associated with acute abdominal pain so that a patient with a mildly raised serum amylase in association with acute abdominal pain is not necessarily suffering acute pancreatitis. Abdominal trauma, not necessarily involving the pancreas, may result in an increased amylase; a significant minority of patients who receive abdominal surgery have a transient rise during the post-operative period.

Amylase is cleared from the blood by the kidneys, so that patients in acute or chronic renal failure typically have slight to moderate increases in serum amylase. A moderate to marked increase is often a feature of diabetic ketoacidosis, a condition discussed in Chapter 3. Disease of, or damage to, the parotid glands where salivary amylase is produced may result in an increase in serum amylase. Examples include infection with the mumps virus, maxillofacial surgery and parotid gland irradiation.

Finally, raised serum amylase is a feature of a rare and entirely benign condition called macroamylasaemia, in which amylase circulates in serum in the form of macromolecular aggregates of amylase or bound to serum proteins. Because they are so large these macromelcules cannot pass across the glomerular membrane of the kidneys and are not excreted in urine; instead they accumulate in serum.

Table 12.1 provides a summary of the principle causes of raised serum amylase.

Table 12.1   Principal causes of raised serum/plasma amylase.

- Acute pancreatitis
- Chronic pancreatitis
- Renal failure
- Diabetic ketoacidosis
- Intestinal obstruction
- Perforated peptic ulcer
- Acute cholecystitis
- Abdominal trauma
- Mumps
- Macroamylasaemia

Case history 18

Mrs Campbell, a 40 year old pharmacist, arrived by ambulance at the emergency department of her local hospital in considerable pain and distress, looking pale and shocked. The pain, which had only become severe four hours earlier, was localised in the mid-epigastric region; she described it as 'shooting through her back'. She was vomiting. Her temperature was 100°C; blood pressure 90/60 mmHg. and respiratory rate 30/min. During initial examination Mrs Campbell told the admitting doctor that she had been diagnosed as having gallstones and was currently on a weight reduction diet in preparation for cholecystectomy (surgical removal of gall bladder). The doctor suspected Mrs Campbell might be suffering acute pancreatitis. Blood was sampled for U&E, glucose, amylase and full blood count. The laboratory results included:

Serum amylase 1700 U/L
Blood glucose 13.6 mmol/L

Questions

(1) What suggested to the admitting doctor that Mrs Campbell might be suffering acute pancreatitis?
(2) Are the serum amylase and blood glucose normal?
(3) Do the laboratory results support the initial diagnosis?
(4) Why might a patient suffering acute pancreatitis have raised blood glucose?

Discussion of case history 18

(1) Sudden onset of severe abdominal pain is the most common finding in patients with acute pancreatitis; in around a half of cases, this pain is referred to the back. Vomiting is also a common symptom. Mrs Campbell was hypotensive suggesting hypovolaemic shock. Loss of pancreatic secretion into the peritoneal space and haemorrhage due to vessel erosion by pancreatic enzymes, can lead to hypovolaemic shock in acute pancreatitis. Finally acute pancreatitis is a complication of gall bladder disease.

(2) No. Both serum amylase and blood glucose are markedly raised; amylase is more than seven times the upper limit of normal.

(3) Yes, an increase in amylase of this degree is almost diagnostic of acute pancreatitis. Amylase may be raised in a number of non-pancreatic conditions which result in abdominal pain, but very rarely to this degree. Transient hyperglycaemia is sometimes a feature of acute pancreatitis, requiring insulin therapy and regular blood glucose monitoring.

(4) Acute pancreatitis may involve damage to the endocrine (islet) cells of the pancreas, where insulin is produced. Insulin is the principal hormone of blood glucose regulation; a deficiency of the hormone results in raised blood glucose concentration. Islet cells damage may be minimal, in which case normal insulin production and secretion continues and hyperglycaemia does not occur. The stress of the acute illness might also have provoked a rise in epinephrine and cortisol (the so called stress hormones). These hormones oppose the action of insulin and thereby predispose to hyperglycaemia (raised blood glucose).

References

1. Roberts, S., Williams, J. et al. (2008) Incidence and case fatality for acute pancreatitis in England: geographical variation, social deprivation, alcohol consumption and aetiology – a record linkage study, *Aliment Pharmacol Ther*; 28: 931–41.
2. Frossard, J.-L., Steer, M. et al. (2008) Acute pancreatitis, *Lancet*, 371: 143–52.

Further reading

Despins, L., Kivlahan, C. and Cox, K. (2005) Acute pancreatitis: diagnosis and treatment of a potentially fatal condition, *Am J Nursing*, 105: 54–7.

Harper, S. and Cheslyn-Curtis, S. (2011) Acute pancreatitis, *Ann Clin Biochem*, 48: 23–37.

Holcomb, S. (2007) Stopping the destruction of acute pancreatitis, *Nursing 2007*, 37: 42–7.

CHAPTER 13

DRUG OVERDOSE: PARACETAMOL AND SALICYLATE

Key learning topics

- Therapeutic value and safety of paracetamol and aspirin
- Mechanisms of toxicity in paracetamol and aspirin overdose
- Signs and symptoms of paracetamol and aspirin overdose
- Plasma paracetamol/salicylate used to assess overdose severity
- Plasma paracetamol/salicylate used to monitor overdose treatment
- Principles of treatment in paracetamol and aspirin overdose

Clinical laboratory staff members are often requested to analyse blood or urine samples for the presence of specific drugs. Such analyses are valuable in two usually separate clinical contexts: deliberate or accidental drug overdose; and therapeutic drug monitoring. Chapter 14 is concerned principally with the latter, whilst this chapter is concerned with how laboratory measurement of serum or plasma concentration of salicylate and paracetamol contributes to the care of patients who have, or are suspected of having, taken a deliberate or accidental acute overdose of aspirin (acetylsalicylic acid) or paracetamol (called acetaminophen in the US). Despite government initiatives to restrict over the counter sales[1], paracetamol remains the most common medicinal drug to be taken in overdose, accounting for a half of all drug overdose related attendances at UK hospital emergency departments[2]. If not promptly treated paracetamol overdose can cause potentially fatal liver damage; it is the most common cause of acute liver failure and necessity for liver transplantation. It has been estimated that paracetamol overdose is the sole or contributory cause of death for around 500 people every year in England and Wales[3] and the sole cause of death for 100–150 people. Overdose with aspirin is less common but still accounts for 5–7% of drug overdose related hospital admissions and is solely responsible for around 30–40 deaths in the UK each year[4].

Understanding Laboratory Investigations: A Guide for Nurses, Midwives and Healthcare Professionals, Third Edition. Chris Higgins.
© 2013 John Wiley & Sons, Ltd. Published 2013 by John Wiley & Sons, Ltd.

Clinical use of aspirin and paracetamol; safety of therapeutic dose

Both aspirin and paracetamol are analgesics and antipyretics, that is they reduce pain and body temperature. They are frequently self-prescribed for the relief of temporary symptoms associated with minor viral infections (e.g. influenza, colds etc.) and for the relief of headaches and minor muscular aches and pains. Aspirin has two further major pharmacological properties: at high dose (>3 g/day) it has anti-inflammatory effect and at lower dose (75–300 mg/day) an anti-thrombotic (anti-blood clotting) effect. These two properties have determined that long-term prescription of aspirin is useful in the treatment of chronic inflammatory conditions like arthritis, and for the prevention of myocardial infarction and strokes among high-risk patients. The efficacy of regular aspirin among the general adult population for primary prevention of myocardial infarction and strokes has been proposed but remains controversial. There is accumulating evidence that long-term aspirin use may protect against many common cancers[5]; that evidence is now particularly strong and, to all intents and purposes, proven with respect to colorectal (bowel) cancer[6,7].

The maximum recommended dose of paracetamol for adults and children over the age of 12 years is two 500 mg tablets, with an interval of at least four hours between doses. No more than eight tablets should be taken in 24 hours (i.e. a maximum dose of 4 g/day). Children aged 6–12 years should be given no more than half the adult maximum single and total 24 hour dose, and children aged 1–5 years no more than a quarter of the adult maximum dose. So long as these dosing recommendations are not exceeded, paracetamol has no adverse effect and is a remarkably safe drug, even if used for a prolonged period.

Long-term aspirin use, even at prescribed therapeutic doses, is less safe. In common with other non-steroidal anti-inflammatory drugs (NSAIDs), long-term aspirin use is associated with irritation of the stomach wall lining (gastric mucosa) and the risk of gastrointestinal bleeding and stomach ulcers. Patients with a history of peptic ulcer or an increased tendency to bleed are not prescribed aspirin. Some patients on long-term, high dose aspirin therapy may experience some of the symptoms of acute overdose (see later), even if they are taking what for others is a safe therapeutic dose. There is evidence that aspirin use among children with a viral infection precipitates a serious life-threatening condition known as Reyes syndrome. For this reason aspirin is not recommended for use in children. The recommended dose for analgesic and antipyretic effect is one to two 325 mg tablets every four hours; no more than 12 tablets in 24 hours should be taken. For anti-inflammatory effect, that dose has to be increased to around two 500 mg tablets, usually every six hours. Just 75–150 mg/day is sufficient for anti-thrombotic effect.

Paracetamol

Absorption, metabolism and acute toxicity

Paracetamol is quickly absorbed from the gastrointestinal tract to blood over a period of 30 minutes to 2 hours for a therapeutic dose. A small amount (up to 5%)

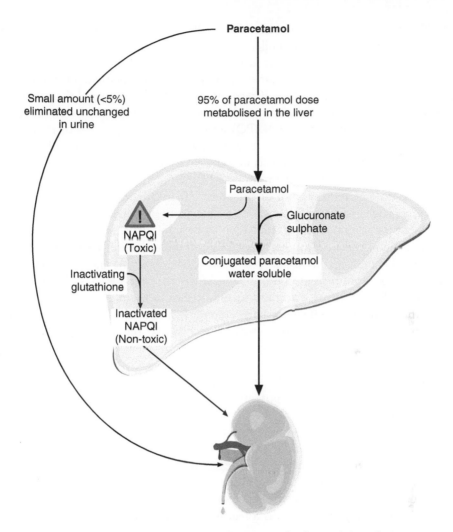

Figure 13.1 Metabolism of paracetamol NAPQI=**N-a**cetyl-**p**-benzo**q**uinonei̇mine.

is eliminated unchanged in urine, but the remainder is metabolised in the liver (Figure 13.1). Like most other drugs, paracetamol must be made more water soluble for appreciable elimination in urine. This is achieved in the liver, by synthetic conjugation (joining) of paracetamol with sulphate, glucuronate, glycine and phosphate. The resulting water-soluble conjugates of paracetamol are non-toxic. Around 90% of an ingested paracetamol dose is eliminated safely via urine in this way. The rest of the paracetamol (5–10% of an ingested dose) is oxidised in the liver, to a highly reactive and toxic free radical called N-acetyl-p-benzoquinone imine (NAPQI). It is NAPQI that is responsible for the toxic effects of paracetamol. At normal paracetamol dose the liver is able to inactivate this potentially damaging NAPQI by reaction with a substance called glutathione, which is synthesised in the liver. The product of the reaction between NAPQI and glutathione is non-toxic and is eliminated safely in urine and bile.

If there were no limit to the rate at which the liver could synthesise glutathione, then paracetamol would not be harmful, no matter how much had been taken, but unfortunately this is not the case. If recommended dose is exceeded the production of NAPQI increases, but the ability of the liver to synthesise the inactivating glutathione cannot keep pace, and NAPQI accumulates in liver cells, disrupting cellular mechanisms and eventually causing liver cell death (necrosis)[8]. Without prompt treatment, liver cell necrosis becomes extensive, leading to acute liver failure. At this stage liver transplantation may be the only treatment option.

A single dose of paracetamol of between 150–200 mg/kg is sufficient to cause liver cell damage in adults. This means that for an adult weighing an average 70 kg, just 10 g of paracetamol (i.e. 20 tablets) may be significant. Twelve grams (24 tablets) can be fatal and without treatment 25 g (50 tablets) is inevitably fatal. Certain drugs (notably the anticonvulsants phenytoin, carbamazepine and phenobarbitone) and alcohol result in increased production of the enzymes responsible for NAPQI production. Thus patients who have taken alcohol or these drugs are particularly susceptible to the toxic effects of paracetamol. Malnourished individuals are also more than normally susceptible because they have reduced liver glutathione reserves.

Signs and symptoms of acute overdose
The early symptoms of even potentially fatal paracetamol overdose are non-specific and unremarkable. For the first 24 hours, nausea and vomiting are the only symptoms and these may be absent; loss of consciousness is not an early feature. Signs and symptoms of extensive liver cell damage including jaundice, abdominal tenderness, continuing nausea and vomiting begin to develop in the 24–36 hours after overdose. Deterioration in liver function over the next few days leads to acute liver failure in the most severe cases. Drowsiness, and eventually coma (hepatic encephalopathy), is a feature of paracetamol overdose only at this late stage.

Principles of overdose treatment
So long as treatment is initiated early enough (i.e. within 12 hours of overdose), a complete recovery can be expected, even after a potentially fatal dose of paracetamol. Because of the speed at which paracetamol is absorbed from the intestine, efforts aimed at reducing absorption of paracetamol, including gastric administration of activated charcoal are only likely to be effective if begun within an hour or two of the overdose. The main treatment is early IV administration of the paracetamol antidote: N-acetylcysteine (NAC). In the body NAC is converted to glutathione, the substance required for inactivation of NAQI, the toxic metabolite of paracetamol. NAC is successful in preventing liver damage if administered within 12 hours of the overdose. Although less effective after 12 hours, some benefit can be gained by administration up to 24 hours, or even 72 hours in some cases, after overdose.

Aspirin

Absorption, metabolism and acute toxicity

Absorption of aspirin from the gastrointestinal tract is dependent on the amount and formulation of the drug. Therapeutic doses of regular (non-enteric coated) aspirin are absorbed rapidly within two hours. Larger quantities (overdose) of regular aspirin however inhibit gastric emptying with a resulting delay of up to six hours in intestinal absorption. Enteric coated formulations of aspirin are designed to be impervious to the acid content in the stomach and only begin to dissolve after arrival in the alkaline medium of the small intestine; such formulations may take up to 12 hours to be completely absorbed.

After absorption, aspirin is rapidly hydrolysed to salicylic acid (salicylate). This is the substance responsible for the acute toxicity as well as many of the therapeutic effects of aspirin. Before salicylate can be eliminated in urine it must first be conjugated with glycine to form salicyluric acid, or glucuronate to form phenolic glucuronides, but the enzymes for these detoxifying reactions become rapidly saturated at even therapeutic blood levels. As a consequence, salicylate accumulates in tissues in a dose dependent manner. Increased serum salicylate concentration is associated with increased stimulation of respiratory centre in the brain and thereby hyperventilation, which results in increased carbon dioxide elimination and respiratory alkalosis (Chapter 7). Salicylate at toxic levels has an effect on cellular metabolism which results in hyperpyrexia, sweating and abnormally high production of metabolic acids. Along with salicylate, itself an acid, these acids accumulate in blood causing metabolic acidosis. Salicylate causes increased permeability of the vasculature in the lungs, predisposing to the development of pulmonary oedema in salicylate overdose, particularly among smokers and the elderly. Finally salicylate can adversely affect normal control of blood glucose concentration; overdose of aspirin may result in hypoglycaemia (low blood glucose) or reduced levels of glucose in the brain, (neuroglycopaenia) despite normal blood glucose levels. Mild toxicity arises after a single dose of around 150 mg/kg body weight, whereas severe toxicity is associated with a single dose of greater than 500 mg/kg. For an adult of average weight (70 kg) then, just 20 tablets of 500 mg or 30 tablets of 325 mg are sufficient for mild toxicity.

Signs and symptoms of acute toxicity

Salicylate poisoning is more likely to be associated with early symptoms than paracetamol poisoning. Mild to moderate poisoning commonly causes nausea, vomiting and tinnitus, with loss of hearing. Patients are usually hyperventilating, hyperpyrexial and sweating. Dehydration secondary to vomiting, sweating and hyperventilation is usually a feature, particularly in severe poisoning. Blood gas analysis reveals disturbance of acid-base homeostasis (respiratory alkalosis or metabolic acidosis or combined disturbance). Acidaemia (low blood pH) is a poor prognostic sign because it enhances salicylate entry into tissue cells; entry of salicylate into brain cells causes additional neurological symptoms including confusion, delerium and extreme agitation. Loss of consciousness may occur, but is rare.

Principles of overdose treatment

There is no antidote for the treatment of aspirin overdose, as there is for paraceta-mol overdose. Treatment instead is based on three main objectives:

- Preventing further absorption of aspirin from the gastrointestinal tract.
- Increasing urinary elimination of salicylate.
- Correcting dehydration and deranged blood chemistry (acid-base and electrolyte disturbances, and hypoglycaemia if present).

The delay in intestinal absorption of high dose aspirin, especially enteric coated formulation means that oral administration of activated charcoal is more likely to be effective in reducing absorption than is the case in paracetamol overdose, although, of course, the sooner it is started, the more effective it will be. Urinary elimination of salicylate is increased if urine is made alkaline (pH >7.5) and urine output increased. This is achieved by administration of large volumes of sodium bicarbonate. Such treatment has the additional advantage of making blood more alkaline and thereby inhibiting the entry of salicylate into cells. Removal of salicy-late from blood by haemodialysis or peritoneal dialysis may be considered in the most severe cases. Dextrose may be added to any IV fluid used to correct fluid and electrolyte disturbance since there is evidence that, even if blood glucose is normal, the brain is depleted of glucose in moderate to severe salicylate poisoning.

Laboratory measurement of salicylate and paracetamol

Patient preparation

No particular patient preparation is necessary.

Timing of sample

The time of blood sampling and the time of the overdose (if known) must be recorded on the accompanying request card. Because of varying rates of paraceta-mol absorption, it is impossible to accurately interpret a paracetamol result of a sample taken less than four hours after an overdose. Blood sampling should there-fore be delayed until four hours have elapsed since paracetamol was taken. In all cases of salicylate poisoning it is useful to know the peak concentration. This can only be found by repeat sampling (every three hours) until a reduction in concen-tration is detected.

Sample requirements

Around 5 ml of venous blood is required for paracetamol and salicylate estimation. Analysis can be performed on either serum or plasma. If local policy is to use serum, blood must be collected into a plain (without additives) tube. If local policy is to use plasma, blood must be collected into a tube containing the anticoagulant, lithium heparin.

Transport of samples

The results of paracetamol and salicylate estimation are required for immediate patient management and therefore samples must be considered urgent and transported to the laboratory without delay.

Interpretation of paracetamol result

There seems to be no universal agreement about units of measurement for paracetamol; some laboratories report paracetamol in traditional units (mg/L or μg/ml); note that 1 mg/L = 1 μg/ml. Other laboratories use the SI unit of measurement (mmol/ml or mmol/L); note 1 mmol/ml = 1000 mmol/L.

To convert paracetamol concentration expressed in mg/L to paracetamol concentration expressed in mmol/L, divide by 151.

A potentially dangerous interpretation is possible if units are confused. Interpretation of paracetamol results depends crucially on knowing the approximate time of overdose. Figure 13.2 is a widely used nomogram, which allows assessment of the severity of overdose, and therefore risk of liver injury, based on the paracetamol concentration in relation to the time in hours since the overdose. For example, it can be seen from the graph in Figure 13.2 that a paracetamol concentration of 80 mg/L four hours after an overdose indicates that liver damage is extremely unlikely. However the same paracetamol result in a blood sample taken 12 hours after an overdose indicates that without antidote (N-acetylcysteine) treatment, severe, possibly fatal liver damage can be expected.

The graph highlights two important features of paracetamol toxicity. First it is not possible to accurately determine the severity of a paracetamol overdose, based on a serum paracetamol derived from blood sampled less than four hours after an overdose; a repeat sample would be advisable in these circumstances. Secondly any measurable amounts of paracetamol in serum 24 hours or later after an overdose indicate a poor prognosis especially as antidote treatment at this late stage is unlikely to be very effective in halting liver cell damage.

Interpretation of salicylate result

Again there is no consensus between laboratories concerning units of measurement. Most laboratories use either mg/L or mg/dl. Note: a salicylate concentration of 10 mg/dl = 100 mg/L.

Patients on long-term high dose aspirin therapy for chronic inflammatory conditions such as rheumatoid arthritis typically have a serum salicylate concentration of 25–35 mg/dl (i.e. 250–350 mg/L). These levels are rarely associated with any symptoms

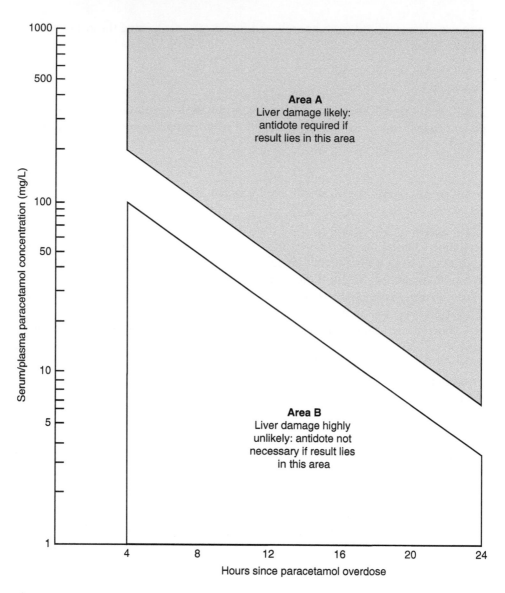

Figure 13.2 Interpretation of paracetamol result following overdose.
Notes: 1. If result lies between areas A and B, antidote treatment is normally only considered necessary if patient has also taken alcohol or certain other drugs that increase the toxicity of paracetamol. 2. It is not possible to interpret a result if blood is sampled less than four hours after overdose.

of acute toxicity. Mild to moderate toxicity occurs with peak salicylate concentration in the range 35–80 mg/dl (300–800 mg/L) whilst peak levels greater than 80 mg/dl (800 mg/ml) are associated with severe toxicity; around 5% of patients admitted to hospital with this level of toxicity do not survive. Serum salicylate levels provide an approximate and useful guide to the severity of a particular overdose but are not as reliable in this regard as serum paracetamol is in cases of paracetamol overdose. The clinical condition of the patient and the blood gas and electrolyte results are as important as plasma salicylate results for assessment of prognosis and clinical care planning. However some general points can be made. Nearly all symptomatic patients, even those with mild toxicity will be given activated charcoal. The likelihood that a patient will require alkalinisation of urine increases as the serum salicylate increases beyond 50 mg/dl. Finally haemodialyis is usually reserved for those patients whose serum salicylate is in excess of 80 mg/dl, although it may be considered the treatment of choice for all patients who have significant loss of renal function.

A rise in serum salicylate during treatment may indicate continuing salicylate absorption and/or failure to adequately increase urine elimination. A decline in serum salicylate concentration is used to confirm that treatment aimed at increased urinary elimination of salicylate has been effective. Sometimes however a reduction in serum concentration merely reflects haemodilution, if high volume fluids have been infused.

Case history 19

Andrew Roberts, a 23 year old university student, became depressed having failed his final examinations. Following an alcoholic binge he returned to his flat, took 18 paracetamol tablets and fell asleep. On waking, early the next morning, some six hours after taking the tablets, he was feeling sick and extremely regretful about taking the tablets. Worried about the possible effects, he rang the local hospital accident and emergency department for advice.

Question

What would your advice be?

Discussion of case history 19

Andrew had taken 9 g of paracetamol, well in excess of the maximum recommended single dose, which is 1 g. Assuming an average body weight of 70 kg, 9 g represents a dose of 9000/70 mg/kg (i.e. 129 mg/kg). Liver damage is unlikely if a single dose of <150 mg/kg has been taken. However, the fact that Andrew also took alcohol must be taken into account, because alcohol increases production of the enzymes necessary for oxidation of paracetamol to the toxic metabolite NAPQI. The toxicity of paracetamol is increased if alcohol has been taken. It would be wise for Andrew to attend casualty urgently so that his serum paracetamol can be checked.

Case history 19 (continued)

Andrew accepted the advice given by A&E staff. Within the hour he arrived at the hospital and was seen immediately by the casualty officer who took blood for serum paracetamol estimation, some eight hours after taking the tablets. The laboratory telephoned back the result:

Serum paracetamol – 42 mg/L.

Questions

(1) Would it have been advisable for Andrew to have received activated charcoal on arrival?
(2) What is the significance of the paracetamol result?

Discussion of case history 19 (continued)

(1) Paracetamol is absorbed from the gastrointestinal tract within a few hours of ingestion. It is unlikely that there would have been any paracetamol remaining in Andrew's stomach by the time he arrived in A&E. Charcoal administration would have been ineffective at this late stage.

(2) The significance of the paracetamol result is revealed by reference to the nomogram (Figure 13.2) that relates serum paracetamol, time since overdose and risk of significant liver disease. It is evident from the nomogram that Andrew was not at risk of liver damage and did not require antidote therapy. His physical health was considered not at risk.

References

1. Hawton, K., Simkin, S. et al. (2004) UK legislation on analgesic packs before and after study of long term effects, *BMJ*, 329: 1076–80.
2. Greene, S., Dargan, P. and Jones, A. (2005) Acute poisoning: understanding 90% of cases in a nutshell, *Postgrad Med J*, 81: 204–16.
3. Morgan, O., Griffiths, C. and Majeed, A. (2005) Impact of paracetamol pack size restrictions on poisoning from paracetamol in England and Wales, *J Public Health*, 27: 19–24.
4. Wood, D., Dargan, P. and Jones, A. (2005) Measuring plasma salicylate concentrations in all patients with drug overdose or altered consciousness: is it necessary?, *Emerg Med J*, 22: 401–3.
5. Rothwell, P.M., Fowkes, F.G., Belch, J.F. et al. (2011) Effect of daily aspirin on long-term risk of death due to cancer: analysis of individual patient data from randomized trials, *Lancet*, 377: 31–41.
6. Garcia-Albeniz, X. and Chan, T. (2011) Aspirin for the prevention of colorectal cancer, *Best Practice and Research: Clinical Gastroenterology*, 25: 461–72.
7. Burn, J., Gerdes, A-M., Macrae, F. et al. (2011) Long-term effect of aspirin on cancer risk in carriers of hereditary colorectal cancer: an analysis form the CAPP2 randomised controlled trial, *Lancet*, 378: 2081–7.
8. James, L., Mayeux, P. and Hinson, J. (2003) Acetaminophen-induced hepatotoxicity, *Drug Metabolism and Disposition*, 31: 1499–506.

Further reading

Farley, A., Hendry, C. and Napier, P. (2005) Paracetamol poisoning: physiological aspects and management strategies, *Nursing Standard*, 19(38): 58–64.
Ferner, R., Dear, J. and Bateman, D. (2011) Management of paracetamol poisoning, *BMJ*, 342: 968–72.
O'Malley, G. (2007) Emergency department management of the salicylate poisoned patient, *Emerg Med Clin N Amer*, 25: 333–46.

CHAPTER 14

THERAPEUTIC DRUG MONITORING: LITHIUM, DIGOXIN AND THEOPHYLLINE

Key learning topics

- The concept of therapeutic drug monitoring
- Pharmacological action and clinical use of lithium, digoxin and theophylline
- Adverse (toxic) effects of lithium, digoxin and theophylline
- How blood values are used to optimise lithium, digoxin and theophylline dose

---

This chapter is concerned with how laboratory measurement of drug concentration in blood helps in determining correct drug dose. Such an approach is either unnecessary or unsuitable for most drug therapies, but for a limited number of drugs including lithium, digoxin and theophylline, measurement of serum or plasma concentration is the preferred method of optimising dosage and preventing dangerous side effects (toxicity). Measuring drug concentration also provides a means of confirming patient compliance. Other drug therapies, not discussed in this chapter, in which therapeutic drug monitoring is useful, include the anticonvulsant drugs carbamazepine, valproate and phenytoin; some drugs used to treat disturbances of cardiac rhythm (e.g. procainamide, quinidine) and a few antibiotics (e.g. gentamicin, vancomycin).

Lithium

Pharmacological action and clinical use

Lithium has proven neuroprotective properties but the precise mechanism of its therapeutic value in psychiatric medicine as a mood stabiliser still remains unclear, 50 years after it was first prescribed. Lithium use is largely confined to the treatment of bipolar disorder[1]. This common long-term mental illness sometimes called manic-depression or affective disorder affects around 1.5–2% of the population

Understanding Laboratory Investigations: A Guide for Nurses, Midwives and Healthcare Professionals, Third Edition. Chris Higgins.
© 2013 John Wiley & Sons, Ltd. Published 2013 by John Wiley & Sons, Ltd.

and is characterised by cyclic episodes of severe depression followed by elation (mania). Normal mood is in the middle of a continuum, which runs from depression at one extreme to mania at the other. Depression is associated with a lack of energy, diminished interest and ability to experience pleasure, along with feelings of despair and pessimism. During the manic phase of bipolar disease however, symptoms are those of an abnormally expansive mood with increased mental and physical energy. Affected patients are hyperactive and have difficulty sleeping. Inflated self-esteem and false optimism are accompanied by flights of fancy and impulsive behaviour. In its most severe form, mania results in thinking that can race so fast that it becomes fragmented. Speech is fast and may be incoherent. Psychotic symptoms, including hallucination, grandiose delusion and illusion, may be a feature of severe acute mania.

Lithium is an anti-manic drug. Although used to treat acute mania and its less severe form, hypomania, among patients presenting with symptoms, the most important use of lithium is to prevent both manic and depressive episodes in patients with bipolar disorder; the result is a marked reduction in mood swings. Patients may need to take lithium for many years in order to remain well. Unfortunately, for unknown reasons, some patients with bipolar disease do not respond to lithium therapy. Lithium may also be used in conjunction with anti-depressant drugs to treat severe depression not associated with bipolar disease (unipolar depression) that does not respond to anti-depressant drugs alone.

Adverse side effects

All drugs have unwanted side effects and lithium is no exception. Lithium can affect kidney function, causing a condition known as nephrogenic diabetes insipidus, which is characterised by increased urine flow (polyuria) and resulting increased thirst (polydipsia). The thyroid gland of patients on long-term lithium therapy may become under active, with resulting symptoms of hypothyroidism (Chapter 10). This may contribute to the weight gain that is often associated with lithium use. Patients on long-term lithium therapy should have regular (six monthly) thyroid function tests, and serum creatinine estimation to assess renal function. Special caution should be taken in prescribing lithium during pregnancy, as there is increased risk of congenital malformation of the developing foetus associated with lithium use, particularly during the first three months of pregnancy. Lithium is eliminated from the body almost entirely by the kidneys in urine. For this reason the potential for lithium toxicity is greater in older patients, whose renal function is reduced, and patients with kidney disease. To avoid adverse effects, such patients may need a lower dose of lithium than those with normally functioning kidneys.

Why and when to measure serum lithium

The lithium dose required for treatment or prevention of manic symptoms (called the therapeutic dose) is very close to that which results in toxicity. In common with all three drugs discussed in this chapter, lithium is said to have a low 'therapeutic index' or narrow 'therapeutic window'. Fortunately there is a well-defined therapeutic range for serum lithium, providing a means of checking that sufficient drug is being administered for maximum therapeutic effect, consistent with minimum risk of toxic side effects. Serum lithium is checked initially after five to seven days on initial prescription dose. If serum concentration is below the therapeutic range, dose is increased, and if higher than therapeutic range, dose is decreased. Once a safe and effective maintenance dose has been established, serum lithium should be checked every week for four weeks and then every three months. Urgent blood testing is however necessary if any signs or symptoms of toxicity arise and in cases of deliberate overdose (parasuicide).

Patients suffering bipolar disease may be reluctant to take their lithium regularly once initial symptoms of mania have subsided; they may falsely believe that they do not require lithium, and stop taking tablets without consultation with their doctor. Measuring serum lithium provides a means of confirming that patients are continuing with their medication.

Digoxin

Principle pharmacological action and clinical use

Digoxin, which is derived from digitalis, a compound extracted from the leaves of the foxglove plant (*digitalis lanata*) is used in the treatment of heart disease. Digoxin inhibits the enzyme (ATPase) required for action of the sodium-potassium pump, present in the membrane of all cells, which maintains the distribution of sodium and potassium between cells and surrounding extracellular fluid (Chapter 3). The net effect of reduced sodium-potassium pump activity (and therefore digoxin administration) is an increase in sodium and calcium concentration within cells and a decrease in concentration of cellular potassium. It is the increase in calcium concentration within the muscle cells of the heart that accounts for the positive inotropic (increased force of cardiac muscle cell contraction) effects of digoxin. Apart from its positive inotropic effects, digoxin also indirectly affects (via vagal stimulation) the pacemaker cells of the sino-atrial (SA) and atrio-ventricular (AV) nodes in the heart that propagate electrical signals necessary for normal heart rate and rhythm.

For many years digoxin – in combination with diuretics – was the mainstay drug prescribed for all patients with chronic heart failure, a common condition among the elderly that is discussed in Chapter 9. With the introduction of a more effective drug regime (ACE inhibitors and β-blockers plus diuretic), digoxin is now used more selectively. It is used for that sub-set of patients, around a third, whose heart failure is complicated by co-exisiting atrial fibrillation, the most common cardiac arrhythmia. Digoxin is also used for heart failure patients whose symptoms are worsening or not improving despite optimal dose of ACE inhibitor, β-blocker and diuretic. In patients without heart failure, digoxin use is confined to those with atrial fibrillation.

Toxic (unwanted) side effects

Symptoms of digoxin toxicity include nausea, vomiting, diarrhoea and loss of appetite. Abnormal cardiac rhythms, which may result in either slowing of the heart rate (bradycardia) or increased heart rate (tachycardia), are common; in severe overdose these may be life threatening. Disturbances of normal vision, including blurring of vision and loss of ability to distinguish some colour combinations, may occur. Mental effects include confusion and restlessness; rarely digoxin toxicity can precipitate acute psychoses. The primary effect of digoxin on the sodium-potassium pump determines that digoxin toxicity may be accompanied by raised serum potassium.

Most digoxin is normally eliminated from the body unchanged, by the kidneys, in urine. Patients with diminished kidney function (the elderly and those with renal disease) cannot eliminate digoxin as efficiently as those with normal kidney function and are therefore at greater risk of digoxin toxicity. Abnormally low concentration of serum potassium (hypokalaemia), often the result of diuretic therapy, potentiates digoxin toxicity. A low serum magnesium and raised serum calcium has a similar effect.

Why and when measure serum digoxin

Routine monitoring of serum digoxin levels for all patients receiving digoxin is not considered necessary. However the test is useful in certain clinical situations. Like lithium, digoxin has a low therapeutic index. The serum level required for therapeutic effect is close to that which results in toxic symptoms so that digoxin toxicity is relatively common. Unfortunately many of the signs and symptoms of mild to moderate toxicity are non-specific and may even be due to the underlying disease, which digoxin is being used to treat. The only sure way of making or excluding the diagnosis of digoxin toxicity is to measure serum digoxin concentration. A request for blood digoxin level may be made following a poor clinical response to a standard digoxin dose. If the result is below the therapeutic range an increased dose may be safely prescribed. Finally the test can be used to assess patient compliance.

Theophylline

Principle pharmacological action and clinical use

Theophylline is a naturally occurring substance related to caffeine, which is found in the leaves of the tea plant. Although the mechanism of its action is poorly understood, theophylline has three important pharmacological effects: stimulation of cardiac muscle, relaxation of smooth muscle (notably respiratory muscles) and stimulation of the central nervous system. It also has anti-inflammatory effect. The principal clinical use of theophylline, which is derived from its effect on smooth muscle in the lung, is as a bronchodilator and anti-inflammatory agent in the treatment of asthma and chronic obstructive pulmonary disease (COPD).

Asthma is a very common condition of the lungs that affects close to 10% of all children and adults in the UK. It is characterised by episodic attacks of airway constriction. Between attacks patients are usually quite well but during attacks, which may be triggered by any number of factors including respiratory infection, environmental irritants (chemical fumes, smoke etc), exercise and even in some cases laughter, the bronchial airways constrict, become inflamed and produce abnormal amounts of mucus. These result in the common symptoms associated with an asthma attack: cough, wheeze and increased breathlessness. In its most severe manifestation, an asthma attack can cause respiratory failure in which normal gas exchange of oxygen and carbon dioxide is sufficiently compromised to threaten life. Although prompt hospital admission and treatment can be life saving, asthma is the cause of around 1000 premature deaths each year in the UK.

Theophylline may be given orally as part of the ongoing drug treatment of chronic asthma to prevent attacks, and is also administered intravenously in the form of aminophylline (a salt of theophylline) for the emergency treatment of acute asthma attacks. Theophylline acts directly to relax the smooth muscles of the bronchi effectively dilating or 'opening' the airway. The bronchodilator effect of theophylline is more pronounced if the airway is already constricted, as it is in patients with asthma.

Apart from asthma theophylline is also used in the treatment of chronic obstructive pulmonary disease. A quite separate property of theophylline, the ability to stimulate the respiratory centres in the central nervous system, is thought to be the reason for its effectiveness in the treatment of apnoea of prematurity. Affected premature babies suddenly stop breathing for 20 seconds or more, threatening brain function with risk of permanent brain damage. Both the frequency and duration of these so-called apnoea attacks are reduced with theophylline treatment.

Toxic (unwanted) side effects

Many patients experience minor adverse effects of theophylline therapy, and for this reason the drug is usually only prescribed for the prevention of asthma attacks, after other anti-asthma drugs have failed. Nausea, vomiting and loss of appetite are the most common signs of mild toxicity. Headache, insomnia, nervousness and increased irritability reflect the effect of theophylline on the central nervous system (CNS). Whilst many patients may experience both gastrointestinal and CNS effects when they first take theophylline, a tolerance is usually acquired and symptoms disappear. Theophylline is a gastrointestinal irritant that can reactivate peptic ulcers. In addition to the gastrointestinal and CNS symptoms, marked toxicity may result in palpitations, increased heart rate and abnormal heart rhythms (usually sinus tachychardia). Cardiac arrest can occur in patients given a single large dose of theophylline (aminophylline) to control an acute asthma attack. Convulsions and loss of consciousness can occur during marked toxicity. Although rare, severe toxicity can be fatal.

Certain diseases (e.g. liver disease, chronic heart failure and any condition associated with persistent fever) cause a decrease in the rate that theophylline can be eliminated from the body and a consequent increase in serum theophylline to a concentration normally associated with toxic symptoms. Asthmatic patients with these additional problems require a lower dose than normal and careful monitoring if they are to avoid the effects of theophylline toxicity. Conversely smokers eliminate theophylline more efficiently than non-smokers so require a higher dose to achieve the same therapeutic effect. Toxicity may arise after quitting smoking if dose is not reduced. Many drugs, including alcohol and some antibiotics, reduce theophylline elimination, thereby increasing toxicity at a given dosage. A full drug history must be taken into account when prescribing theophylline.

Why and when to measure serum theophylline

Theophylline has a low therapeutic index: the serum concentration required for therapeutic effect is close to that which results in toxic symptoms. Although the serum level for therapeutic effect has been established, the dose required to attain this therapeutic level varies, so that all patients should have their serum concentration checked during initiation of therapy. Typically dose is increased in small increments until serum concentration is within the therapeutic range. Once an effective and safe dosing regime has been established, serum concentration need only be checked at six monthly or yearly intervals. More frequent monitoring may be considered in the following types of patients whose ability to eliminate theophylline might be diminishing. All these patient types have an increased risk of theophylline toxicity:

- Elderly patients.
- Patients with concurrent liver disease (cirrhosis, hepatitis).
- Patients with concurrent congestive heart failure.
- Acutely ill patients (e.g. those receiving intensive care).
- Those patients being prescribed some additional drugs.

All patients presenting with signs of toxicity should have serum concentration checked to decide whether a reduction in dose or even temporary withdrawal of the drug is warranted.

Patients who seem to be failing to respond to theophylline might require a larger dose. If serum concentration is below the therapeutic range an increase in dose may be warranted.

Laboratory measurement of serum lithium, digoxin or theophylline

Patient preparation

No particular patient preparation is necessary.

Sample requirements

Around 5 ml of venous blood is required. This should be collected into a plain glass (without additives) tube.

Timing of sample

The concentration of any drug in blood varies in relation to the time of the last dose, so that timing of sample collection is vital for accurate interpretation of routine therapeutic drug monitoring results.

- Blood for lithium should be sampled at 12 hours after the last dose.
- Blood for digoxin should be sampled at six hours after the last dose
- Blood for theophylline should be sampled at one to two hours after the last dose.

If a patient is exhibiting signs of toxicity or a deliberate overdose is suspected, an urgent test result may be required. In these circumstances it is clearly not appropriate to wait before sampling blood, but it is important to record the time that the sample was taken and the time of the last dose or overdose, if known.

Interpretation of results

Serum lithium

Therapeutic range for those with symptoms of acute mania – 0.8–1.5 mmol/L.
Therapeutic range for maintenance dose to *prevent* symptoms – 0.5–1.0 mmol/L.

The objective is to maintain serum concentration within the therapeutic range. Patients actually suffering symptoms of acute mania can tolerate slightly higher doses of lithium than those without symptoms; hence the different therapeutic ranges. Once acute symptoms have passed and the patient is stabilised, a maintenance dose must be prescribed which results in a serum concentration within the lower therapeutic range.

Symptoms of mild toxicity (vomiting, diarrhoea, nausea and coarse tremor) usually arise as serum concentration rises above 1.5 mmol/L, although a minority of patients may experience these symptoms of lithium toxicity when serum concentration is less than 1.5 mmol/L. More symptoms including confusion, dizziness, tinnitus, irregular heart rate and blurred vision are associated with serum levels above 2.0 mmol/L. Loss of consciousness and fatality can occur in severe overdose (serum lithium >2.5 mmol/L) if treatment to eliminate lithium is not urgently initiated.

Serum digoxin

Therapeutic range – 0.8–2.0 µg/L (1.0–2.6 nmol/L).

Symptoms of toxicity are usually associated with serum digoxin concentration greater than 2.3 µg/L (3.0 nmol/L). However some patients (e.g. those with hypokalaemia, hypomagnesaemia, hypercalcaemia and thyroid disease) have increased sensitivity to the effects of digoxin and symptoms of toxicity might be present at concentration below 2.3 µg/L, and may even occur at concentration within the therapeutic range. So long as causes of increased sensitivity can be excluded, then serum digoxin level within the therapeutic range indicates that any symptoms suggestive of digoxin toxicity are unlikely to be due to digoxin; another cause must be sought and there is no real justification for reducing dose. Conversely the finding of a serum digoxin concentration below the therapeutic range in a patient who is not responding clinically as expected provides objective evidence that the patient is not receiving a sufficiently high dose.

Serum theophylline

Therapeutic range for asthma/COPD treatment – 10–20 mg/L (55–110 μmol/L). Therapeutic range for apnoea of prematurity – 8–20 mg/L (28–44 μmol/L).

The objective is to maintain serum concentration within the therapeutic range. A serum concentration below the therapeutic range indicates current dose is unlikely to be effective and a serum concentration above the therapeutic range results in unwanted side effects (toxicity). Mild to moderate toxicity is associated with serum concentration in the range (i.e. 20–30 mg/L). Severe toxicity with seizures and life-threatening cardiac arrhythmias do not usually occur until serum concentration is in excess of 165 mmol/L (i.e. 30 mg/L).

Case history 20

Mr Anderson is 75 years old. He was first suspected of having a failing heart ten years ago, when he noticed that he was becoming breathless on climbing stairs. Over the next year or two his condition worsened. He became breathless when lying flat, making it difficult to sleep without additional pillows and he developed ankle oedema. His prescription included digoxin and an oral diuretic. Although he required increasing amounts of diuretics to control oedema, his symptoms were relieved and he became much more physically active, until a month ago when his condition deteriorated. Immediately prior to hospital admission he was unable to perform any physical activity, preferring to sleep downstairs propped in a chair rather than make the effort of climbing the stairs at night, and his ankles were so swollen with oedema, he was unable to wear shoes. Despite a loss of appetite his body weight had been rising with progressive accumulation of oedema fluid. On admission, Mr Anderson's serum digoxin was 1.7 μg/L (2.2 nmol/L) and his serum potassium 3.6 mmol/L. Over the next two days he was given large oral doses of the diuretic frusemide to remove accumulating fluids; by day three of admission this had resulted in a 12 kg fall in body weight. Mr Anderson's body weight was now normal, but he felt nauseous, retched frequently, felt very weak and complained of a headache; he became increasingly drowsy. As these are all signs of digoxin toxicity, blood was sampled for serum digoxin; urea and electrolytes requests were made at the same time. The laboratory reported the following results:

Serum Digoxin   – 1.6 μg/L (2.1 nmol/L)
Serum Potassium   – 2.4 mmol/L
Serum Creatinine   – 110 mmol/L

Questions

(1) Did digoxin results either at the time of admission or three days later indicate that Mr Anderson might be receiving too much digoxin?

(2) Are serum potassium results normal?

(3) Why might Mr Anderson be suddenly suffering from digoxin toxicity despite no increase in dose for the past five years?

Discussion of case history 20

(1) Both digoxin results are within the therapeutic range. The deterioration in Mr Anderson's heart prior to hospital admission cannot be attributed to failure on his part to continue with his digoxin medication. Serum digoxin results do not indicate digoxin toxicity, rather they indicate that he was receiving an appropriate digoxin dose.

(2) The normal range for serum potassium is 3.6–5.0 mmol/L. On admission then, Mr Anderson's serum potassium was at the low end of the normal range but after diuretic therapy on day three of admission, his potassium level was markedly reduced.

(3) The water diueresis, induced by administration of frusemide which Mr Anderson urgently required, was accompanied by increased losses of potassium in urine. This is a well-documented side effect of some diuretic therapies. Since before this treatment, serum potassium was already at the low end of the normal range, possibly due to low dietary potassium intake because of loss of appetite, this increased loss of potassium in urine sent Mr Anderson's serum potassium plummeting; he became severely hypokalaemic. Reduced serum potassium concentration potentiates the toxicity of digoxin, so that, as in Mr Anderson's case, symptoms of toxicity appear despite the fact that serum digoxin is within the therapeutic range. Treatment of digoxin toxicity in this case is based not on withdrawal of digoxin, which might exacerbate Mr Anderson's underlying heart failure, but on restoring serum potassium to a level within the normal range by administration of potassium supplements.

References

1. Mahli, G., Adams, D. and Berk, M. (2009) Is lithium in a class of its own? A brief profile of its clinical use, *Australian and New Zealand J Psychiatry*, 43: 1096–104.
2. Mittal, M., Chockalingam, P. and Chockalingham, A. (2011) Contemporary indications and therapeutic implications for digoxin use, *American J Therapeutics*, 18: 280–7.

Further reading

Barnes, D. (2003) Theophylline – new perspectives for an old drug, *Am J Respir Crit Care*, 167: 813–18.

Dunne, F. (2010) Lithium toxicity: the importance of clinical signs, *Br J Hosp Med*, 71: 206–10.

Jefferson, J. (1998) Lithium, *BMJ*, 316: 133.

Shaw, M. (2004) The role of lithium clinics in the treatment of bipolar disorder, *Nursing Times*, 100: 42–6.

The Digitalis Investigation Group (1997) The effect of digoxin on mortality and morbidity in patients with heart failure, *New Eng J Med*, 336: 525–33.

PART 3

Haematology Tests

FULL BLOOD COUNT – 1: RED BLOOD CELL COUNT, HAEMOGLOBIN AND OTHER RED CELL INDICES

Key learning topics

- Production, function and fate of red blood cells (erythrocytes)
- Structure and function of haemoglobin
- Defining red cell indices – haematocrit (PCV), MCV and MCHC
- How patient haemoglobin level is used to confirm anaemia
- Principle causes and consequences of anaemia
- How red cell indices help in establishing cause of anaemia

Of all laboratory blood tests, the full blood count (FBC) is the most frequently requested, reflecting the wide range of both common and less common disturbances of health that may be associated with abnormality in FBC results. It is not one test, but a panel of tests including a count of each of the three cellular or formed elements of blood: red cells (erythrocytes), white cells (leucocytes) and platelets (thrombocytes). In this first of two chapters that focus on the FBC, we consider the red cell count and several other tests included in the FBC which all relate to red cell function. All these tests (listed in Table 15.1) are used primarily to identify those patients who are anaemic; they also help in elucidating the cause of that anaemia. In Chapter 16 we consider the significance of the total and differential white cell count, whilst the platelet count will be dealt with in Chapter 17, which focuses on tests of blood coagulation.

Blood film

For this test blood is spread in a thin film on a glass microscope slide, then stained with dyes and examined under the microscope. A blood film report includes the

Understanding Laboratory Investigations: A Guide for Nurses, Midwives and Healthcare Professionals, Third Edition. Chris Higgins.

Table 15.1 Tests included in a full blood count (FBC) that relate to red blood cells.

Name of test (common abbreviation)	What is measured	Unit of measurement
Red blood cell (RBC) count	The number of red blood cells	Number of thousand million (i.e. 10^9) red cells in 1 litre of blood (10^9/L)
Haemoglobin (Hb)	Concentration of the protein haemoglobin in blood	Number of grams in 100 ml of blood (g/dl)
The red cell indices:		
Packed cell volume (PCV) [or Haematocrit (Ht)]	The percentage of total blood volume that is occupied by red cells	Percentage (%)
Mean cell volume (MCV)	The average (or mean) volume of red cells	femtolitre (fl) [Note: 1 femtolitre = 1×10^{-15} L]
Mean cell haemoglobin concentration (MCHC)	The average (or mean) concentration of haemoglobin in red cells	Number of grams of haemoglobin in 100 ml of red cells (g/dl)
Red cell distribution width (RDW)	The variation in red cell volume (expressed as a percentage)	Percentage (%)

details of any abnormalities in appearance and size of red cells. A blood film is usually only prepared and examined if results of the tests in Table 15.1 are abnormal.

Normal physiology

Red cell (erythrocyte) production

Red cells are the most abundant of the three formed elements in blood outnumbering leucocytes (white cells) by around 1000:1 and platelets by 100:1. The process of blood cell production, called haemopoiesis, takes place within the bone marrow. During infancy the bone marrow of all bones have the capacity to manufacture blood cells, but in adulthood this is limited to the bone marrow within the vertebrae, ribs, sternum, skull and pelvis as well as the ends of the long bones, femur and humerus. All blood cells are derived from bone marrow stem cells, which have the potential to differentiate to cells committed to becoming either mature red cells, white cells or platelets. The most primitive of those cells within bone marrow that are destined to become mature red cells is the pro-normoblast (alternative name pro-erythroblast). The pro-normoblast develops by cell division and differentiation through recognisable stages to normoblast (alternative name erythroblast), reticulocyte and finally the mature red cell or erythrocyte (Figure 15.1). This development from stem cell to mature red cell is called erythropoiesis and is characterised by:

- Gradual reduction in cell size.
- Loss of nucleus and therefore ability to divide.
- Loss of internal cell organelles.

The final stage of maturation, reticulocyte to erythrocyte occurs both within the bone marrow and in peripheral blood; normally around 1–2% of the circulating red cell population is reticulocytes. No red cell more primitive than the reticulocyte is normally present in blood.

Mature red cells have a life span of around 120 days. Constant replacement is necessary; on average around 2.3 million red cells are produced every second by the bone marrow throughout life. This production is regulated by erythropoietin, a hormone synthesised in the cells of the kidney (Figure 15.2). In response to a decreasing blood oxygen level, the kidneys release erythropoietin to blood for transport to the bone marrow. Here erythropoietin stimulates erythropoiesis and thereby red cell production. As red cell numbers increase, the oxygen content of blood increases, and kidney production of erythropoietin is stepped down.

Structure and function of red cells

The structure of the mature red cell is well suited to its primary functions: transport of oxygen from the lungs to the tissues and transport of carbon dioxide from tissues to the lungs. Central to this function is haemoglobin, the protein contained

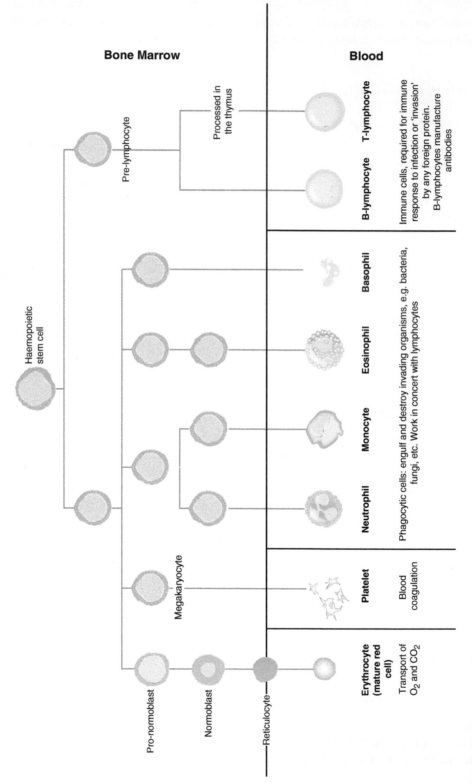

Figure 15.1 Diagrammatic representation of blood cell development.

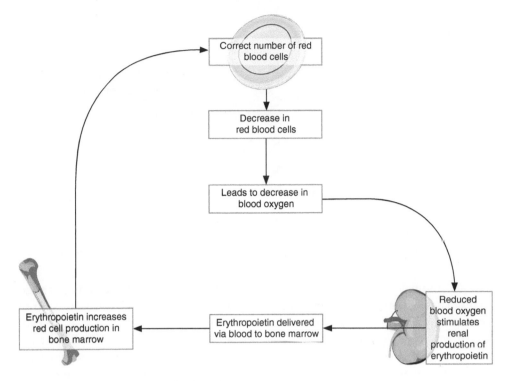

Figure 15.2 Regulation of red cell production.

within red blood cells. Haemoglobin production occurs within the red cell during its development in the bone marrow and is complete before full maturation. Each nearly mature red cell (reticulocyte) leaves the bone marrow with its full complement of 250–300 million molecules of haemoglobin.

Commonly described as a biconcave disc the mature red cell (erythrocyte) can be imagined as a flattened sphere with its sides pushed in. This singular shape allows the largest surface area for a given volume, providing maximum possible area for oxygen and carbon dioxide gas exchange.

The diameter of the red cell is around 8 μm, twice the diameter of the smallest blood vessels through which it must pass. The membrane is able to deform itself, altering the shape of the red blood cell, so that it can 'squeeze' through the micro-vasculature within tissues, where gases (oxygen and carbon dioxide) are exchanged between blood and tissue cells. Without a nucleus and other internal organelles, the mature erythrocyte may be regarded – albeit simplistically – as little more than a deformable membranous bag, stuffed full of haemoglobin.

Haemoglobin structure and function

Haemoglobin is the oxygen carrying protein pigment present in red cells, which gives blood its colour.

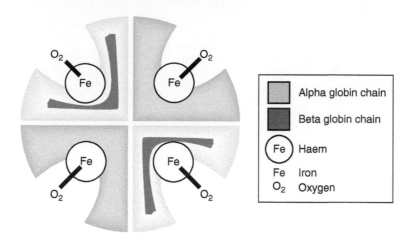

Figure 15.3 Representation of molecular structure of oxygenated adult haemoglobin.

The haemoglobin molecule (Figure 15.3) comprises four folded chains of amino acids. These together form the protein or *globin* portion of the molecule. Each of the four globin sub-units has a much smaller *haem* group attached, and at the centre of each haem group is an atom of iron in the ferrous state (Fe^{2+}). Whilst the structure of the haem group is always the same, the exact sequence of amino acids in the globin sub-units varies slightly, giving rise to four possible globin chains: alpha (α), beta (β), gamma (γ) and delta (δ). Around 97% of adult haemoglobin is haemoglobin A (HbA) comprising 2 α and 2 β globin sub-units. The remaining 3% is HbA2 (2 α and 2 δ globins). In the developing foetus and for the first few months of life, foetal haemoglobin (HbF) is the only haemoglobin produced; HbF is composed of 2 α and 2 γ globin sub-units. The structure of haemoglobin is of more than passing academic interest. There are a large group of inherited disorders of haemoglobin synthesis and structure, collectively known as the haemoglobinopathies. Most are rare, but one, sickle cell disease is relatively common and therefore warrants special attention; they are discussed in Chapter 23.

Haemoglobin transport of oxygen

A very small proportion of oxygen transported in blood is simply dissolved in blood plasma, but most (98–99%) is transported bound to haemoglobin. The necessary oxygen combining property of haemoglobin depends on the single atom of iron present at the centre of each of the four haem groups. An oxygen molecule forms a weak, reversible ionic link with each of these iron atoms in turn; the product of this reaction is oxyhaemoglobin. When all four haem groups are occupied with oxygen the haemoglobin molecule is said to be saturated. The affinity of haemoglobin for oxygen, that is the extent to which it is saturated with oxygen, depends on the amount or partial pressure (P) of oxygen dissolved in the blood plasma in which the red cells, containing haemoglobin are suspended. This is described graphically in the oxygen dissociation curve (see Chapter 7, Figure 7.2). It is clear from the graph in Figure 7.2 that haemoglobin becomes increasingly saturated with oxygen as the partial pressure of oxygen (PO_2) increases. The physiological implications of this relationship are central to the oxygen binding and delivery function of haemoglobin. In the lungs, oxygen in inspired air diffuses from alveoli to blood plasma so that PO_2 of blood here is high (around 95 mmHg). Since this relatively high PO_2 is associated with high haemoglobin affinity for oxygen, haemoglobin quickly (within a few seconds) becomes almost 100% saturated with oxygen. Conversely in the tissues, blood PO_2 is relatively low (only around 40 mmHg) and consequently haemoglobin here has less affinity for oxygen. As a result oxygen is released from haemoglobin and diffuses from blood to tissue cells, where it is required for cell metabolism.

Role of red cell and haemoglobin in the transport of CO_2

Whilst the transport of oxygen from lungs to tissues is almost entirely due to haemoglobin in red cells, the transport of carbon dioxide in the reverse direction is slightly more complex. Carbon dioxide is more soluble in blood plasma than oxygen, so that a significant amount of carbon dioxide is transported simply dissolved in blood plasma. The remainder is transported in two other ways; both mechanisms involve carbon dioxide diffusing from plasma to red cells. Within red cells most carbon dioxide is converted to bicarbonate, and this bicarbonate diffuses from red cells to plasma for transport to the lungs. The rest remains in red cells loosely bound to the haemoglobin that has just released its oxygen to the tissues.

[*Note: The oxygen and carbon dioxide transporting function of haemoglobin is also dealt with in a discussion of respiratory physiology contained in Chapter 7; readers might find it useful to refer to that discussion.*]

Normal red cell destruction

After around 120 days circulating in peripheral blood, red cells are no longer viable and are removed from blood to the reticulo-endothelial (RE) system, as blood passes through the bone marrow, spleen and liver. In these RE sites, the defunct red cell is engulfed by, and internalised to (the process is called phagocytosis) a much larger cell called a macrophage, whose function is controlled destruction of the red cell. Within macrophages the red cell membrane is first degraded, releasing haemoglobin, which is split into its constituent parts: haem and globin. The iron present in haem is recylced for production of new red cells and globin chains are broken down to amino acids, which enter the amino acid pool for synthesis of new proteins. What remains of haem after removal of iron is converted to the yellow pigment bilirubin. This is transported in blood to the liver for further metabolism and eventual excretion, mostly via bile in faeces; a little is excreted as the bilirubin metabolites, urobilin and urobilinogen, in urine.

In health the rate of red cell production in bone marrow matches the rate of red cell destruction in the reticuloendothelial system, so that the number of red cells circulating in peripheral blood remains broadly constant and sufficient to provide all tissue cells with the oxygen they require to survive and function.

Laboratory measurement of FBC

Patient preparation

No particular patient preparation is necessary.

Timing of sample

There are no special timing requirements so blood is best sampled at a time that coinicides with routine transport to the laboratory. Blood for FBC should not be stored longer than 12 hours before transport to the laboratory. FBC is one of those tests that can be performed urgently and out of normal laboratory hours, if necessary. In such circumstances it is essential to telephone the laboratory and transport the blood immediately it has been sampled.

Type of sample

Venous blood is preferable, ideally collected without the use of a tourniquet (if used, a tourniquet should not be left for more than a minute or two before blood is sampled). Capillary blood collection is appropriate if venous blood collection poses difficulty (e.g. in babies and those with 'difficult' veins).

Blood collection bottle

Blood for FBC must be collected into a special tube (usually lavender or pink coloured top) which contains the anticoagulant, K^+EDTA. This both prevents the blood from clotting and preserves the structure of blood cells.

Sample volume

The sample bottles for FBC have a 'line to fill' marked on the label. This is usually 2.5 ml, or 0.5 ml in the case of paediatric sized bottles for capillary blood sampling. This volume will result in the correct ratio of blood to anticoagulant. It is important for accurate result that neither too much nor too little blood is added to these tubes and that anticoagulant and blood are mixed by gentle inversion, as soon as the blood is sampled. Inadequate mixing can result in formation of tiny blood clots, and inaccurate results.

Interpretation of Hb RBC and red cell indices results

Approximate reference ranges

Red blood cell (RBC)
    Adult Males $4.5 - 6.5 \times 10^{12}$/L
    Adult Females $3.9 - 5.6 \times 10^{12}$/L

At birth $3.5-6.7\times10^{12}$/L
Childhood $4.1-5.3\times10^{12}$/L

Haemoglobin (Hb)
   Adult Males   13.5–17.5 g/dl
   Adult Females   11.5–15.5 g/dl
   At birth   14.0–24.0 g/dl
   Childhood   11.0–14.0 g/dl

[Note: In some laboratories and clinical texts the unit of haemoglobin measurement is grams per litre (g/L) rather than grams per deciliter (g/dl). To convert g/L to g/dl, divide by 10. Thus Hb 135 g/L is the same as Hb 13.5g/dl.]

Packed cell volume (PCV) or Haematocrit (Ht)
   Males   40 52%
   Females   36–48%

Mean cell volume (MCV)
   Adults   80–95 fl
   At birth   100–135 fl
   Childhood   71–88 fl

Mean cell haemoglobin concentration (MCHC) – 20–35 g/dl
Red (cell) distribution width (RDW) – 10–15%

Critical values

Haemoglobin   <7.0 g/dl or >20.0 g/dl
PCV (Haematocrit)   <20% or >60%

Terms used to describe red cells

Normocytosis   average size of red cell is normal.
Microcytosis   average size of red cells is smaller than normal.
Macrocytosis   average size of red cells is larger than normal.
Anisocytosis   red cells vary in size more than normal.
Poikilocytosis   red cells vary in shape.
Normochromasia   red cells stain normally indicating they contain normal amount of haemoglobin.
Hypochromasia   red cells appear weakly stained indicating they contain less haemoglobin than normal.

Conditions associated with reduction in RBC, Hb, PCV(Ht)

Anaemia

Anaemia (literally, without blood) is the collection of signs and symptoms that result from reduced oxygen delivery to tissues, due to a decrease in the total number of red blood cells and consequent reduction in haemoglobin concentration of blood. There are many possible causes, so that anaemia is not a disease entity itself, but rather a sign of some underlying disease, which must be identified if treatment of anaemia is to be successful.

Of all the signs and symptoms that may be present in an anaemic patient, the constant sign that is usually used to define anaemia is reduced haemoglobin (Hb) concentration. Diagnosis of anaemia is established if Hb concentration is below the lower limit of the reference range, that is less than 13.5 g/dl for adult males and less than 11.5 g/dl for adult females. In children, who normally have slightly lower levels of Hb, a diagnosis of anaemia is made if Hb is less than 11.0 g/dl. The lower the Hb, the more severe is the anaemia, and anaemia is excluded by the finding of Hb concentration within the reference range (there is an important exception to this, to be explained).

Reduced red cell count and PCV is also a feature of anaemia, although the magnitude of the reduction of red cell count depends not only on the severity of the anaemia, but also its cause. The principle pathological effect of anaemia is reduced delivery of oxygen to tissue cells but the extent to which this causes symptoms, depends on several factors including:

- **Severity of the anaemia:** many patients with mild anaemia, i.e. Hb >10 g/dl have no symptoms, but severe anaemia (Hb <6 g/dl) is almost always associated with symptoms.
- **Speed of onset:** rapid onset of anaemia is more likely to result in symptoms than that which has developed slowly.
- **Co-existing disease:** the normal physiological (compensatory) response to anaemia that ensures, so far as is possible, continued delivery of oxygen to tissues despite reduced Hb concentration is dependent on functioning respiratory and cardiovascular systems. Those with co-existing respiratory and/or cardiovascular disease are particularly vulnerable to the effects of anaemia, and more likely to manifest symptoms.

Signs and symptoms of anaemia

To some extent signs and symptoms depend on the cause of anaemia but there are some that occur irrespective of cause. The principle generalised symptoms of anaemia include:

- Pallor.
- Tiredness and lethargy.
- Shortness of breath, particularly on exertion.
- Dizziness, fainting.
- Headaches.
- Increased heart rate (tachycardia), palpitations.

The absence of symptoms does not preclude anaemia; many mildly anaemic individuals remain asymptomatic, particularly if anaemia has developed slowly (chronically) and there has been time for induction of compensatory mechanisms that help to ensure oxygen delivery to tissues despite reduced oxygen carrying capacity of blood.

Causes of anaemia

Whilst Hb, RBC and PCV measurement all help in identifying those patients who are anaemic and in assessing the severity of anaemia, they provide little information about cause.

Anaemia may be caused by:

- Significant acute blood loss (haemorrhage), e.g. trauma, surgery, postpartum haemorrhage (PPH).
- Deficiency of iron (required for Hb production); this is the most common cause of anaemia and is discussed further in Chapter 18.
- Anaemia is a common complication of chronic inflammatory disease (e.g. rheumatoid arthritis), chronic infectious disease (e.g. tuberculosis) and malignant disease (cancer). Because there is a common mechanism (inflammation) that gives rise to the anaemia in all these conditions, it is called anaemia of chronic disease (ACD). ACD is the second most common cause of anaemia after iron deficiency, and the most common cause in the elderly. (The elderly represent the age group most likely to be suffering the underlying chronic/malignant diseases.) A distinguishing feature of ACD is that it is almost invariably mild in nature, with Hb rarely being less than around 9–10 g/dl.
- Deficiency of vitamins B12 and/or folate that are both required for production of red cells. Pernicious anaemia accounts for most cases of anaemia in this group, but the whole group is discussed further in Chapter 18.
- Chronic kidney disease (CKD). Inadequate production of erythropoietin (required for regulation of red cell production) is the main cause of the anaemia that commonly occurs in those with CKD.
- Some diseases are associated with an increased rate of red cell destruction, such that despite maximal red cell production by the bone marrow, the number of circulating red cells declines; anaemia is the inevitable consequence. Haemolytic anaemia, the name given to anaemia that results from increased red cell destruction, is a feature of a number of conditions including: sickle cell disease, transfusion reaction, haemolytic disease of the newborn, malaria and lead poisoning. Very rarely, haemolytic anaemia can be an adverse effect of prescribed drugs, most commonly the cephalosporins (a class of antibiotics). A distinguishing feature of haemolytic anaemia is that it can result in jaundice, a condition that is discussed in some detail in Chapter 11.
- Rarely, anaemia can result from damage to, or defect in, bone marrow stem cells and consequent reduced bone marrow production of red cells (and all other blood cells). This is called aplastic anaemia which can be due to an inherited defect, or much more commonly acquired as a result of exposure to radiation, some drugs, toxic chemicals or viruses. No cause can be identified in many cases.
- Reduced bone marrow production of red cells and consequent anaemia is a feature of malignant diseases of bone marrow such as leukaemia and myeloma.
- Prematurity is a major risk factor for anaemia in the neonatal period for two reasons: decreased red cell production due to inadequate erythropoietin; and

decreased red cell survival (around 35 days rather than the normal 120 days). Additionally, very premature babies require frequent blood testing, which can represent a significant blood loss in the context of their very low total blood volume.

The red cell indices, MCV, MCHC, MCH and RDW, along with microscopic examination of red cells, help in identifying the cause of anaemia. Initially, when investigating the cause of anaemia, MCV is the most useful because all cases of anaemia can be classified according to the average size of red cell (MCV) to one of three groups:

- Microcytic anaemia (low MCV).
- Normocytic anaemia (normal MCV).
- Macrocytic anaemia (raised MCV).

The microcytic anaemias are those that result from iron deficiency and thalassaemia. Some patients whose anaemia is due to chronic disease have a microcytic anaemia, but this is not typical.

Most patients with ACD have a normocytic anaemia. Other causes of anaemia in this normocytic group include acute blood loss (haemorrhage); the haemolytic anaemias; anaemia caused by decreased erythropoietin production (CKD), anaemia caused by damage to bone marrow stem cells (aplastic anaemia) and anaemia, which results from malignant disease of the bone marrow (i.e. the leukaemias etc).

Macrocytic anaemias are confined to those that result from vitamin B12 or folate deficiency.

RDW is helpful in further distinguishing the cause within these three groups; so that, for example, iron deficiency and thalassaemia are both associated with microcytic anaemia. However iron deficiency is associated with a raised RDW, whereas RDW is normal in those with thalassaemia. Similarly RDW is able to distinguish different causes of normocytic anaemia. For example, anaemia of chronic disease is associated with normal RDW whereas haemolytic anaemias are associated with raised RDW. Simply by examining MCV and RDW results of anaemic patients then, it is possible to narrow down the likely cause of anaemia.

The examination of a stained blood smear under the microscope may also be useful because the shape and staining characteristics of red cells from an anaemic patient may give important clues as to cause. For example the red cells of patients with sickle cell anaemia can have a characteristic sickle shape, which gives the condition its name. Relatively small red cells that stain weakly (due to abnormally low concentration of haemoglobin) indicate possible iron deficiency whilst large cells, typically oval in shape indicate anaemia is probably due to deficiency of vitamin B12 or folate. Malarial parasites can be seen in the red cells of a patient with malaria associated anaemia, and anaemia caused by lead poisoning is often evident as abnormal staining of red cells (the abnormality is called basophilic stippling).

Causes of increased red cell count, haemoglobin and PCV (Ht)

Polycythaemia

Polycythaemia (literally many blood cells) is the opposite of anaemia. *Increased* red cell count and haemoglobin concentration is the hallmark of polycythaemia. Since PCV is dependent on the number of red cells, this too is raised in polycythaemia. Polycythaemia may arise as a response to any physiological or pathological condition in which blood contains less oxygen than normal. In response to a low blood oxygen level, the kidney increases erythropoietin production resulting in turn in increased red cell production. This so-called secondary polycythaemia is a feature of:

- Living at high altitude (where inspired air has relatively less oxygen).
- Cigarette smoking (carbon monoxide present in inhaled cigarette smoke binds to haemoglobin, displacing oxygen).
- Chronic lung disease (oxygen transfer from lungs to blood is compromised).
- Cyanotic heart disease (blood is less well oxygenated than normal due to congenital structural defects in the heart).

Primary polycythaemia or polycythaemia vera is a quite separate rare malignant disease of the bone marrow in which bone marrow stem cell proliferation results in marked over-production of red cells (white cell and platelet numbers are also often increased). This huge increase in red cell numbers increases the viscosity (fluidity) of blood and several of the signs and symptoms (headache, increased blood pressure) are related to this increased blood viscosity.

Effect of hydration on RBC, Hb and PCV(Ht)

Measured red cell count, haemoglobin and PCV are all affected by the state of hydration of the patient. Dehydration is associated with increased RBC Hb and PCV simply because plasma volume is reduced. The absolute number of red cells and amount of haemoglobin in blood however remains unchanged. Conversely a patient who has received too much fluid and is overhydrated will have a reduced Hb, red cell count and PCV. This effect of hydration has to be taken into account when interpreting results from patients who are either dehydrated or overhydrated. An increased plasma volume is a normal physiological effect of pregnancy so that pregnancy is associated with gradual decrease in Hb, PCV and RBC, even though absolute numbers of red cells and Hb are normal. Thus a pregnant woman with a slight reduction in Hb, RBC and PCV is not necessarily anaemic. In fact anaemia would not normally be diagnosed during pregnancy if Hb is greater than 10.5 g/dl.

Another anomaly that arises if Hb concentration is being used to define anaemia concerns acute blood loss (haemorrhage). This is associated with equivalent loss of both red cells (containing haemoglobin) and plasma. So despite what might be a significant loss of red cells and contained Hb, Hb concentration, red cell count (concentration) and PCV all remain, initially at least, normal. It is not until compensatory mechanisms (or fluid replacement therapy) have invoked restoration of fluid volume towards normal that anaemia becomes evident in FBC results of a patient who has suffered acute blood loss.

Other causes of a raised mcv

It is worth noting that MCV may be raised in patients who are not anaemic, that is have a normal Hb. The principal causes of an isolated increase in MCV are alcohol abuse and cirrhosis of the liver. An isolated raised MCV in a patient suspected of alcohol abuse is considered objective evidence of continued alcohol use.

The reticulocyte count

As previously discussed reticulocytes are immature red cells. For technical reasons and because it has limited clinical utility, a count of the number of reticulocytes in blood is not included in the routine FBC. It is however offered as a separate test by most laboratories. A brief discussion is appropriate here because its utility is confined to investigation of the anaemic patient – a major focus of this chapter. The sample requirement for reticulocyte count is the same as for FBC (as already discussed).

Approximate reference range

$20–80 \times 10^9/L$
(Some laboratories report reticulocytes as a percentage (%) of the total red cell count in which case the approximate reference range is 0.5–2.0%.)

Interpretation of test result

The clinical value of the reticulocyte count rests on the observation that the normal physiological response to anaemia is to increase bone marrow production of red cells. This increased rate of red cell production is evident as an increased number of immature red cells (reticulocytes) being released to blood from bone marrow, and thereby an increased reticulocyte count. This effect of the physiological response to anaemia is referred to as reticulocytosis. Evidence of reticulocytosis (i.e. increased reticulocyte count) in an anaemic patient implies that the anaemia is not the result of defect in red cell production, but rather the result of either increased red cell destruction (haemolytic anaemia) or acute blood loss (haemorrhage). By contrast a normal or reduced reticulocyte count in an anaemic patient suggests the anaemia is caused by either a deficiency of a nutrient (e.g. iron, vitamins B12 folate) required for red cell production or bone marrow disease that is limiting red cell production.

The reticulocyte count can be used to monitor effectiveness of some anaemia treatments. For example, prescription of iron tablets to a patient with iron deficiency anaemia is associated with a reticulocytosis (increase in reticulocyte count) that begins around five to seven days after the start of treatment. Reticulocytosis provides the first objective evidence that the iron is having the desired effect of increasing bone marrow production of red cells. Clearly absence of such a response suggests the patient is either not taking the tablets or was never iron deficient, and an alternative cause of anaemia should be considered.

Case history 21

Jane Baker, a 32 year old solicitor, attends her GP surgery complaining of feeling 'washed out'. Although normally an active woman, who enjoys horse riding at weekends and regular visits with her children to the local swimming pool, Jane now reports becoming increasingly tired over the past month or two. She feels unable to do much more than a normal day's work. During examination of Jane's eyes, her GP noted a degree of pallor in conjunctival membrane, suggesting anaemia might be the cause her tiredness. No other abnormal signs were detected. He sampled blood for a FBC. The laboratory report, which he received the next day, contained the following results:

Hb – 9.2 g/dl
RBC – 3.8 × 10^{12}/L
PCV – 28%
MCV – 73 fl
MCHC – 20 g/dl
RDW 16%

Questions

(1) What is the laboratory evidence of Jane's anaemia?; is it severe?
(2) Using the red cell indices, classify the anaemia to either:
    (a) microcytic anaemia
    (b) normocytic anaemia
    (c) macrocytic anaemia
(3) Suggest possible causes of the anaemia.
(4) What further test(s) is indicated?

Discussion of case history 21

(1) The haemoglobin (Hb) concentration is used to confirm or exclude anaemia. Jane's Hb is well below the reference range for adult females. This is sufficient evidence to make a diagnosis of anaemia. An Hb of 9.2 g/dl indicates that Jane is moderately anaemic; anaemia is usually considered severe only if Hb is less than 6.0 g/dl. Although not required to make a diagnosis, both PCV and RBC results are low, reflecting anaemia.

(2) The MCV (mean cell volume) is a measure of the average size of red cells. Jane's MCV is reduced which means that her red cells are, on average, smaller than normal; her anaemia is microcytic in nature.

(3) Almost all cases of microcytic anaemia are due to:
- iron deficiency,
- thalassaemia (an inherited disorder of haemoglobin synthesis found particularly in those of Mediterranean descent), or
- particularly severe anaemia of chronic disease (infection, inflammation, malignancy).

Of these, iron deficiency is by far the most common, and thalassaemia the least common. Since Jane has no medical history of chronic disease, iron deficiency is the most likely cause of her anaemia. The RDW result provides supportive evidence for such a diagnosis since it is usually raised in iron deficiency and normal in both thalassaemia and anaemia of chronic disease.

(4) A serum iron and serum ferritin test (Chapter 18) will confirm the diagnosis of iron deficiency anaemia. As will be made clear in Chapter 18 there are many causes of iron deficiency. If iron deficiency is confirmed, Jane may require further investigation to establish the cause of the deficiency in her case.

Further reading

Aster, R. (2010) Adverse drug reactions affecting blood cells, *Handbook of Experimental Pharmacology*, 196: 57–76.

Buttarello, M. and Plebani, M. (2008) Automated blood cell counts – state of the art, *Am J Clin Pathol*, 130: 104–16.

Frewin, R., Henson, A. and Provan, D. (1997) ABC of clinical haematology: iron deficiency anaemia, *BMJ*, 314: 360–3.

Hoffbrand, A. and Moss, P. (2011) Erythropoiesis and general aspects of anaemia. In: *Essential Haematology* 6th edn, Wiley-Blackwell.

Kaferele, J. and Strzoda, C. (2009) Evaluation of macrocytosis, *Am Fam Physician*, 79: 203–8.

Weatherall, D.J. (1997) ABC of clinical haematology: the hereditary anaemias, *BMJ*, 314: 492–6.

CHAPTER 16

FULL BLOOD COUNT – 2: WHITE CELL COUNT AND DIFFERENTIAL

Key learning topics

- Function of the five different kinds of white cell
- Defining a total and differential white cell count
- Defining some white cell related terms
- Causes and consequences of increased white cell count
- Causes and consequences of decreased white cell count
- A brief introduction to leukaemia – a malignant disease of white cells

In this second of two chapters devoted to the most commonly requested blood test – the full blood count (FBC) – we consider one element of it: the white blood cell count (WBC). Unlike the mature red cell population, which is homogenous in nature, the white cell (leucocyte) population is heterogeneous, composed as it is of five morphologically and functionally distinct populations. These are: neutrophils, eosinophils, basophils, monocytes and lymphocytes. The total WBC is the sum of all of these white cell types, whilst the differential WBC or 'diff' is a count of each of the five types. An increase in white cell numbers is a very common feature of disease, which can be attributed to one of several pathological processes, including the big three: infection, inflammation and malignancy. A reduced white cell count, which is much less common, implies a reduction in immunity and therefore high risk of infectious disease.

Normal physiology

In common with all other formed elements in blood, white cells (leucocytes) are derived from the pluripotent stem cell present in bone marrow (see Chapter 15, Figure 15.1). Mature white cells have a limited life span so that constant bone

Understanding Laboratory Investigations: A Guide for Nurses, Midwives and Healthcare Professionals, Third Edition. Chris Higgins.
© 2013 John Wiley & Sons, Ltd. Published 2013 by John Wiley & Sons, Ltd.

marrow production is necessary throughout life. An increase in bone marrow production of white cells is part of the body's normal (inflammatory) response to any insult to the body (i.e. any tissue injury, whatever the cause). The purpose of the inflammatory response is to contain and control injury, to eliminate potential pathogens (bacteria, viruses, fungi, protozoa, parasitic worms) and initiate healing and tissue repair. As key players in the inflammatory response white cells must leave the blood and enter the tissues. Although, as we shall see, each type of white cell has a different and well-defined job to do in the overall process of inflammation, they operate in concert, communicating via a range of chemical messengers called cytokines.

Neutrophils

Comprising 40–70% of the total white cell population, the neutrophil is the most abundant of all white cells in blood. The mature neutrophil has a multi-lobed purple staining nucleus and dark blue staining granules in the cytoplasm. It has a diameter of about 15 μm, around twice that of a red cell. The function of these cells is to enter the tissues and kill invading bacteria. On release from the bone marrow, mature neutrophils spend only around eight hours in the blood stream and the rest of their four to five day maximum life span in the tissues. Chemicals called chemotactic factors released from bacteria and other cells (including basophils, macrophages and lymphocytes, explained further) attract neutropils to the site of tissue infection or inflammation. In the tissues, neutrophils surround and engulf bacteria by a process called phagocytosis (destruction). Once inside the neutrophil, bacteria are killed by the action of enzymes and highly reactive free radical chemicals produced within the darkly staining granules of the neutrophil cytoplasm. Pus, the yellowish fluid that oozes from some bacterially infected sites, is a visible reminder of neutrophil function. It is largely composed of dead and dying neutrophils, bacterial debris and other cellular detritus produced during the fight against infection caused by pyogenic bacteria.

Eosinophils

Although much fewer in number, comprising only 0.2–5% of total white cell population, eosinophils have similarities, both in appearance and function, to neutrophils. The nucleus of the eosinophil is like the neutrophil, lobed in appearance, though whereas the neutrophil nucleus is multi-lobed, the eosinophil nucleus has just two lobes. The granules of the eosinophil cytoplasm stain orange-red in contrast to the dark blue of the neutrophil, due to the presence of chemicals peculiar to the eosinophil. Like neutrophils, eosinophils are capable of phagocytosis, although it seems unlikely that they have a role in the killing of bacteria. Instead they target foreign material too large for normal neutrophil mediated phagocytosis. For example, they bind to parasitic worms and inflict damage by releasing enzymes, and then phagocytose the products of this enzymic destruction. Their main function then is protection against infection by organisms larger than bacteria and viruses. Eosinophils are recruited to the site of inflammation caused by allergic reactions, such as the airways of allergic asthma and hay fever sufferers. Chemicals released from 'activated' eosinophils at these sites contribute to the pathogenesis of allergic inflammatory disease.

Basophils

These are so few in number that they are only rarely seen during microscopical examination of blood. They have a multi-lobed nucleus that is hidden by dense dark blue staining granules. Basophils migrate into tissues where they mature to mast cells. When activated, mast cells release many chemical mediators of the inflammatory response, which include a chemotactic factor that attracts neutrophils, histamine a chemical which dilates blood vessels, increasing the blood flow to damaged areas, and heparin, an anticoagulant required to begin the process of repair to damaged blood vessels.

Monocytes

The monocyte is the largest blood cell and has a lobulated nucleus, with a usually clear (non-granulated) voluminous cytoplasm. After a short period of 20–40 hours circulating in the blood, these phagocytic cells migrate to the tissues where they mature to cells called macrophages. Macrophages phagocytose and kill foreign organisms in the same way that neutrophils do but have a second important role in processing and presenting foreign proteins or antigens (derived from bacteria etc.) to T-lymphocytes for initiation of a cell mediated immune response (discussed further). Macrophages also have an important physiological role in the controlled destruction of red cells when they are no longer viable. This is discussed in Chapter 15.

Lymphocytes

Between 20% and 40% of the circulating white cell population are lymphocytes; these are the second most abundant type of white cell in blood. Like all other blood cells they are derived from the bone marrow, but a proportion undergo further processing within the thymus; these are thymus dependent lymphocytes or T-lymphocytes, which comprise around 70% of all circulating lymphocytes. Most of the remaining 30% are B-lymphocytes. There is an additional small population of non-B, non T-lymphocytes called natural killer (NK) lymphocytes. The routine lymphocyte count is the sum of these three types.

Like all other white cells, lymphocytes are required for immunity (protection) from infection. B-lymphocytes differentiate to plasma cells, which produce antibodies. These are proteins that bind specifically with complementary proteins called antigens. Micro-organisms (bacteria, viruses etc.) all have specific surface proteins which act as antigens. Antibody binding of these surface antigens prevents bacteria and viruses from invading tissue cells. Furthermore antibody coated bacteria are much more easily phagocytosed (destroyed) by neutrophils and macrophages. Antibodies can also bind to, and thereby neutralise, bacterial toxins.

Although antibodies are effective in the process that leads to destruction of microbes outside cells, they cannot enter cells and therefore have no effect on the microbes harbouring within cells. The body's defence against these depends largely on NK- lymphocytes and T-lymphocytes.

T-lymphocytes can 'recognise' and destroy tissue cells that are infected, thereby preventing further spread. Since all viruses must infect cells in order to replicate, and many bacteria parasitise body cells, this so called cell mediated immunity invoked by the T-lymphocyte is a vital component of the body's defence against infection. T-lymphocytes (and NK-lymphocytes) also have the capacity to recognise and kill cancerous cells, so are part of the body's defence against cancer.

An important feature of lymphocyte mediated immunity, whether it be B-lymphocyte (i.e. antibody) mediated or T-lymphocyte (i.e. cell) mediated is that, unlike all other white blood cells, both classes of lymphocytes have the capacity to 'remember' an invading organism, so that the response to a subsequent encounter is greater and more rapid. This so called 'acquired' immunity explains why we seldom suffer more than once from a particular infection. First exposure provides increased immunity from subsequent infections with the same organism. The function of NK-lymphocytes is not dependant on this 'acquired' immunity mechanism, but in common with non-lymphocyte white blood cells (neutrophils, eosinophils, basophils and monocytes), they are part of what is known as the body's 'innate' immunity, that is the immunity we are born with.

Laboratory measurement of full blood count

Interpretation of WBC and diff results

Approximate reference ranges
Total white blood cell (WBC) count:
    Adult males $3.7–9.5\times10^9$/L
    Adult females $3.9–11.1\times10^9$/L
Differential white cell count:

Neutrophils (40–75% of total white cells)	$2.5–7.5\times10^9$/L
Lymphocytes (20–40% of total white cells)	$1.5–4.0\times10^9$/L
Monocytes (2–10% of total white cells)	$0.2–0.8\times10^9$/L
Eosinophils (1– 5 % of total white cells)	$0.04–0.44\times10^9$/L
Basophils (<1% of total white cells)	$0.01–0.10\times10^9$/L

At birth the total white cell count is very high ($9–26\times10^9$/L). This falls sharply to around $5–18\times10^9$/L during the first two months of life and to normal adult levels by 12–15 years of age.

Critical values

White blood cell count (WCC) $<2\times10^9$/L or $>30\times10^9$/L.

Terms used in interpreting results

Polymorphonuclear cells (polymorphs)	literally 'many shaped nucleus' cells, refers to all white blood cells with a lobed nucleus ie neutrophils, eosoinophils, and basophils. Lymphocytes and Monocytes are non-polymorphs because they have a more regular shaped nucleus.
Granulocytes	all white cells with visibly staining granules in the cytoplasm (i.e. neutrophils, eosinophils and basophils.) Lymphocytes and monocytes are non-granulocytes.
Agranulocytosis	complete or near absence of granulocytes in blood.
Phagocytes and non-phagocytes	phagocytes are cells that are able to phagocytose foreign material (bacteria etc.). Neutrophils, eosinophils, basophils and monocytes are all phagocytes. Lymphocytes do not have this ability; they are non-phagocytes.
Leucocytosis	an increase in total white cell count.
Neutrophilia, eosinophilia, basophilia	a selective increase in neutrophil, eosinophil and basophil count respectively.
Lymphocytosis	an increase in lymphocyte count.
Leucopaenia	a reduced total white cell count.
Neutropaenia	a reduced neutrophil count.
Lymphopaenia	a reduced lymphocyte count.
Pancytopaenia	a reduction in all blood cells (red cells, white cells and platelets).

Terms used to describe white cells when viewed under the microscope

Increase in band forms	band cells are slightly immature neutrophils recognisable by the non-segmented shape of the nucleus. Normally only 3% of total neutrophils in peripheral blood are of this sort. An increase implies the bone marrow is increasing white cell production in response to infection or inflammation.
Shift to left	an alternative term to 'increase in band cells' denoting increase in immature neutrophils in peripheral blood.
Blast cells	primitive white cells never normally seen in peripheral blood. Their presence almost always indicates an acute haematological malignancy (e.g. acute leukaemia).

Causes of an increase in total white cell numbers

General considerations

An increase in white cell numbers (leukocytosis) occurs most commonly as a result of infection, inflammation or indeed any significant tissue damage. Since the role of white cells is to defend the body against infection it is entirely appropriate that numbers should increase under these circumstances. This so called benign or reactive leukocytosis must be distinguished from the much less common and entirely inappropriate leukocytosis that may be a feature of haematological malignancies, including the leukaemias.

The leukaemias are a group of malignant diseases of the bone marrow, characterised by the unregulated proliferation of one sort (a clone) of immature white blood cell at the expense of normal blood cell production. Nearly all cases can be classified to one of four groups depending on whether the clinical course of the disease is rapid (acute) or slow (chronic) and whether the immature cancerous cells are derived from the myeloid bone marrow cells (which normally mature to neutrophils, eosinophils basophils or monocytes) or lymphoid bone marrow cells (which normally mature to lymphocytes). The four main types of leukaemia then are: acute myeloid leukaemia (AML), chronic myeloid leukaemia (CML), acute lymphoblastic leukaemia (ALL) and chronic lymphoid leukaemia (CLL). Some of the distinguishing features of the four sorts of leukaemia are outlined in Table 16.1. Since in all cases normal blood cell development is impaired, anaemia (due to deficiency of normal red cells), impaired blood coagulation with increased tendency to bleed (due to low platelet count) and high risk of infection (due to reduced numbers of normal white cells) can be features of all leukaemias.

Whether it be benign (reactive) or malignant, leukocytosis is usually the result of a predominant, although not necessarily entirely selective, increase in one of the five types of white cell. The differential count thus provides clues as to the cause of an increased total white cell count. A more detailed account of the cause of increased white cell numbers will be given focusing on each type of white cell in turn.

Causes of increased neutrophil count (neutrophilia)

Neutrophilia is the most common derangement of white cell numbers.

Reactive neutrophilia is a feature of:

- Most acute bacterial infections. Particularly high (up to 50×10^9/L) in pyogenic (pus forming) infections, e.g. those caused by *Staph* and *Strep* bacterial species.
- Non-infective acute inflammation (e.g. rheumatoid arthritis, inflammatory bowel disease etc.).
- Tissue damage (surgery, trauma, burns, myocardial infarction).
- Solid tumours, e.g. lung cancer (an appropriate response to the tissue necrosis (death) which accompanies tumour growth).
- Extreme physical exercise.
- Pregnancy and labour of pregnancy.

Table 16.1 Some features of the four main types of leukaemia.

In the context of all malignant disease leukaemia is rare, accounting for just 2% of all cancers. Close to 7500 new cases of leukaemia are diagnosed annually in the UK – around 80% of these can be attributed to one of the four main types

Acute myeloblastic leukaemia (AML)	Acute lymphoblastic leukaemia (ALL)	Chronic myeloid leukaemia (CML)	Chronic lymphocytic leukaemia (CLL)
Most common of the two types of acute leukaemia (around 2000 new cases in the UK each year). Can occur in childhood but most are more than 50 years at diagnosis.	Around 550 new cases each year In the UK – 80% of cases occur in children. Peak incidence at age 2–3 years. This is by far the most common type of leukaemia in childhood and is the most common childhood cancer.	Around 550 new cases each year in the UK – practically all adults. Rare in childhood. Incidence increases with advancing years – most aged more than 50 years at diagnosis.	Most common type of leukaemia – around 3600 new cases each year in the UK – nearly all adults. Incidence increases with advancing years – most aged more than 50 years at diagnosis.
French-American-British (FAB) classification based on appearance of abnormal white cells allows identification of eight sub-types (M0–M7).	French-American-British (FAB) classification based on appearance of abnormal white cells allows identification of three sub-types (L1–L3).	No FAB classification - no subtypes. CML differs from all other leukaemias in that a single genetic lesion (the abnormal 'Philadelphia' chromosome) is responsible in practically all cases.	No FAB classification.
Rapidly fatal without treatment.	Rapidly fatal without treatment.	Disease typically progresses slowly over a period of several years. Later a rapidly progressive (acute) phase may intervene.	Disease typically progresses slowly over a period of several years.
May or may not be acutely ill at the time of diagnosis. Symptoms include tiredness and lethargy due to anaemia. Fever/infection due to low numbers of mature functioning white cells. Bruising and increased tendency to bleed due to reduced platelets.	Typically acutely ill at the time of diagnosis. Symptoms include tiredness and lethargy due to anaemia. Fever/infection due to low numbers of mature functioning white cells. Bruising and increased tendency to bleed due to reduced platelets. Infiltration of central nervous system (CNS) is common, resulting in severe headache and vomiting.	Not usually acutely ill at the time of diagnosis - in fact often asymptomatic. Most common symptom is tiredness and breathlessness on exertion due to slowly progressive anaemia. Easy bruising due to reduced platelet numbers. There may be a history of weight loss and right sweats is common.	A significant minority (20–25%) are symptom free at the time of diagnosis when the disease is identified by chance FBC testing. This symptom free period may last for several years. Symptoms when they eventually occur similar to CML.

(Continued)

Table 16.1 (Cont'd)

In the context of all malignant disease leukaemia is rare, accounting for just 2% of all cancers. Close to 7500 new cases of leukaemia are diagnosed annually in the UK – around 80% of these can be attributed to one of the four main types

Acute myeloblastic leukaemia (AML)	Acute lymphoblastic leukaemia (ALL)	Chronic myeloid leukaemia (CML)	Chronic lymphocytic leukaemia (CLL)
Initial treatment is with chemotherapy delivered IV (combination of three cytotoxic dugs). Bone marrow (stem cell) transplantation may be considered. AML is a curable condition but cure rates are low (20–30%). Temporary remission from disease however is the norm. In general younger patients have a far better prognosis in terms of 5 year survival rates (50–60% in those aged less than 50 years and 5–10% in those aged >75 years)	Initial treatment with chemotherapy delivered IV (a combination of three or four cytotoxic drugs). Radiation therapy for CNS disease treatment or prevention. Bone marrow (stem cell) transplant considered if chemotherapy fails. The majority (80–90%) of affected children cured. Very young (those aged less than 1 year) and adults fair less well. Cure rates for these age groups closer to 30%.	First line drug treatment with a tyrosine-kinase inhibitor, usually Imatinib (Glivec) delivered orally. Bone marrow (stem cell) transplantation may be considered if this fails. Since introduction 10 years ago Imatinib and its relative drugs have greatly improved the prospects for patients. A small minority (10%) might actually be cured by this drug, and 90% survive with normal quality of life for at least seven years.	No treatment necessary until onset of symptoms. Chemotherapy/radiotherapy is standard treatment for those who need it. Bone marrow (stem cell) transplant may be appropriate for some patients in whom it can effect a cure. Prognosis highly variable. Some survive more than 20 years, others just a year.

Malignant cause of neutrophilia
Chronic myeloid leukaemia. The total white cell count is very high, usually greater than 50×10^9/L and sometimes up to 500×10^9/L. These cells are predominantly immature (of the myeloid series) with increased numbers of neutrophils.

Causes of increased lymphocyte count (lymphocytosis)
Reactive lymphocytosis is a feature of:

- Infectious mononucleosis (glandular fever). This acute infectious disease caused by the Epstein-Barr virus is the most common cause of an isolated marked lymphocytosis. Most cases occur among teenagers and young adults. Symptoms include sore throat, fever, extreme tiredness, nausea and headache. Swollen and tender lymph nodes of the throat and neck are usual. Lymphocyte count rises a few days after symptoms appear and may peak very high (in the range $10–30\times10^9$/L) before gradually returning to normal over the following month or two. The diagnosis is confirmed by the finding of a positive Paul-Bunnell test. This is a blood test designed to detect specific antibodies produced as a result of infection with the Epstein-Barr virus.
- Other less common viral infections that are usually associated with lymphocytosis include: cytomegalovirus, early stages of HIV infection, viral hepatitis, rubella, mumps and chicken pox.
- Chronic bacterial infection. Although bacterial infections are usually associated with neutrophilia rather than lymphocytosis, bacterial infections which are long standing (chronic) in nature are characterised by lymphocytosis. The most common chronic bacterial infection is tuberculosis.
- Other miscellaneous infections: whooping cough (caused by the bacteria *Bordetella pertussis*) and toxoplasmosis (caused by the protozoan, *Toxoplasma gondii*).

Malignant causes:

- Chronic lymphoblastic leukaemia. The total white cell count is usually raised (often very high, in the range $50–100\times10^9$/L). Most of these cells are mature (but non functional) lymphocytes. Severe lymphocytosis (i.e. $>50\times10^9$/L) in an older person is most likely due to CLL.
- Some cases of non-Hodgkin's lymphoma (a haematological malignant disease originating in lymph nodes).

Cause of increase in eosinophil count (eosinophilia)
Eosinophillia is much less common than either neutrophilia or lymphocytosis. Principle causes are:

- Parasitic worm infections (e.g. tapeworm, hookworm, strongyloides, schistosoma etc.).
- Allergic diseases (e.g. hay fever, eczema, allergic asthma, food sensitivity).
- Sometimes raised in Hodgkin's lymphoma.

Causes of increase in basophils and monocyte counts

An increase in the numbers of either of these cells is rare. Basophil numbers are raised in chronic myeloid leukaemia. Monocytosis may be a feature of TB, subacute bacterial endocarditis and other chronic bacterial infections.

Causes of a reduction in white cell numbers (leukopaenia)

General considerations

A reduction in total white cell numbers is much less common than an increase; it is never 'appropriate' in the same way an increase in white cell numbers often is. A reduced white cell count is almost always the result of decrease in either neutrophils or lymphocytes, or both.

Low neutrophil count (neutropaenia)

- A slight neutropaenia is a feature of some viral infections (mumps, influenza, viral hepatitis, HIV etc.). The combination of a low neutrophil count and raised lymphocyte count (see earlier) explains why in some viral illnesses the total white cell count may remain normal despite reduction in neutrophil numbers.
- Overwhelming bacterial infection. In rare cases of extreme infection the bone marrow is unable to replace neutrophils at a sufficiently rapid rate.
- Aplastic anaemia, a condition of damage to, or defect of, bone marrow stem cells and consequent marked reduction in blood cell production. The condition is associated with not only potentially life threatening severe neutropaenia, but failure to produce adequate numbers of all blood cell types (red cells, white cells and platelets). The condition can arise as a result of an inherited (genetic) defect or much more commonly is acquired by exposure to any one of a range of drugs, some chemical (organic) toxins or some viruses. Over exposure to radiation (including that used therapeutically and diagnostically) can cause aplastic anaemia.
- Acute leukaemia – malignant blood cells proliferate at the expense of normal blood cell development, with resulting neutropaenia.
- Many solid malignant tumours spread (metastasise) to the bone where they infiltrate and suppress normal bone marrow blood cell production. Neutropaenia may therefore be a feature of advanced cancer.

Causes of reduced lymphocyte count

- AIDS. Human immunodeficiency virus (HIV-1), which causes AIDS, exerts its devastating effects by specifically infecting T-lymphocytes. The virus replicates within T-lymphocytes causing cell death, so that AIDS is characterised by progressive T-lymphocyte destruction and resulting lymphocytopaenia.
- Autoimmune destruction of lymphocytes is the cause of the lymphocytopaenia, which is a common feature of systemic lupus erythematosus (SLE).
- A slight decrease in lymphocyte numbers often accompanies some acute inflammatory conditions; examples include pancreatitis, appendicitis and Crohn's disease.
- Influenza virus infection.
- Burns, surgery and severe trauma.

• A profound deficiency of lymphocytes is a feature of several very rare congenital disorders discovered at birth. These include DiGeorge's syndrome in which, due to failure of thymus development, babies are born with no T-lymphocytes. A lack of both B- and T-lymphocytes is a feature of severe combined immunodeficiency syndrome (SCID).

Clinical consequences of abnormal white cell numbers

Increased bone marrow production of white cells is a component of the body's normal inflammatory response to injury and infection, so that an increase in white cell numbers is physiological and usually has no deleterious consequences. In some cases of leukaemia however, the white cell count rises so high ($>100 \times 10^9$/L) that the sheer numbers of white cells reduces the fluidity of blood, making it more viscous. This condition known as hyperleukocytosis is associated with sludging of white cells in the microvasculature of any organ tissue, compromising blood flow; it is a life threatening medical emergency.

A reduction in white cell numbers leaves affected patients at risk of infection. This becomes clinically evident as neutrophil count drops below 1×10^9/L, when bacterial infections of the mouth and throat particularly occur. Without adequate numbers of protective neutrophils these infections fail to resolve, causing ulceration. Those with neutrophil counts of less than 0.5×10^9/L are at high risk of death from uncontrolled bacterial infection. Even normally harmless bacteria, present on the skin or in the environment, pose a serious threat to life for these patients; who require careful barrier nursing to minimise the risk of infection.

A severe reduction in lymphocyte numbers compromises the immune response leaving affected patients also at high risk of infection from bacterial, viral and fungal infection. The life threatening opportunistic infections and rare cancers commonly suffered by HIV/AIDS patients prior to effective antiviral therapy, are a result of severe reduction in T-lymphocyte numbers.

Case history 22

James Herron, a 14 year old boy, was admitted to the local hospital A&E department, via his GP with severe central abdominal pain. James had been vomiting before admission and was slightly pyrexial (temp 38°C) on admission. Physical examination and symptoms suggested that James was suffering acute appendicitis. The admitting doctor sampled blood for urgent U&E and FBC.

The following FBC results were telephoned to A&E, 30 minutes later.

Hb	13.1 g/L
PCV	42%
RBC	5.1×10^{12}/L
WBC (total)	18.1×10^9/L
Neutrophils	12.8×10^9/L
Lymphocytes	2×10^9/L
Monocytes	0.7×10^9/L
Eosinophils	0.2×10^9/L
Basophils	$<0.1 \times 10^9$/L

Questions

(1) Are there any abnormalities in these results?

(2) Would you expect abnormalities in FBC results in a patient with acute appendicitis?

Discussion of case history 22

(1) Yes. There are two abnormal results. James has a slightly raised total white cell count due to an increase in neutrophil numbers (neutrophilia).

(2) Yes. Appendicitis is acute inflammation of the appendix. Any active inflammatory disease process is likely to be associated with an increase in neutrophil numbers. Such an increase is found in the vast majority of cases of acute appendicitis and therefore provides further evidence to support the provisional diagnosis made on the basis of physical examination, reported history and symptoms. A slight decrease in lymphocyte numbers is also sometimes a feature of acute appendicitis.

Further reading

Borregard, N. (2010) Neutrophils, from marrow to microbes, *Immunity*, **33**: 657–70.

Christenson, R., Henry, E., Jopling, J. et al. (2009) The CBC: reference ranges for neonates, *Seminars in Perinatology*, **33**: 3–11.

Hoffbrand, A. and Moss, P. (2011) *Essential Haematology*, 6th edn, Wiley-Blackwell.

CHAPTER 17

TESTS OF HAEMOSTASIS: PLATELET COUNT, PROTHROMBIN TIME (PT), ACTIVATED PARTIAL THROMBOPLASTIN TIME (APPT),THROMBIN TIME (TT) AND D-DIMER

Key learning topics

- Defining haemostasis
- Platelets and their role in haemostasis
- The blood clotting cascade – its role in haemostasis
- Fibrinolysis and D-dimer production
- What is being measured in the prothrombin time test
- Causes/consequences of increased platelet count
- Causes/consequences of decreased platelet count
- Venous thromboembolism (VTE) and its prevention
- Role of D-dimer test in diagnosis of VTE

Blood loss following blood vessel injury is minimised by the capacity of blood to form a physical plug at the site of the vessel injury. The complex physiological process that ensures this life preserving property of blood is called haemostasis. Blood must retain its ability to quickly form a physical plug of coagulated blood at the site of vessel injury, preventing undue blood loss, whilst remaining fluid and free of coagulated blood within undamaged vessels. Disturbance of this fine balance, a feature of many disease processes, can result in either an increased tendency to bleed if the coaguablity of blood is less than normal, or formation of a blood clot (thrombus) within patent undamaged blood vessels, if coagulability is abnormally increased.

Understanding Laboratory Investigations: A Guide for Nurses, Midwives and Healthcare Professionals, Third Edition. Chris Higgins.

Four of the five blood tests discussed in this chapter, platelet count, prothrombin time (PT), activated partial thromboplastin time (APPT) and thromboplastin time (TT) are primarily used in the first line investigation of patients who are suspected of suffering disease associated with an increased tendency to bleed, whilst the D-dimer test is used in the assessment of patients suspected of suffering thrombotic disease, that is disease associated with increased tendency of blood to coagulate and form thrombi inappropriately within patent blood vessels.

Patients suffering, or at high risk of suffering, thrombotic disease are treated with anticoagulant drugs that artificially decrease the coagulability of blood. Two of the blood tests considered in this chapter, prothrombin time (PT) and activated partial thromboplastin time (APPT) are routinely used to monitor this anticoagulant therapy.

Normal physiology

The sequence of events that leads to formation of a stable fibrin plug and cessation of bleeding (haemostasis) following blood vessel injury is described in Figure 17.1.

The first physiological response to blood vessel injury is local vasoconstriction, which reduces blood flow to the injured site thereby minimizing to some extent blood loss. Vessel injury also initiates two further physiological responses. The first is platelet adhesion and aggregation with formation of a physical plug of platelets at the site of vessel injury, and the second is initiation of the so called clotting cascade which results in production of the structural protein, fibrin. Fibrin strands join together (polymerise) and the fibrin polymers cross-link. The effect is a growing linked mesh of fibrin forming around and between aggregating platelets, which both stabilizes and gives mechanical strength to the somewhat fragile platelet plug.

Normal haemostasis is crucially dependent then on two factors:

- adequate numbers of normally functioning platelets and
- normally functioning blood clotting cascade.

In order to understand the defects of haemostasis associated with disease and how the results of the five blood tests are applied, it is helpful to examine platelets and the clotting cascade in a little detail.

Platelet production, structure and function

Like the other formed elements or cells that circulate in blood, platelets (alternative name thrombocytes) are derived from the stem cells of the bone marrow (see Chapter 15, Figure 15.1). A proportion of stem cells differentiate by stages within the bone marrow to megakaryocytes. Platelets are produced within the cytoplasm of these cells. Still within the bone marrow, platelets are released from mature megakaryocytes and pass from bone marrow to blood. Each megakaryocyte produces around

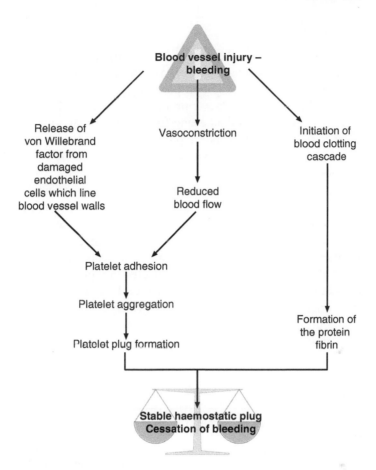

Figure 17.1 Overview of haemostasis.

4000 platelets. Platelets have a lifespan of just ten days in blood so that constant bone marrow production is necessary. With a diameter of 1–2 mm, platelets are far smaller than either red cells or white cells. Like mature red cells, they have no nucleus.

The principle function of platelets is to plug 'holes' in vessel walls caused during injury. The first stage in this process is adhesion of platelets to the wall of the damaged vessel. This adhesion is facilitated in part by a protein called von Willebrand factor, which is released from injured endothelial cells that line the internal surface of blood vessels. Adhesion proteins present on the surface of passing platelets bind to von Willebrand factor which itself is bound to proteins present on the surface of damaged endothelial cells. Following adhesion, platelets secrete many substances that modulate both the clotting cascade (explained further) and further platelet function. Among these are substances (e.g. ADP and thromboxane A_2) which both induce platelets to stick to each other (aggregate) and swell in size. This process, called aggregation, continues until the mass of aggregated swollen platelets is sufficiently large to plug the damaged vessel.

Blood clotting cascade

As platelets are aggregating at the site of vessel injury, fibrin is being produced locally by the blood clotting (coagulation) cascade. This is a series of reactions in which specific proteins present in blood plasma, called clotting factors, are activated in sequence. Each activated factor promotes activation of the next and so on down the cascade; the final product being fibrin. These reactions are enzymic in nature. In their inactive state factors are pro-enzymes (i.e. have no enzymic activity). Enzymic action converts proenzymes (unactivated factors) to active enzymes (activated factors). Whilst most clotting factors are pro-enzymes/enzymes, some are not actually enzymes but substances that are required for some enzymic actions to occur. Thirteen clotting factors (Table 17.1) have been identified, numbered by convention in Roman numerals in the order in which they were first discovered. The once postulated Factor VI is no longer thought to exist.

The convention is that activated factors are distinguished from their inactive counterparts by the subscript 'a' and this is reflected in Figure 17.2, which is a simplified account of current understanding of the blood clotting cascade. The cascade comprises the intrinsic and extrinsic pathway, which both result in activation of Factor X. The route from activated Factor X to fibrin production is referred to as the common pathway.

Table 17.1 Blood clotting factors.

Factor	Alternative name(s)	Notes
Factor I	Fibrinogen	Precursor of fibrin – synthesised in the liver
Factor II	Prothrombin	Pro-enzyme – synthesised in the liver
Factor III	Tissue factor Tissue thrombloblastin	Protein present in all tissues
Factor IV	Calcium	Inorganic ion co-factor
Factor V	Labile factor	Protein co-factor synthesised in the liver
Factor VI	Once proposed but no longer thought to exist	
Factor VII	Proconvertin Stable factor	Pro-enzyme – synthesised in the liver
Factor VIII	Antihaemophilic factor	Protein – co-factor
Factor IX	Christmas factor	Pro-enzyme – synthesised in the liver
Factor X	Stuart factor	Pro-enzyme – synthesised in the liver
Factor XI	Plasma thromboplastin antecedent	Pro-enzyme
Factor XII	Hageman factor Contact factor	Pro-enzyme
Factor XIII	Fibrin stabilising factor	Pro-enzyme

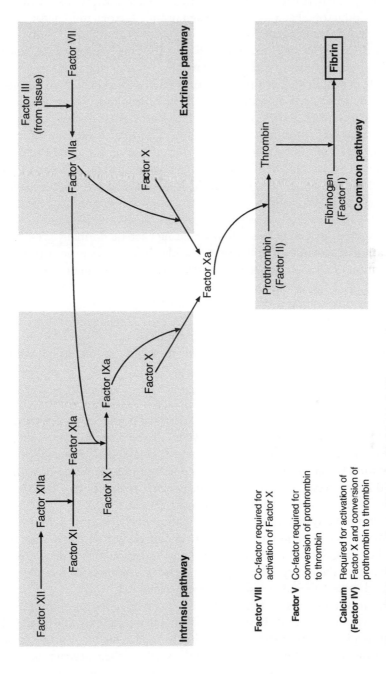

Figure 17.2 Generation of fibrin by the blood clotting cascade.

The intrinsic pathway is initiated when Factor XII is activated by contact with proteins within blood vessel endothelial cells, that are exposed as a result of vessel wall injury. Activated Factor XII then activates Factor XI, which in turn activates Factor X. Co-factors, Factor VIII (antihaemophilic factor) and Factor IV (calcium) are required for this last reaction.

The extrinsic pathway is initiated by Factor III. This is a substance called thromboplastin, found in most tissues and released to blood during tissue injury. Factor III activates Factor VII, which in turn activates Factor IX. In the final common pathway, activated Factor X activates Factor II (prothrombin) to the active thrombin, which in turn converts fibrinogen (Factor I) to fibrin. Factor V is a cofactor required for conversion of prothrombin to thrombin. The final formation of cross-linked fibrin polymers from fibrin (monomers) is dependent on activated Factor XIII.

Most of the factors of the blood clotting cascade including Factor I (fibrinogen), Factor II (Prothrombin), Factors V, VII, IX, X, XI and XII are synthesised in the liver and released to blood in their inactive form. The liver synthesis of Factors II (prothrombin), VII, IX and X is crucially dependent on vitamin K. Vitamin K is derived from two sources, diet and vitamin K synthesising bacteria normally present in the gut.

Formation of fibrin by the clotting cascade depends then on adequate plasma concentration of **all** clotting factors, which in turn is dependent on:

- Normally functioning liver (for their synthesis).
- Adequate dietary source of vitamin K.
- Normal bacterial flora in the gastrointestinal tract.
- Normal gastrointestinal absorption of dietary and non-dietary vitamin K.

Breakup of a blood clot – fibrinolysis

The fibrin-platelet 'plug' is a temporary structure produced in response to blood vessel injury to limit blood loss. It must eventually be degraded for healing to occur. A process called fibrinolysis is responsible for this degradation. Fibrinolysis also serves to limit fibrin clot growth so that it does not impede blood flow through the damaged blood vessel, and also limits the growth of tiny fibrin clots that are continuously being formed in patent undamaged vessels.

The fibrinolytic system thus keeps coagulation in check. It is useful to reflect that the fibrin clot is a dynamic structure in a state of growth or dissolution depending on whether coagulation or fibrinolysis is in ascendancy. When the clot is no longer needed because the injury is healing, or if a clot is beginning to form in an undamaged blood vessel, fibrinolysis should be in ascendancy.

Central to the process of fibrinolysis is a protein called plasminogen, which is synthesised in the liver and circulates in blood. Here it binds to fibrin, thereby being incorporated into a fibrin clot as it is being formed. This incorporation of plasminogen means that all blood clots contain the seeds of their destruction.

In common with factors of the clotting cascade, plasminogen is an inactive proenzyme so has no effect within the clot until it is converted in a controlled manner to the active enzyme, plasmin. On activation, plasmin enzymically cleaves the cross-linked fibrin polymers. The product of plasmin action is a heterogenous collection of cleaved fragments of fibrin that are swept in the blood stream from the currently dissolving fibrin clot. The cleaved fragments are collectively called fibrin degradation products (FDP), and among them is one kind of FDP called D-dimer, so called because it comprises two linked fragments (a dimer) from a part of the fibrin molecule called the D domain. Because they retain the cross linking that is peculiar to the structure of the fibrin within a fibrin clot, the presence of D-dimer in blood is objective evidence of current fibrin clot formation/degradation.

Laboratory measurement of platelet count, PT, APPT, TT and D-dimer

A platelet count is one of the tests included in a FBC. Laboratory measurement and sample requirements for FBC are discussed in Chapter 15. This section is concerned only with PT, APPT, TT and D-dimer.

Patient preparation

No particular patient preparation is necessary.

Timing of sample

Blood for PT, APPT, TT and D-dimer may be sampled at any time. However the proteins of the clotting cascade are not well preserved in a blood sample and falsely abnormal PT, APPT and TT results can occur if blood is not tested within four to six hours of sampling. This period can be extended to 15 hours if the sample is stored in a refrigerator at 4°C. Samples more than 15 hours old are not suitable for analysis.

Sample requirements

The tests are performed on plasma, the fluid that remains when all cellular elements are removed from anticoagulated blood. The blood must be collected into a tube containing the anticoagulant sodium citrate (usually a light blue top), which also preserves blood clotting proteins (factors). The volume required (usually 5 ml) is indicated on the bottle; it is important that neither more nor less than the volume indicated is added to the bottle. Gentle inversion to mix blood with the anticoagulant is essential. It is inadvisable to sample blood for these tests via an indwelling catheter, since heparin flushes are often used to keep these lines patent; falsely abnormal results will be obtained if blood samples are contaminated with heparin.

What do tests of blood coagulation measure?

Whilst it is clear that a platelet count is simply a measure of the number of platelets present in blood and the D-dimer test is a measure of the concentration of the protein D-dimer in blood plasma, it might be less obvious what is being measured by the three other tests considered in this chapter. Prothrombin time (PT), activated partial thromboplastin time (APPT) and thrombin time (TT) all test the ability of blood to generate fibrin by the blood clotting cascade. In essence, they all measure the time taken for a sample of patient's blood plasma to form a fibrin clot in a test tube, after addition of a reagent that initiates the clotting cascade. Results are expressed in time (seconds). In the case of the prothrombin time test, commercially produced thromboplastin (Factor III) is added to the patient's plasma. This is the clotting factor that initiates the extrinsic pathway, so that prothrombin time is a test specifically of the extrinsic and common pathways; a deficiency of any factor or factors of these two pathways (i.e. Factors X, VII, V, prothrombin and fibrinogen) will result in an abnormally prolonged time for a fibrin clot to form (i.e. PT will be raised).

In a similar way, by adding only an initiator of the intrinsic pathway to patient's plasma, the APPT tests only the intrinsic and common pathways. In this case, an abnormally prolonged result indicates a deficiency of one or more of those factors required by the intrinsic and common pathways.

Finally, for the thrombin time test, thrombin is added to patient's plasma. This is a test specifically of the final stages of the common pathway: fibrinogen to fibrin. An abnormally prolonged thrombin test indicates a deficiency of Factor I (fibrinogen).

So long as PT, APPT and TT are all normal, it can be assumed that there is a sufficiency of all coagulation (clotting) factors in the patient's blood. As such, the normal results provide evidence that in the event of vessel injury the clotting cascade would work normally and perform its haemostatic function adequately.

Interpretation of results

Approximate reference ranges

Platelet count	$150-400 \times 10^9$/L
Prothrombin time (PT)	10–14 seconds
Activated Partial Thromboplastin Time (APPT)	30–40 seconds
Thrombin Time (TT)	14–16 seconds
D-dimer	<500 ng/ml

[Caution: The D-dimer reference range varies greatly due to significant differences in methodology between laboratories.]

Critical values

Platelet Count	$<40 \times 10^9$/L or $>1000 \times 10^9$/L
Prothrombin Time	>30 seconds
Activated Partial Thromboplastin Time	>78 seconds

Terms used in interpretation

Thrombocytes	alternative name for platelet.
Thrombocytopaenia	reduced platelet count, that is $<150 \times 10^9/L$.
Thrombocytosis	increased platelet count, that is $>400 \times 10^9/L$.
Thrombosis	formation of a blood clot within a blood vessel.
Haemophilia	a pathological state of decreased blood coagulability and therefore increased tendency to bleed.
Thrombophilia	a pathological state of increased blood coagulability and therefore increased tendency to form blood clots (thrombi) inappropriately within patent blood vessels.

Causes of decreased platelet count

Reduction in platelet numbers can be caused by:

- Reduced bone marrow production of platelets.
- Increased rate of platelet destruction.
- Increased rate of platelet consumption.

Reduced bone marrow production of platelets and resulting severe decrease in platelet numbers (may be less than $50 \times 10^9/L$) is a feature of aplastic anaemia, acute leukaemia, cytotoxic drug therapy and radiotherapy. Megaloblastic anaemia, that is anaemia invariably caused by deficiency of vitamins B12 or folate (Chapter 18), is also associated with decreased bone marrow production of platelets, although not usually severe. Secondary spread of primary cancer to the bone marrow can result in reduced platelet production so that a reduced platelet count is sometimes a feature of advanced cancer.

Immune thrombocytopaenic purpura (ITP) is the most common cause of **increased platelet destruction**. This relatively common disorder, which affects both adults and children but predominantly middle aged/elderly women, results from production of autoantibodies against a patient's platelets. The cause of this autoantibody production is not known. In most cases the condition arises in otherwise well individuals, but it can be a secondary complication of some other primary disorder; these include systemic lupus erythematosus (SLE), infection with HIV and chronic lymphocytic leukaemia. Autoantibodies bind to platelets resulting in their premature removal and destruction within the reticuloendothelial system. Platelet lifespan is reduced from the normal ten days to just a few hours in this condition. Bone marrow production cannot keep pace with this rate of destruction and the reduction in platelet numbers is severe, in the range $10–50 \times 10^9/L$. A similar mechanism (antibody-mediated platelet destruction) is the cause of the reduced platelet count that sometimes complicates recovery from some viral infections (e.g. chicken pox and measles) in childhood.

Increased platelet consumption is a feature of disseminated intravascular coagulation (DIC), a not uncommon complication of many serious/critical conditions including: sepsis; severe tissue damage sustained during trauma or major surgery; obstetric emergencies such as pre-eclampsia/eclampsia and placental abruption; and incompatible blood transfusion. DIC is characterised by abnormal (inappropriate) activation of clotting cascade and platelet aggregation within blood vessels (i.e. thrombosis). The result is depletion of both platelets and clotting factors leaving these already very sick patients at risk of severe, even fatal, haemorrhage. The micro-thrombi formed during DIC may block blood vessels causing widespread ischaemic damage that may be sufficiently severe for progress to multi-organ failure.

The anticoagulant heparin and many other commonly used drugs can induce production of destructive antibodies directed at platelets with resulting increased platelet destruction. Drugs that may result in a reduction in platelet numbers include some anti-inflammatories, antibiotics (penicillin, suphonamide) and some diuretics (frusemide, acetazolamide).

Causes of increased platelet count

An increase in platelet numbers, termed thrombocytosis, is a feature of those malignant disorders of the bone marrow, collectively called the myeloproliferative disorders that are characterised by abnormal proliferation of myeloid stem cells. The myeloproliferative disorders in which an increase in platelet numbers can be expected include chronic myeloid leukaemia (around a third of all cases), polycythaemia vera (around a half of all cases) and essential thrombocythaemia (all cases).

A mild to moderate increase in platelet numbers (usually between 400 and 1000×10^9/L) is a relatively common phenomenon among acutely ill patients. The raised platelet count reflects bone marrow stimulation induced by blood loss, infection or tissue injury. It is termed secondary thrombocytosis to distinguish it from the thrombocytosis due to the primary bone marrow diseases already described. The conditions that might be associated with secondary thrombocytosis include: severe tissue injury due to major surgery or trauma; acute and chronic infection; malignancy; chronic inflammatory conditions such as rheumatoid arthritis or Crohn's disease and chronic iron deficiency anaemia.

Surgical removal of the spleen (where platelets are normally sequestered when they are no longer viable), results in particularly high platelet count.

Consequences of abnormality in platelet numbers

Since platelets are required for normal haemostasis, patients with a reduced platelet count are at increased risk of excessive bleeding. Spontaneous bleeding may occur if platelet count falls below 50×10^9/L. Potentially fatal haemorrhage almost inevitably occurs if count falls below 5×10^9/L. An increased tendency to bleed due to platelet deficiency has several clinical manifestations, including increased menstrual blood loss (menorrhagia), easy or even spontaneous bruising, bleeding gums, nose bleeds (epistaxis), petechial (tiny pinpoint) haemorrhages into the skin giving a red rash like appearance and purpura. Widespread purple/brown discoloration of skin (ecchymosis), akin to bruising, occurs due to haemorrhage into tissues.

An increase in platelet numbers carries with it the theoretical risk of increased coagulability of blood (thrombophilia) and resulting thrombosis. In practice this risk of thrombosis is certainly not real until platelet count rises well in excess of $1000 \times 10^9/L$ and in any case a direct link between severe thrombocytosis and increased risk of thrombosis is disputed.

Causes of increased PT, APPT and TT

An increase in any of these tests indicates a deficiency of one or more clotting factors. Deficiency may be congenital (i.e. inherited) or, much more commonly, acquired as a result of disease or anticoagulant drug therapy.

Haemophilia A, which accounts for around 85% of all the many known inherited blood clotting defects, is the most common inherited blood clotting deficiency. The defect is in the gene that codes for production of Factor VIII (also called anti-haemophilia factor). This is the co-factor required for activation of Factor X by Factor IXa (Figure 17.2). The result of the genetic defect is a marked deficiency or complete absence of Factor VIII and severely impaired blood clotting. Without Factor VIII replacement therapy, affected patients are at risk of life-threatening haemorrhage. Chronic episodic bleeding into joints and resulting joint pain and deformity can lead to permanent disability for those not treated effectively. The extrinsic and common pathways are intact in the patient with haemophilia A so that PT and TT are normal. APPT (a test of the intrinsic pathway) however is abnormally prolonged. Haemophilia B (Christmas disease), a less common but equally devastating inherited defect of the clotting cascade in which the deficiency is of Factor IX rather than Factor VIII, also causes raised APPT.

Since many clotting factors are synthesised in the liver, multiple factor deficiency is a feature of liver disease (acute and chronic hepatitis, cirrhosis etc.). PT, APPT and TT may all be increased in severe liver disease, although a raised TT is less usual. Of the three, PT is the most sensitive marker of liver disease and is routinely used as a test of liver function both in its detection and to monitor progress.

The production of several factors of both the intrinsic and extrinsic pathway is dependent on vitamin K, so that deficiency of vitamin K is associated with an increase in both PT and APPT. Newborn babies are at risk of vitamin K deficiency, and thereby a bleeding abnormality called haemorrhagic disease of the newborn. This provides the rationale for the routine prophylactic administration of vitamin K to babies at the time of birth.

Adult vitamin K deficiency usually only arises as result of impaired absorption from the gastrointestinal tract. Absorption of the fat-soluble vitamin K is dependent on the bile salts contained in bile so that diseases that may be associated with poor absorption of vitamin K include those that result in obstruction of the bile tract (e.g. gall stones, cancer of the head of pancreas) and pancreatitis.

Dietary deficiency of vitamin K may occur in malnourished adults. Antibiotic use can be associated with deficiency because it affects the balance of normal gut flora, and therefore bacterial production of vitamin K. Whatever the cause, vitamin K deficiency is associated with an increase in PT and APPT; TT is normal.

Consumption and resulting deficiency of several clotting factors is a feature of the abnormal coagulation within blood vessels that characterises DIC (already discussed). PT, APPT and TT are all raised in DIC; the increase in TT is particularly marked.

Clotting factors are not well preserved in stored blood so that those patients who receive massive blood transfusion (i.e. total blood volume replaced) are paradoxically at increased risk of haemorrhage because the blood that is being transfused is relatively deficient of clotting factors. Increased PT, APPT and TT may all be evident in the patient who has received massive blood transfusion.

Consequences of increased PT, APPT AND TT

An increase in any or all of these tests implies a deficiency of one or more clotting factors, reduced blood coagulability and therefore a greater than normal risk of excessive bleeding.

Causes of increased D-dimer

Since, as already discussed, D-dimers are a product of thrombus degradation it is to be expected that markedly increased D-dimer concentration is a feature of thrombotic disease. Additionally, D-dimer is raised – often to a lesser extent – in a range of other diseases, in which for one reason or another, blood is in an abnormally pro-coagulant state. The list of common conditions associated with increased D-dimer is thus long (Table 17.2) and it is not difficult, after consideration of this list, to appreciate that the majority of hospitalised patients have increased D-dimer.

The D-dimer test has proven of greatest value in the assessment of patients suspected of suffering two common related thrombotic diseases: deep vein thrombosis (DVT) and pulmonary embolism (PE), which together are known as venous thromboembolism (VTE). Before addressing the way D-dimer is used in the diagnosis of VTE, we will consider the condition itself and the national co-ordinated strategy aimed at its prevention. Prevention of VTE is now considered an imperative of safe patient care that is led by specialist nurses and involves most hospital nurses[1].

Venous thromboembolism (VTE)

Although thrombi (blood clots) can form in any part of the venous system, the most common site for clinically significant thrombi formation is in the deep veins that pass through the muscles of the legs. Typically, DVT originates in the veins of the calf muscles. The thrombus may be asymptomatic and resolve without clinical effect due to the physiological 'clot busting' action of the fibrinolytic system already described.

Alternatively, a DVT may persist and grow causing symptoms that include calf muscle pain and tenderness, along with swelling and reddening of the affected area.

Table 17.2 Non-exhaustive list of conditions that can be associated with increased D-dimer.

Arterial thrombotic diseases
Myocardial infarction (MI)
Stroke
Limb ischaemia
Atrial fibrillation

Venous thrombotic disease
Deep vein thrombosis (DVT)
Pulmonary embolism (PE)

Other
Disseminated intravascular coagulation (DIC)
Severe infection/sepsis
Severe inflammation
Systemic inflammatory response syndrome (SIRS)
Surgery/trauma (extensive tissue damage)
Sickle cell crisis
Cancer (any malignant disease)
Acute kidney disease (AKI)
End stage renal disease
Aortic dissecting aneurysm
Heart failure
Severe liver disease (cirrhosis)
Pre-eclampsia and eclampsia
Normal pregnancy
Use of thrombolytic drugs

DVTs can extend proximally up the venous system to the knee, thigh and pelvis causing pain and so on at these sites. The larger the thrombus grows, and the further it extends, the greater is the risk of the potentially life-threatening consequence of DVT, PE.

PE occurs in patients with DVT when a thrombus or thrombus fragment breaks free and is swept away in the venous system to the right side of the heart, and onwards via the pulmonary artery to the vasculature of the lungs, where it eventually becomes lodged at some point in the pulmonary arterial tree, obstructing blood flow to a portion of lung. Technically, a thrombus or thrombus fragment that moves from its original site is called an embolus or more accurately a thromboembolus, and the process of movement through the vascular system is called thromboembolism.

The consequences of PE are variable and depend to a great extent on the site of the pulmonary vascular blockage, that is the area of lung that is deprived of blood by the blockage. Worst case scenario involves an embolus sufficiently large to block a major pulmonary artery with resulting extensive pulmonary infarction, cardiovascular collapse and sudden death before treatment (clot busting drugs) can be administered. This is rare (only around 5% of PE cases result in sudden death).

More commonly in patients with PE, a medium or small pulmonary vessel is blocked. PE signs and symptoms include: sudden onset of breathlessness, coughing up blood (haemoptysis), chest pain, cyanosis and hypotension. In any particular patient the presence and severity of these symptoms will broadly reflect the size of the area of lung that is inadequately perfused. Occlusion of very small pulmonary vessels may have no symptomatic effect, so that PE can be clinically silent.

Current understanding of the pathophysiology of VTE is based on the notion that thrombi form in veins for one or more of three reasons, collectively known as Virchow's triad. They are:

- Reduced blood flow (slow blood flow promotes clot formation).
- Increased blood coagulability.
- Injury or disease mediated damage to the endothelium that lines the internal surface of blood vessels.

The relative importance of each of these three causative factors for development of VTE varies between individuals. Virchow's triad helps to explain some of the many known risk factors that predispose to, or provoke, VTE (Table 17.3).

So, for example, one of the most widely publicised provoking triggers for VTE is long-haul air travel. This particular VTE risk factor arises from travellers having to sit for prolonged periods and the resulting immobilisation reducing blood flow up the veins of the leg. Blood clots (thrombi) are more likely to form in blood that is flowing sluggishly (first element of Virchow's triad), so this explains why long-haul air travellers are at higher than normal risk of DVT. The risk is greater for those immobilised long-haul air travellers who are among the 1 in 20 of the population who also have an inherited defect (e.g. Factor V Leiden) that increases the coagulability of blood (second element of Virchow's triad) or have recently suffered trauma or disease that has damaged the endothelium of blood vessels (third element of Virchow's triad).

Given the long list of possible risk factors, the cause of VTE varies greatly between patients, but in one way or another Virchow's triad is usually always satisfied.

VTE prevention

The extent of the health problem posed by VTE was highlighted in a House of Commons report published in 2005[2] which revealed that PE following DVT was responsible for close to 30 000 deaths in hospital each year in the UK, which represents 10% of all hospital deaths. With acknowledgement that treatment strategies directed at preventing VTE are highly effective, most of these deaths were judged to be preventable. The report sparked a nationally co-ordinated strategy for VTE prevention that is now being implemented.

Recently published national guidelines for VTE prevention[3] recommend that all patients admitted to hospital be assessed for risk of VTE at the time of admission. All those judged to be at risk as a result of this assessment should be treated to prevent VTE. There are broadly two kinds of preventative treatments: mechanical and pharmaceutical. Mechanical VTE prophylaxis involves the use of compression stockings or similar device that promote blood flow through the veins of the leg (this is addressing the first of Virchow's triad). Pharmaceutical prophylaxis – which addresses the second of Virchow's triad – involves the use of an anticoagulant drug (heparin or

Table 17.3   Risk factors that predispose to, and provoke venous thromboembolism (VTE).

Chronic Predisposing Factors

Inherited defects that increase blood coagulability

Factor V (Leiden)

This is an inherited defect in the gene that codes for production of clotting Factor V. The resulting abnormal Factor V is not effectively degraded so its action persists inappropriately, leading to excessive growth of fibrin clots. This defect is common, affecting 5% of the population and is significant in close to a third of all VTE cases.

Factor II (G20210A mutation)

This is an inherited defect in the gene that codes for production of Factor II (prothrombin). It results in excessive production of prothrombin and thereby excessive growth of fibrin clots. Affects around 2–3% of population

Inherited deficiency of natural anticoagulant proteins

The normal function of these blood borne proteins is to inhibit specific steps of the clotting cascade and thereby control fibrin clot formation. This control is lost in those with these individually rare inherited protein deficiencies.

Acquired predisposing factors

- increasing age
- obesity
- lupus anticoagulant
- varicose veins
- cancer
- oestrogen therapy (oral contraceptives, HRT)
- chronic medical conditions (e.g. heart failure, COPD)
- previous VTE episode

Acute triggers – provoking factors

- surgery, particularly orthopaedic surgery
- hospitalisation (bed bound (immobilised))
- trauma (particularly that involving fracture of leg or pelvis)
- intravascular device, e.g. venous catheter
- long haul travel (immobilised)
- acute medical conditions (e.g. myocardial infarction, severe infection)
- pregnancy

---

heparin derivative) that artificially decreases the coagulability of blood. This is contraindicated for patients at high risk of bleeding, so all patients at risk of VTE should also have an assessment of bleeding risk before pharmaceutical prophylaxis is administered. The guidelines[3] include the detail of how risk should be assessed, as well as the detailed application of both kinds of prophylactic treatment to specific patient groups, and other more general aspects of care that impact on VTE risk.

The use of D-dimer in the diagnosis of DVT/PE

D-dimer concentration is increased in patients with DVT and PE. Since it is also raised in many other conditions (Table 17.2) it is not possible to make a definitive diagnosis of DVT or PE on the basis of a positive (increased) D-dimer test. However so consistent is the finding of a positive D-dimer test in patients with DVT/PE that it is possible to reliably exclude DVT/PE if D-dimer test is negative, and this is the basis for the routine use of D-dimer test.

A definitive diagnosis of DVT/PE requires imaging evidence of a blood clot (thrombus) in a deep vein. Imaging is expensive, time consuming and ideally reserved only for those in whom there is very strong suspicion of DVT/PE. A negative D-dimer test in a patient with clinical details that are not highly suggestive of DVT/PE provides sufficient evidence to exclude the diagnosis without imaging. So the real value of the D-dimer test is to significantly reduce the number of patients that need be submitted for expensive imaging tests.

Monitoring anticoagulation therapy

One of the principle uses of the prothrombin time (PT) and activated partial thromboplastin time (APPT) tests is to monitor the anticoagulation therapy used in the treatment and prevention of VTE and other potential thromboembolic conditions.

The aim of anticoagulation therapy is to artificially decrease the coagulability of blood thereby preventing thrombi formation and reducing growth of existing thrombi. Heparin, administered intravenously or subcutaneously, is used for the treatment of existing DVT functions in this regard by inhibiting the action of several activated factors of the extrinsic pathway; it also impairs platelet function. To prevent further DVT episodes in a patient who has suffered DVT, long-term oral anticoagulant warfarin is prescribed. Warfarin operates by inhibiting the action of vitamin K in production of vitamin K dependent factors.

Of course reducing the coagulability of blood carries with it the risk of increased bleeding, so that anticoagulation therapy must be carefully monitored to ensure maximum level of anticoagulation consistent with minimum risk of excessive bleeding. Heparin is monitored using APPT and warfarin is monitored using the PT test. In the case of heparin use, dose is adjusted so that APPT is 1.5–2 times the normal value.

Warfarin, prothrombin and INR

As we have seen, when PT is used to investigate a suspected coagulation defect results are expressed in time (seconds). This is not the case when PT is used to monitor warfarin therapy. Instead, the international normalised ratio (INR) is used. The INR provides a way of expressing PT results to take account of the differing activity of commercially prepared tissue thromboplastin used in the test. This ensures that prothrombin results are more directly comparable and provides a more accurate control of warfarin therapy. The INR is defined as the patients PT in seconds, divided by the mean of the PT reference range, raised to the power of the international sensitivity index (ISI) of the particular thromboplastin being used:

$$\text{Patient's INR} = \left(\frac{\text{Patient's Prothrombin Time(secs)}}{\text{Mean Normal Prothrombin Time(secs)}} \right)^{\text{ISI}}$$

Warfarin dose is adjusted so that the INR is maintained within a therapeutic range, which depends on the precise clinical reason for prescribing warfarin. For most patients the INR must be maintained within the range 2–3. In some circumstances increased level of anticoagulation is required in which case the therapeutic INR range is 3–4.5. If INR rises above the prescribed range (i.e. 2–3 or 3–4.5) dose must be adjusted downwards. All patients on long-term warfarin therapy should have their INR checked at regular (2–3 week) intervals.

Advances in technology have allowed the development of portable analysers for monitoring warfarin therapy. These allow anticoagulant monitoring outside the laboratory, either in clinics or primary care centres, where analysis is performed by nurses. In some anticoagulant clinics nursing staff are not only analysing patient samples but interpreting results and adjusting warfarin dose. The success of this arrangement has been demonstrated in several studies that have shown that a nurse specialist anticoagluant service is as effective as a haematology consultant run service, in maintaining therapeutic control among patients receiving warfarin[4]. Some studies[5,6] have demonstrated the feasibility of patients themselves taking control of their own blood testing and dose management. Just as some diabetic patients monitor their own blood glucose and adjust insulin dose accordingly, so too some patients can successfully self-manage their long-term anticoagulation therapy, thereby avoiding the inconvenience of frequent hospital appointments.

Case history 23

Amy Waters had to retire prematurely from her physically demanding job in 2002, when she was just 52 years old, because of worsening rheumatoid arthritis. Two years later she was given a hip replacement to increase her mobility. Post-operative recovery was complicated by an infection and on the tenth day following surgery she suddenly became extremely breathless. Understandably panicked, Amy also reported chest pain. During physical examination, the orthopaedic SHO noted some swelling of the left calf which Amy described as slightly tender when touched. A diagnosis of pulmonary embolus secondary to DVT in her left leg was eventually made. For the next few days Amy was given a continuous intravenous infusion of heparin and the breathlessness quickly resolved. After heparin was withdrawn Amy was prescribed warfarin tablets. She was eventually discharged home feeling well and delighted with her new hip. She was given a prescription to continue her daily dose of warfarin and asked to attend the haematology outpatients clinic every three weeks for a blood test.

Questions

(1) What blood test did Mrs Waters need?
(2) Why did she need this test?
(3) How long would she have had to continue to attend out-patients for this test?
(4) It seems much less likely that if Mrs Waters was given a hip replacement now, rather than in 2004, she would suffer the same postoperative complication. Why is this?
(5) What blood test is helpful in the diagnosis of DVT and PE? How is it helpful?

Discussion of case history 23

(1) The blood test required is prothrombin time (PT) reported as INR.

(2) Mrs Waters was receiving long-term oral anticoagulation therapy in the form of warfarin tablets to prevent recurrence of DVT/PE she suffered during post operative recovery. This drug decreases the tendency of the blood to coagulate by inhibiting the production of several clotting factors (proteins) required for blood coagulation. The drug carries with it the risk of increased bleeding (haemorrhage) and so must be carefully monitored to ensure that the dose given continues to give the maximum protection against thrombus formation consistent with minimum risk of haemorrhage.

(3) Mrs Waters continued to have her prothrombin time checked at regular intervals for the duration of time she was receiving warfarin. In the event this was for six months and she has had no recurrence of VTE since stopping warfarin therapy. If she does have a recurrence then warfarin and regular testing would be resumed, most likely for a much longer period.

(4) Strategies aimed at prevention of DVT/PE among hospital patients are much more rigorously applied now than was the case in 2004. All hospital patients are now assessed for risk of venous thromboembolism at the time of admission. Simply by virtue of the elective procedure (hip replacement) that Mrs Waters was about to undergo she would have been identified as 'at risk'. Her underlying chronic condition, rheumatoid arthritis would have been identified as one that increases that risk. She would now receive both mechanical and pharmaceutical prophylaxis within hours of her operation (subject to pre-operative assessment of bleeding risk), and would be encouraged to drink sufficiently to avoid postoperative dehydration. Mobility would also be encouraged as soon after the operation as possible, and she would be educated before discharge about how she can contribute to avoidance of VTE during convalescence. All these measures ensure that it is much less likely that Mrs Waters would suffer post-operative VTE if she received a hip replacement today.

(5) The D-dimer test. The D-dimer test is almost always positive (raised) in patients with DVT and PE so provides evidence in support of the diagnosis. Since the test is also positive in a range of other conditions it cannot be used alone to make the diagnosis. A negative (normal) D-dimer result is strong evidence to exclude a diagnosis of DVT/PE.

References

1. Collins, R., MacLellon, L., Gibbs, H. et al. (2010) Venous thromboembolism prophylaxis: the role of the nurse in changing practice and saving lives, *Austr J Adv Nursing*, 27: 83–9.
2. House of Commons Health Committee (2005) The prevention of venous thromboembolism in hospitalised patients, The Stationery Office.
3. National Institute for Health and Clinical Excellence NICE (2010) NICE Guideline 92: Venous thromboembolism: reducing the risk, National Institute for Health and Clinical Excellence.
4. Connor, C., Wright, C. and Fegan, C. (2002) The safety and effectiveness of a nurse led anticoagulant service, *J Adv Nursing*, 38: 407–15.
5. Heneghan, C., Ward, A., Perera, R. et al. (2012) Self monitoring of oral anticoagulation: systematic review and meta analysis of individual patient data, *Lancet*, 279: 322–34.
6. Bloomfield, H., Krause, A. and Greer, N. (2011) Meta-analysis: effect of patient self testing and self management of long term outcome anticoagulation on clinical outcomes, *Ann Intern Med*, 154: 472–82.

Further reading

Chines, D., Bussel, J. et al. (2004) Congenital and acquired thrombocytopaenia, *Hematology* (Am Society of Hematology Education Program book), 1: 390–406.

Glicksman, H. (2004) You're hurt and bleeding; how do you spell relief?, available at: http://www.arn.org/docs/glicksman/eyw_040501.htm.

Griesshammer, M., Bangerter, M. and Sauer, T. (1999) Aetiology and clinical significance of thrombocytosis: analysis of 732 patients with an elevated platelet count, *J Int Med*, 245: 295–300.

Lankshear, A., Harden, J. and Simms, J. (2010) Safe practice for patients receiving anticoagulant therapy, *Nursing Standard*, 24: 47–55.

Oldenburg, J., Dolan, G. and Lemm, G. (2009) Haemophilia care then, now and in the future, *Haemophilia*, 15: Suppl. 1: 2–7.

Kempher, K. and Little, J. (2004) Assessment of red blood cell and coagulation laboratory data, *AACN Clin Issues*, 15(4): 622–37.

Rowswell, H. and Law, C. (2011) Reducing patients risk of venous thromboembolism, *Nursing Times*, 107: 12–14.

Slusher, K. (2010) Factor V Leiden: a case study and review, *Dimensions of Crit Care Nursing*, 29: 6–10.

Tripodi, A. (2011) D-Dimer testing in laboratory practice, *Clinical Chemistry*, 57: 1256–62.

CHAPTER 18

LABORATORY INVESTIGATION OF ANAEMIA: SERUM IRON, TOTAL IRON BINDING CAPACITY, SERUM FERRITIN, SERUM B12 AND FOLATE

Key learning topics

- Iron metabolism and role of iron in red blood cell function
- Dietary source of vitamins B12 and folate
- Gastrointestinal absorption of vitamins B12 and folate
- Vitamin B12 and red cell production
- Causes of iron deficiency
- Causes of vitamin B12/folate deficiency
- How blood tests are used to diagnose iron deficiency anaemia
- How blood tests are used to diagnose anaemia caused by deficiency of vitamin B12 and/or folate

---

The means by which the results of full blood count (FBC) identify those patients who are anaemic was discussed in Chapter 15. It was emphasised that anaemia is not a single disease, but rather a syndrome with many possible causes. Successful treatment of anaemia depends crucially on identifying its cause. It will be remembered that tests included in the full blood count (most notably the MCV) suggest possible causes of anaemia, but further testing is necessary. The principle use of the five tests described in this chapter is to confirm the cause of anaemia.

Deficiency of iron is the most common cause of anaemia in the UK and around the world. World Health Organisation (WHO) best estimates suggest that 1.62 billion people are anaemic, that is 25% of the world population, and iron deficiency is the cause in around half of these cases[1]. In developed countries like the UK around 2–5% of the adult (non-pregnant) population have iron deficiency anaemia[2]. Prevalence is higher among pregnant women.

Understanding Laboratory Investigations: A Guide for Nurses, Midwives and Healthcare Professionals, Third Edition. Chris Higgins.
© 2013 John Wiley & Sons, Ltd. Published 2013 by John Wiley & Sons, Ltd.

Measurement of the serum or plasma concentration of serum iron, total iron binding capacity (TIBC) and ferritin together provide the means of confirming a diagnosis of iron deficiency anaemia. Similarly measurement of the serum or plasma concentration of the vitamins B12 and folate provides the means of identifying those patients who are suffering so called megaloblastic anaemia. As we shall see anaemia is not the only condition in which abnormality in results of these five tests can be expected.

Normal physiology

Function of iron and iron metabolism

The oxygen delivery function of haemoglobin (Hb) contained within red cells is dependent on the presence of iron in the haem part of haemoglobin (see Chapter 15, Figure 15.3). Oxygen forms a reversible weak link with the single atom of iron in each of the four haem groups contained in the Hb molecule. Iron is thus essential for Hb production and function. The muscle protein, myoglobin and the function of some enzymes are also dependent on iron, although compared with the role of iron in Hb, these are of much less clinical significance.

Around 70% of the approximately 4–5 g of iron present in the body is contained in the Hb in circulating red cells (see Chapter 18, Figure 18.1). A little is contained in another much less abundant oxygen carrying protein called myoglobin, but most of the rest is stored in tissues (principally the liver but also the spleen and bone marrow). In these storage 'compartments' iron is contained within the proteins ferritin and haemosiderin. Some ferritin is present in the plasma part of blood and the concentration of ferritin in plasma is a reliable indicator of the body's total iron tissue stores. Just 3–4 mg (i.e. 0.1% of total body iron) circulates in blood plasma, where it is bound to the transport protein transferrin. It is the concentration of this transferrin bound fraction of total body iron that is measured in the serum iron test.

Iron is well conserved by the body. When red cells die at the end of their 120 day life span, the iron they contain is returned via blood to body stores for bone marrow production of new red cells. Since iron is protein bound and therefore cannot be filtered from blood at the glomerulus, very little iron is excreted in urine; the only significant loss is that contained in surface epithelial cells constantly shed from the body; just 1 mg/day is lost from the body via this route. Since most of the body's iron is contained within red cells, blood loss represents a potential route for significant iron depletion. For example, normal menstruation is associated with a loss of around 15 mg of iron every month. When this is taken into account, healthy pre-menopausal women lose on average 1.5–2 mg of iron a day. To replace these minimal losses and maintain normal iron stores, at least 1 mg of iron in the case of healthy children, adult men and post-menopausal women, and up to double this in the case of pre-menopausal women, must be absorbed every day from diet. In fact a normal well balanced diet contains approximately 10–15 mg of iron/day. The principal sources of dietary iron are meat (particularly red meat) and fish, green leafed vegetables and breakfast cereals. Vitamin C increases the availability for

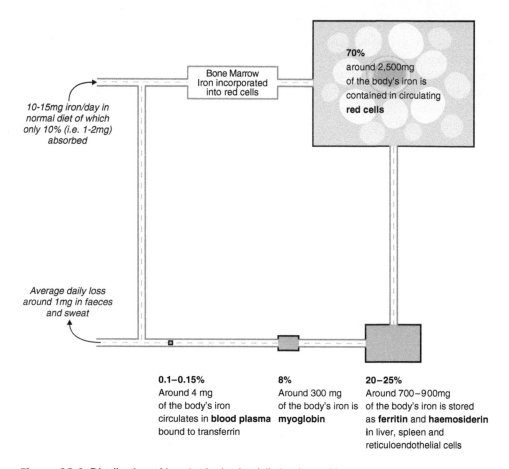

Figure 18.1 Distribution of iron in the body: daily intake and loss.

absorption of the iron present in vegetables and cereals. Absorption of dietary iron occurs in the upper small intestine (duodenum). Just 10% of available dietary iron is normally absorbed, sufficient to replace daily losses. It is vital for good health that iron stores remain replete but not overloaded with iron because, as we shall see, too much iron can be as damaging to health as too little iron. Since there is no control of the iron lost from the body, control of iron body stores depends crucially on the control mechanisms of dietary iron absorption. Absorption of dietary iron is minutely adjusted to meet the body's requirements at the time. Hepcidin, a hormone synthesised in the liver is the key regulator of this dietary iron absorption. Excess dietary iron is not absorbed and passes from the body in faeces.

Function and metabolism of vitamins B12 and folate

Vitamins are a group of organic substances of widely differing chemical structure that are essential, albeit in tiny amounts, for life. They cannot be synthesised by the human body (vitamin D is an exception) and our only source is the food we eat. Most vitamins of the B group, which includes both B12 (alternative name cobalamin) and folate (alternative name folic acid), function as essential co-enzymes or co-factors in the enzymic reactions of cellular metabolism.

Specifically, B12 and folate are both required for the action of key enzymes involved in the synthesis of deoxyribonucleic acid (DNA) during cell division. Tissues characterised by rapid cell turn over and consequent unremitting cell division are particularly dependent on intact DNA synthesis and therefore vitamins B12 and folate. Bone marrow is one such tissue: blood cell production by the bone marrow continues minute by minute throughout life and an adequate supply of B12 and folate is essential for the continuing normal production of blood cells. Although essential for several other cellular enzyme reactions, the role of B12 and folate in the cell division required for normal production of blood cells is the one that is of prime clinical significance.

Both B12 and folate are naturally synthesised only by bacteria, and we obtain them by eating animal and plant foods that are naturally contaminated with these bacteria. The principal dietary source of vitamin B12 is meat (liver is a particularly rich source), fish and dairy products. Vegetables do not contain B12. Folic acid is present in green leafy vegetables; liver is a rich source. Most breakfast cereals and a few other processed foods are fortified with B12 and/or folate. The minimum adult daily requirement for B12 is 1.5 µg and for folate 200 µg. A normal healthy diet provides well in excess of the minimum requirement of B12, but only just twice the amount of folate required.

The acidity of gastric juice is vital for release of B12 from foods in the stomach prior to absorption lower down the gastrointestinal tract. Additionally, for absorption to occur B12 must first be bound to so called intrinsic factor, a peptide (small protein) produced by the gastric parietal cells. Thus functioning gastric parietal cells that line the stomach wall and produce both the hydrochloric acid and intrinsic factor present in gastric juice are essential to absorption of B12. Once bound to intrinsic factor, B12 is absorbed to blood via cells that line the lower (distal) end of the small intestine (the ileum). Absorbed B12 is transported in blood to bone marrow and other cells, bound to the transport protein, transcobalamin. The body has considerable capacity to store large reserves of vitamin B12 in the liver, sufficient in fact to remain in normal health for several years on an entirely vitamin B12-free diet.

Absorption of folate

Absorption of folate is less complex. It is absorbed higher up the small intestine than B12 at the jejenum and is transported in blood to bone marrow and other folate requiring tissues, either in its free form or bound to albumin.

Like vitamin B12, folate is stored principally in the liver. However folate stores are sufficient to last only a few months on a folate-free diet.

Normal production of red cells in the bone marrow is dependent then on:

- A healthy diet containing sufficient B12 and folate.
- Production of gastric acid and intrinsic factor by the stomach, for absorption of B12.

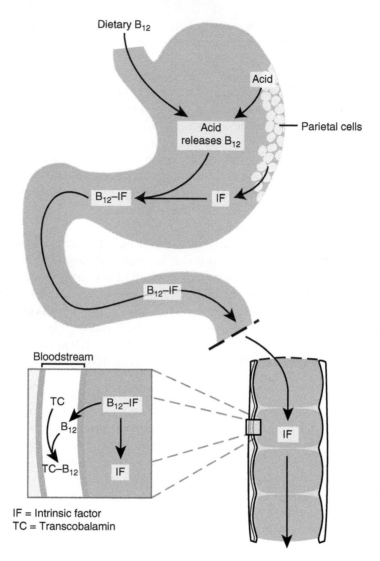

Figure 18.2 Absorption of vitamin B12.

- Normal absorption at the ileum (i.e. functioning gastrointestinal tract).
- Adequate production of the transport protein transcobalamin.

Laboratory measurement

With few exceptions the tests described in this chapter should be reserved for those patients in whom anaemia has been demonstrated by FBC (see Chapter 15). The mean cell volume (MCV) result indicates which of these tests are most appropriate. A reduced MCV indicates probable iron deficiency anaemia, in which case serum iron, total iron binding capacity and serum ferritin are appropriate. If MCV is raised then B12 and folate should be measured first.

What is being measured

Serum/plasma iron – this is the concentration of the small proportion of total body iron that circulates in the plasma part of blood bound to transferrin; it does not include the iron contained in red cells or that contained in ferritin.

Total iron binding capacity (TIBC) – this is a test performed on plasma or serum and is essentially a measure of the amount of transferrin available for iron to bind to. Remember, all the iron being transported in blood around the body is bound to transferrin.

Serum ferritin – ferritin is the protein in which iron is stored in tissues; a very small proportion escapes from tissues to blood. The concentration of ferritin in blood serum is a reliable indicator of total iron stores.

Serum B12 and **folate** – the concentration of vitamin B12 and folate in serum. A low result indicates deficiency.

Red cell folate – concentration of folate in red cells. A low result indicates deficiency.

Patient preparation

No particular patient preparation is necessary.

Timing of sample

No particular timing is required. It is best practice to collect blood at a time to coincide with routine transport to the laboratory.

Sample requirements

Around 5 ml of venous blood is sufficient for iron, TIBC and ferritin. Most commonly serum is used, in which case blood should be collected into a plain tube containing no anticoagulant. Blood for red cell folate must be collected into a tube containing the anticoagulant EDTA (lavender coloured top) bottle. A further 5 ml of venous blood is required for serum B12 and folate (collected into a plain tube containing no additive).

Interpretation of results

Approximate reference ranges

Serum Iron   10–30 µmol/L
Serum TIBC   40–75 µmol/L

Serum ferritin   10–300 µg/L

Serum B12   of the order 150–1000 ng/L but values vary according to methodology; consult local laboratory

Serum Folate   of the order 150–700 µg/L but values vary; consult local laboratory

Conditions associated with abnormal results of either serum iron, TIBC or ferritin

These are:

- Iron deficiency anaemia.
- Chronic infection, inflammation malignancy (anaemia of chronic disease, ACD).
- Iron overload.

Iron deficiency anaemia

Causes

In particular patients there may be more than one cause: iron deficiency anaemia is frequently multifactorial. The many possible causes can be addressed under the four main headings:

- Insufficient iron in the diet, poor nutrition.
- Increased loss of iron (in blood) from the body.
- Inadequate absorption of dietary iron.
- Increased demand for iron.

It is unusual for poor diet to be the sole cause of iron deficiency in developed countries, although a diet relatively deficient of iron (e.g. high proportion of 'junk' food) may be a contributory factor in some cases. Poor nutrition is however a major cause of iron deficiency in most areas of the developing world.

The most common cause among adults in developed countries like the UK is chronic blood loss. Red cells contain 70% of the body's iron, and blood loss represents a significant iron deficit. So long as iron tissue stores are replete, a single acute episode of even severe blood loss will not cause iron deficiency. However chronic blood loss, that is the continuous or regular loss of small amounts of blood over a prolonged period, will slowly exhaust iron stores. Chronic excessive menstrual blood loss (menorrhagia) is the most frequent cause of iron deficiency anaemia among non-pregnant, pre-menopausal women.

Chronic blood loss from the gastrointestinal tract, which may go unrecognised for many months or even years, as blood is lost imperceptibly in faeces, is a feature of a number of relatively common but serious diseases of the gastrointestinal tract. These include ulcerative colitis; cancer of oesophagus, stomach and colon; and stomach ulcers. Aspirin and some other non-steroidal anti-inflammatory drugs irritate the gastric lining of the stomach sufficiently to cause low grade bleeding in some people. For this reason long-term aspirin use is associated with a risk of iron deficiency anaemia. Together these gastrointestinal conditions associated with chronic blood loss account for most cases of iron deficiency anaemia among adult males and post-menopausal women. Some diseases of the gastrointestinal tract cause iron deficiency by reducing absorption of dietary iron. Foremost among these is coeliac disease (gluten sensitivity). This is an autoimmune disease, confined to genetically predisposed individuals, that is provoked by eating foods containing gluten (a protein constituent of wheat). It results in inflammatory damage to the mucosal lining of the small intestine that impairs absorption of many diet derived nutrients, including iron. Coeliac disease is common (affects 1–2% of the population) but currently remains under diagnosed. Iron deficiency anaemia can be a presenting sign, and coeliac disease has in recent years emerged as one of the more common causes of iron deficiency anaemia. A gluten-free diet (the standard treatment for coeliac disease) is effective in eradicating iron deficiency anaemia in such cases. Chronic inflammatory bowel conditions (Crohn's disease and ulcerative colitis) are also associated with reduced iron absorption and consequent high risk of iron deficiency anaemia. Surgical removal of the stomach (gastrectomy) is associated with reduced absorption of iron.

Colonisation of the stomach with the bacterium *Helicobacter pylori* is very common, and usually benign. In some people however it leads to gastritis and gastric ulcers. In others it can cause iron deficiency anaemia. The mechanism is unclear but reduced absorption of iron is likely. Antibiotic treatment aimed at eradication of *Helicobacter pylori* might be an effective treatment for iron deficiency anaemia in these cases[3].

Increased red cell production is one of the many physiological changes that occur during pregnancy. To accommodate this around two to three times the normal amount of iron is required. This increased demand for iron can lead to iron deficiency if iron stores are not replete, and iron deficiency anaemia is a not uncommon complication of late pregnancy[4]. Increased demand for iron during growth contributes to the iron deficiency that can occur in malnourished babies and children.

In all cases of iron deficiency anaemia, a cause should be sought no matter what the severity because it may be a presenting sign of serious underlying gastrointestinal or gynaecological disease. The advice of recently published guidelines[2] is that all patients with unexplained iron deficiency anaemia, no matter what the severity, should be screened for coeliac disease using a blood test (serum IgA-tTG) that detects a causative autoantibody (the tissue transglutaminase antibody).

All those with unexplained iron deficiency anaemia should also have urine tested for the presence of blood (haematuria), a signal of possible bladder cancer. In addition upper and lower gastrointestinal tract investigation (e.g. barium meal, endoscopic examinations) should be considered for all male patients and all female patients over the age of 50 (post-menopausal) to identify disease associated with chronic gastrointestinal bleeding or inflammation that might explain the anaemia.

Symptoms

In addition to the general symptoms of anaemia already listed, patients with iron deficiency anaemia may exhibit some other specific symptoms of iron deficiency which include:

- Glossitis (inflammation of the tongue).
- Angular cheilosis (ulceration of lips at the corners of the mouth).
- Changes to nails (unusually brittle; may become spoon shaped – indented (koilonychia)).

Results of blood testing

Serum ferritin concentration reflects iron stores, so that a reduction in serum ferritin is evident before anaemia develops, during the period of progressive iron store depletion. By the time that iron stores are totally depleted, when signs and symptoms of iron deficiency anaemia begin to occur, serum ferritin concentration is extremely low or undetectable. Serum iron is usually reduced, but may remain at the low end of the reference range. Serum total iron binding capacity is always raised.

Typical blood results in iron deficiency anaemia are:

- Serum iron usually reduced, in the range 5–10 µmol/L (may be at the low end of the reference range).
- Serum TIBC raised (i.e. greater than 75 µmol/L).
- Serum ferritin greatly reduced (usually undetectable, i.e. <5 µg/L).

Chronic inflammation and infection

As outlined in Chapter 15, many patients with chronic infectious or inflammatory disease as well as those with malignant disease may become mildly to moderately anaemic (it is unusual for Hb to fall lower than 9 g/dl in such cases).

This is called anaemia of chronic disease (ACD). Although ACD is not the result of iron deficiency (iron stores are not depleted), it is associated with disturbance of iron metabolism that is reflected in blood test results. Serum iron concentration is usually reduced, as it is in iron deficiency anaemia. However in contrast to iron deficiency anaemia, serum TIBC is reduced and serum ferritin is either normal or in some cases increased. Since a deficiency of iron is not the problem, iron supplements are of little use to these patients. Indeed such treatment may be harmful by putting them at risk of iron overload. Instead treatment is directed at the underlying condition; as this resolves, or is ameliorated anaemia may itself lessen. Other treatment options include recombinant erythropoietin injections.

To summarise, patients with chronic infections (e.g. TB, bacterial endocarditis, pneumonia etc.) and chronic inflammation (e.g. rheumatoid arthritis, SLE, Crohn's disease etc.) as well as some cancer patients may be anaemic. The severity of anaemia reflects the severity of the underlying disorder.

ACD is associated with:

- Reduced serum iron concentration.
- Reduced serum TIBC.
- Normal or raised serum ferritin concentration.

Iron overload

In the physiological state all iron in the body is bound to a protein (Hb in red cells, ferritin in storage compartments and transferrin in blood plasma). In this state it is non-toxic. However free (unbound) iron is toxic. There is a finite amount of each of the 'protective' binding and storage proteins, and once they are saturated with iron, any additional iron in cells exists in its toxic-free (unbound to protein) state. Free iron is toxic because it promotes production of highly reactive free radicals that disrupt normal cell structure and function. Unchecked this can lead to tissue damage. Tissues affected in disease caused by chronic iron overload include:

- Pancreas – fibrosis of pancreas leading to diabetes.
- Liver – cirrhosis and eventual liver failure, liver cancer.
- Heart – arrhythmias, heart failure.
- Gonads – impotence.
- Joints – severe joint pain (similar to arthritis).

Causes

Hereditary haemachromatosis. Those with this genetically determined disease absorb increased amounts of available iron in diet, 3–4 mg/day instead of the normal 1–2 mg. There is no physiological means of increasing iron excretion so iron accumulates at the rate of 0.5–1.0 g/year. In late middle age when first clinical effects of iron overload occur, total body iron may be in the range 20–40 g rather than normal 4–5 g. Around one in ten of us carry a single copy of the defective gene (it is the most common inherited genetic defect). Only inheritance of the defective gene from both parents (i.e. two copies of the defective gene) results in the most severe form of haemachromatosis, which leads to diabetes, cirrhosis etc. Other causes of iron overload include repeated blood transfusion and inappropriate iron therapy. One unit of blood contains around 250 mg of iron in red cells, 100 times the daily requirement. Patients whose treatment includes repeated blood transfusion over a prolonged period (e.g. those suffering thalassaemia and sickle cell disease) are particularly at risk of iron overload.

Blood test results

The blood test results of those with iron overload are, as might be expected, the opposite of those associated with iron deficiency. No matter what the cause, iron overload is associated with:

- Raised serum iron.
- Reduced serum TIBC.
- Raised serum ferritin.

Conditions associated with reduced B12 and folate results

Megaloblastic anaemia

Megaloblastic anaemia is a term applied to all those anaemias in which due to impaired DNA synthesis there is abnormal development of blood cells in the bone marrow. Impaired DNA synthesis results in production of large (mega) immature (blast) red cells, many of which do not develop to maturity and die within the bone marrow. There is thus a marked reduction in the number of circulating red cells, hence the anaemia. Some of those red cells that do survive and appear in peripheral blood are larger than normal, often characteristically oval in shape. Large red cells in peripheral blood are called macrocytes, so the term macrocytic anaemia is sometimes used as an alternative name for megaloblastic anaemia, although the terms are not, strictly speaking, synonomous. The effect of impaired DNA synthesis is not confined to red cells, numbers of both white cells and platelets may be reduced in those with severe megaloblastic anaemia. With a few very rare exceptions, the cause of the impaired DNA synthesis that leads to megaloblastic anaemia is vitamin B12 and/or folate deficiency.

Causes of vitamin B12 or folate deficiency

The causes can be summarised under the following headings:

- Dietary deficiency.
- Failure to absorb B12 due to inadequate production of intrinsic factor.
- Failure to absorb either B12 or folate due to gastrointestinal disease.
- Increased demand for B12 and folate during pregnancy.

Dietary deficiency of B12 is rare except among strict vegetarians (vegans) who eat no dairy products. Dietary deficiency of folate is more common; in fact it is the most common cause of folate deficiency. Unlike vitamin B12, folate in food can be destroyed by cooking, and the normal dietary intake is close to the minimum required. Dietary deficiency of folate is quite common among chronic alcoholics; this combined with effects of alcohol on folate metabolism, render this group particularly susceptible to folate deficiency. The infirm elderly, whose diet is often not well balanced and may be deficient of folate, are considered another group at risk of dietary deficiency of folate.

The most common cause of vitamin B12 deficiency is failure to absorb the vitamin due to lack of intrinsic factor. The specific type of megaloblastic anaemia that results from lack of intrinsic factor is known as pernicious anaemia. Those with pernicious anaemia are unable to produce intrinsic factor because of damage (autoimmune in nature) to the parietal cells of the stomach lining, where intrinsic factor is produced. The condition tends to run in families and is often associated with other autoimmune diseases (e.g. thyroid disease, Addison's disease, coeliac disease and Type 1 diabetes). Absorption of folate is not affected in pernicious anaemia.

Patients with pernicious anaemia must be given B12 by injection, as that given by the oral route cannot be absorbed.

Partial and total gastrectomy can of course also result in reduced production of intrinsic factor.

Various gastrointestinal diseases associated with inflammatory or other damage to areas where B12 and folate are normally absorbed can result in reduced absorption and vitamin deficiency. Surgical removal of areas of the gastrointestinal tract (e.g. jejunal or ileal resection) can lead to either B12 or folate deficiency. Patients receiving such surgery may be given regular injections of B12 and folate to prevent anaemia developing. Pregnancy is associated with increased demand for B12 and folate. A deficiency at around the time of conception and during the first weeks of pregnancy is associated with increased risk of giving birth to a baby with serious neural tube defects such as spina bifida. This provides the rationale for the well-publicised advice to women contemplating pregnancy and newly pregnant women to take folic acid supplements.

Symptoms of megaloblastic anaemia

Whether they are caused by dietary deficiency or poor absorption of B12 or folate, the resulting symptoms may include:

- General symptoms of all anaemias.
- Mild jaundice.
- Glossitis (inflamed tongue).
- Angular cheilosis (sores at the corner of the mouth).

Patients with B12 deficiency, but less commonly those with folate deficiency, may also suffer a progressive condition of the nervous system called sub-acute combined degeneration of the cord. Those with this additional effect of B12 deficiency may present with any of a range of neurological/cognitive symptoms including:

- Paraesthesia (abnormal sensation, e.g. numbness, tingling in fingers and toes).
- Gait ataxia, resulting in difficulty in walking.
- Increased irritability.
- Memory loss.
- Depression.
- Rarely, personality change and other overt psychiatric problems.

These neurological/psychiatric symptoms of B12 deficiency may be present with or without signs and symptoms of anaemia.

Blood test results

Serum B12 is usually reduced in pernicious anaemia and all other cases of megaloblastic anaemia and neuropathy caused by deficiency of B12. In some cases the serum level remains at the low end of the reference range, causing some diagnostic difficulty. Serum folate is usually normal but may be slightly raised. Red cell folate by contrast is either normal or low in cases of B12 deficiency.

In cases of megaloblastic anaemia caused solely by folate deficiency, serum B12 is normal, but as might be expected both serum and red cell folate are reduced. Red cell folate is considered a more reliable test of folate status because serum folate may be low in some illnesses (e.g. severe liver and kidney disease) despite normal folate status.

Case history 24

Jane Baker is a 32 year old solicitor who is being investigated by her GP because of increasing tiredness of several months duration (see case history 21). The results of an FBC demonstrate she is anaemic and that the anaemia may be due to iron deficiency. Jane's GP takes a further sample of blood for iron studies and prescribes a course of iron tablets. Three days later the following laboratory report is received at the GP surgery:

Serum Iron	9 µmol/L
Serum TIBC	113 µmol/L
Serum Ferritin	<5 µg/L

Questions

(1) Are the results normal?
(2) What is ferritin and why is its concentration in blood serum measured in patients who are suspected of being iron deficient?
(3) What do the results indicate?
(4) Why might further investigation be necessary?

Discussion of case history 24

(1) No. Serum iron and ferritin are both abnormally reduced and serum TIBC is raised.

(2) Ferritin is a water-soluble molecule composed of an outer protein shell enclosing an iron core. Each ferritin molecule contains 4000–5000 atoms of iron and this iron constitutes around 20% of its weight. Most of the body's ferritin is in tissue cells (liver, spleen, bone marrow) where its function is iron storage. A small fraction circulates in blood plasma where its concentration reflects total iron body stores. Reduction in serum ferritin concentration, as iron stores become progressively depleted, is the first objective evidence of iron deficiency. Reduction in serum ferritin concentration occurs before iron is sufficiently depleted to affect haemoglobin production and therefore occurs before symptoms of iron deficiency anaemia occur. Serum ferritin remains low or undetectable until iron stores are replete.

(3) Reduced serum iron and increased serum TIBC in association with undetectable levels of ferritin in blood serum is the typical pattern of results expected in iron deficiency anaemia. There can be no doubt that Mrs Bishop is iron deficient and requires the iron supplements her doctor prescribed.

(4) A diagnosis of iron deficiency should be followed by investigation of its cause. Why has Mrs Bishop become iron deficient? In a woman of reproductive age like Mrs Bishop, the most common cause is menorrhagia (increased loss of iron in menstrual blood) – which itself may require further investigation – but this is by no means the only cause of iron deficiency. Current guidelines[2] suggest that a woman of Mrs Bishop's age with unexplained iron deficiency anaemia should be offered, in the first instance, a blood test (serum IgA-tTG) to screen for coeliac disease. Her urine should also be tested for the presence of blood to screen for malignancy of the renal tract.

Case history 25

Mr Sandhu had been in good health all his life until, at the age of 45, he began to suffer symptoms of depression and anxiety. Over the following ten years he had three episodes of depression/anxiety, which were treated with anti-depressant drugs (fluoxetine and a benzodiazepine). Although there was partial recovery from each episode and drugs were withdrawn, residual symptoms remained. Ten years after the first episode, Mr Sandhu's residual symptoms worsened and became more frequent. He also became increasingly forgetful and complained of increased tiredness and fatigue. He began to have daytime drowsiness and reported a weight loss of 10 kg at this time. Despite more intensive antidepressant drug therapy there was no improvement over a period of six months, indeed his mental/neurological health deteriorated and a psychiatric consultation at this time, when Mr Sandhu was exhibiting signs suggestive of hypomania/mania, resulted in a diagnosis of bipolar disorder and prescription of the psychoactive drug, valproate. This had no beneficial effect.

Eventually, some 10.5 years after first becoming unwell, Mr Sandhu was admitted to hospital for full neurological/psychiatric assessment. At this time he had significant neurological deficit, was unable to balance, swayed while walking and exhibited sluggish reflexes. His memory/cognition was impaired (mini-mental status examination, MMSE, score was 16/30 and his measured IQ was just 67). He was disoriented to time and place. The diagnoses considered as a result of this assessment included dementia and bipolar affective disorder.

As part of the assessment blood was sampled from Mr Sandhu for a range of tests. Among the results returned from the laboratory were the following:

Haemoglobin (Hb)	6.5 g/dl
Mean Cell Volume (MCV)	105 fl
Serum B12 98.5 ng/L	(reference range 211–911 ng/L)
Anti-parietal cell antibodies	positive

Questions

(1) Are Hb and MCV results normal? If not what do they indicate?
(2) Mr Sandhu was diagnosed as suffering pernicious anaemia. From what you know of this condition, how did results of the four blood tests contribute to making the diagnosis?
(3) What treatment do you think was initiated as a result of the diagnosis?
(4) As a result of the treatment Mr Sandhu's neuropsychiatric symptoms resolved. What does this case study tell about the function of B12 beyond red cell formation?

Discussion of case history 25

(1) No. Hb is markedly reduced and MCV is increased (see Chapter 14 for normal values). Reduced haemoglobin is diagnostic of anaemia. Increased MCV indicates red cells are on average larger than normal – macrocytic. Together these results indicate that Mr Sandhu had quite severe macrocytic anaemia.

(2) Pernicious anaemia is caused by slowly progressive autoimmune mediated damage to the lining of the stomach (the gastric mucosa). This includes damage to the gastric parietal cells that produce hydrochloric acid and intrinsic factor, both of which are required for absorption of dietary derived vitamin B12. As a consequence of the damage, affected patients become deficient of B12, and because the vitamin is required for bone marrow production of red cells, they become anaemic. The anaemia that results from vitamin B12 deficiency is megaloblastic in nature, meaning many of the red cells are

immature and larger than normal. Mr Sandhu's Hb and MCV results reveal a severe macrocytic anaemia consistent with vitamin B12 deficiency, which was confirmed with the finding of reduced serum B12. The positive result for anti-parietal cell antibodies explains *why* Mr Sandhu became deficient of vitamin B12 because it is evidence of the autoimmune mediated damage to gastric parietal cells that is central to the pathogenesis of pernicious anaemia.

As a result of progressive damage to gastric parietal cells, Mr Sandhu was increasingly less able to produce sufficient intrinsic factor, and therefore increasingly less able to absorb sufficient vitamin B12 for continuing red cell production – hence the anaemia.

(3) Treatment for pernicious anaemia is intramuscular (im) injection of vitamin B12. Initially, Mr Sandhu was given 500 µg hydroxycobalamin (a synthetic form of B12) every day for seven days, then every other day for two weeks. Because those with pernicious anaemia can no longer produce intrinsic factor, and therefore cannot absorb B12 given orally, they require B12 injections for life, typically administered every three months.

Over a period of a few weeks following the start of B12 injections Mr Sandhu's serum B12 and haemoglobin gradually returned to normal and the symptoms of anaemia he had been suffering (extreme fatigue) resolved.

(4) Mr Sandhu's mental/neurological health also improved. Three weeks after the start of vitamin B12 injections his MMSE score improved from 16/30 before treatment to 30/30. He was able to walk normally and unaided. With improved memory and cognition, affective symptoms (those of depression and anxiety) also disappeared. All psychotropic drugs were withdrawn and he was discharged from hospital in good physical and mental health. At a follow up outpatient appointment 15 months later, his measured IQ was 106 and he had remained well. He was now the same sociable, normally functioning man he had been 11 years previously, before he first became unwell.

It is unusual for pernicious anaemia to manifest itself in quite the same way that it did for Mr Sandhu, although it is well established that B12 deficiency can have neurological/psychiatric effect. Clearly vitamin B12 is not only essential for blood cell production, but also for a functioning nervous system. Mr Sandhu's case history, which is based quite closely on an actual one recorded in the medical literature[5], is a reminder that quite serious psychiatric illness can sometimes have a treatable physical cause.

References

1. World Health Organisation (2008) Worldwide prevalence of anaemia 1993–2005, WHO.
2. Goddard, A., James M., Mcintyre, A. et al. (2011) Guidelines for the management of iron deficiency anaemia, *Gut*, 60: 1309–16.
3. Huang, X., Qu, X. and Yan, W. (2010) Iron deficiency anaemia can be improved after eradication of *Helicobacter pylori*, *Postgrad Med J*, 86: 272–8.
4. Milman, N. (2008) Pre-partum anaemia: prevention and treatment, *Ann Hematol*, 87: 949–59.
5. Kate, N. and Grover, S. (2010) Pernicious anaemia presenting as bipolar disorder – a case report and review of literature, *German J Psychiatry*, 13: 181–4.

Further reading

Chanarin, I. (2000) A history of pernicious anaemia. Historical Review, *Br J Haematol*, 111: 407–15.

Kaferle, J. and Strzoda, C. (2009) Evaluation of macrocytosis, *Am Fam Physician*, 79: 203–8.

Milman, N. (2011) Post partum anaemia I: definition, prevalence causes and consequences, *Ann Hematol*, 90: 1247–53.

Milman, N. (2012) Postpartum anaemia II: prevention and treatment, *Ann Hematol*, 91: 143–54.

Pasricha, S-R., Flecknoe-Brown, S., Allen, K. et al. (2010) Diagnosis and management of iron deficiency anaemia – a clinical update, *MJA*, 193: 523–25.

Munoz, M., Garcia-Erce, J. and Remacha, A. (2011) Disorders of iron metabolism Part 1: molecular basis of iron haemostasis, *J Clin Path*, 64: 281–6.

Munoz, M., Garcia-Erce, J. and Remacha, A. (2011) Disorders of iron metabolism Part II: iron deficiency and iron overload, *J Clin Path*, 64: 287–96.

CHAPTER 19

ERYTHROCYTE SEDIMENTATION RATE (ESR) AND PLASMA C-REACTIVE PROTEIN (CRP)

Key learning topics

- Understanding the ESR test
- What factors affect the rate at which red cells sediment
- Causes of increased ESR
- What is C-reactive protein
- Causes of increased plasma CRP concentration
- CRP measurement to assess risk of cardiovascular disease

The principle function of the two tests that are the focus of this chapter is detection and monitoring of inflammatory and infectious disease. Both tests serve essentially the same purpose. Erythrocyte sedimentation rate (ESR), the older and more established of the two, is performed in the haematology laboratory using a whole blood sample. Plasma C-reactive protein (CRP) is an alternative test to the ESR, usually performed in the immunology or clinical chemistry laboratory using a plasma or serum sample. The CRP test has some advantages over the ESR. The diagnostic information that the two tests provide can sometimes be complementary; under these circumstances it is useful to have the results of both tests. We begin with consideration of the ESR.

Erythrocyte sedimentation rate (ESR)

The ESR test is one of the oldest and simplest tests still performed in clinical laboratories, and is based on a very visible phenomenon, familiar to all those who have collected blood. If a blood sample, collected into a tube containing an

Understanding Laboratory Investigations: A Guide for Nurses, Midwives and Healthcare Professionals, Third Edition. Chris Higgins.
© 2013 John Wiley & Sons, Ltd. Published 2013 by John Wiley & Sons, Ltd.

anticoagulant, is left undisturbed then the red cells (erythrocytes) gradually fall or sediment to the bottom of the container, leaving the clear straw coloured, plasma fluid above. At the end of the nineteenth century, physicians investigated this phenomenon and discovered that the red cells in a blood sample taken from healthy volunteers sediment slowly, but that the cells in a blood sample taken from those suffering a range of disease sediment much faster. From these observations the ESR test was born.

Despite minor modifications, measurement of ESR has remained essentially unchanged since its introduction nearly a hundred years ago. A narrow bore tube of standard length is filled with anticoagulated blood and placed in a vertical position. The tube is left undisturbed for a defined time (usually one hour). During that time the erythrocytes sediment leaving an increasingly large column of clear plasma above. After one hour has elapsed the distance from the top of the tube to the interface between clear plasma and red cells is measured. This distance is the ESR expressed in millimetres per hour. In short the ESR is the distance in millimetres red cells fall in one hour.

Normal physiology: what affects red cell sedimentation?

Although apparently simple, the rate at which erythrocytes sediment is a complex phenomenon, which even now is not entirely understood. Clearly red cells fall due to gravity, because they have a greater density then the plasma in which they are suspended. Red cells have a net negative charge due to the presence of membrane bound proteins on their surface. This electrostatic force tends to make red cells repel each other. This is the situation in health; red cells are for the most part separate and fall individually. If for any reason this tendency of cells to repel each other is overcome, then they aggregate together to form 'rouleaux' (red cells stacked together rather like a pile of coins). Since an aggregation of red cells has greater density than single cells aggregated cells sediment faster. It is this abnormal tendency for cells to overcome their natural repulsion for each other, and aggregate, which explains the increased ESR found in disease. The crucial question is: what makes red cells aggregate? The answer lies in the plasma in which red cells are suspended. Certain proteins in plasma, most notably fibrinogen and immunoglobulins, act as molecular bridges between red cells. When present in high concentration the effect of these proteins is a marked increase in the aggregation of red cells. As will become clear, it is disease states that are associated with abnormally high concentration of these proteins in plasma which most commonly result in a raised ESR.

In addition to the composition of the plasma in which they are suspended the rate at which red cells sediment is also affected by both numbers and shape of red cells themselves. So that, for example, a significant decrease in the number of red cells as occurs in anaemia is associated with an increase in ESR whilst an abnormal increase in red cell numbers (polycythaemia) reduces ESR. The shape of red cells of those suffering sickle cell anaemia is abnormal; these so called sickle cells sediment slower than normal red cells.

Laboratory measurement

Patient preparation

No particular patient preparation is necessary.

Sample timing

Depending on the method being used, a delay of more than a few hours in processing samples can affect results. Samples stored overnight may be unsuitable for analysis. It is therefore best practice to take samples at a time that coincides with routine transport to the laboratory.

Sample requirements

A sample of venous blood is required. Most laboratories provide a specific tube for ESR only (black top) which contains the anticoagulant sodium citrate. The required volume is printed on the label. It is essential that anticoagulant in the bottle is mixed with the blood by gentle inversion.

Interpretation of results

Approximate reference range

Males   1–10 mm/hr
Females   5–20 mm/hr

Causes of a raised ESR

General considerations

ESR increases gradually with age, rising at the rate of around 0.8 mm/hr every five years. From the fourth month of pregnancy ESR usually rises to a peak of 40–50 mm/hr, returning to normal after birth.

ESR is one of the least specific of all laboratory tests. In other words, like a raised temperature or heart rate, a raised ESR occurs in many different sorts of illness. The changes in plasma proteins which give rise to increased red cell aggregation and raised ESR are a feature of any illness associated with significant tissue injury, inflammation, infection or malignancy. Unfortunately, from a diagnostic point of view, in most of these disease states, it is possible for the ESR to be normal. Furthermore it is clear that ESR is occasionally raised in normal healthy individuals. Despite these awkward anomalies that tend to confound interpretation of an ESR result, the ESR continues to be used in clinical practice. In general the higher the ESR the greater is the likelihood of a significant inflammatory, infectious or malignant disease.

Inflammatory disease

The inflammatory response to tissue injury results in abnormal increase in the synthesis of plasma proteins including fibrinogen, which tend to promote rouleaux formation and raise ESR. Potentially then any disease with an acute or chronic inflammatory component may be associated with an increase in ESR. In clinical practice the test is used as supportive evidence of inflammation in the diagnosis of disease associated with chronic inflammation such as rheumatoid arthritis, Crohn's disease and ulcerative colitis. It is frequently used to monitor disease activity in these conditions. A rising ESR in a patient with a known chronic inflammatory condition, such as rheumatoid arthritis, implies that disease activity is continuing or increasing and therefore not responding to current therapy. Conversely a falling ESR indicates reduced inflammation and therefore response to therapy.

Although the ESR has a limited diagnostic role for most diseases with an inflammatory component, because there are other more reliable and specific tests available, there are two related conditions in which ESR is often the only laboratory test that is abnormal. These are temporal arteritis (sometimes called giant cell arteritis) and polymyalgia rheumatica. The first is an inflammatory disease of arteries, usually in the head and neck. The condition is relatively common in the elderly causing general feeling of malaise and tiredness along with severe headaches; sudden blindness may occur if the optic artery is affected. The second is an inflammatory condition affecting muscles causing severe muscle pain and stiffness particularly after resting. The two conditions often appear together in the same patient and both are associated with very high ESR, usually greater than 75 mm/hr, often higher. The ESR gradually returns to normal during treatment with steroids, and the test is used to monitor response to therapy. These are the only conditions in which diagnosis depends on the ESR test.

Infectious disease

Infection may be associated with an increased ESR. In general, bacterial infections tend to result in an increased ESR more frequently than those caused by viruses. Particularly high ESR (i.e. greater than 75 mm/hr) is most frequently found in those suffering chronic infections, for example, TB and sub-acute bacterial endocarditis (infection of valves of the heart), but any bacterial infection, if sufficiently severe, may be associated with very high ESR.

Malignant disease

Many patients suffering cancer of all types have a raised ESR. However, since a significant proportion of cancer patients do not have a raised ESR, the test has no place in cancer diagnosis. In the absence of infectious or inflammatory disease a significant increase in ESR (i.e. >75 mm/hr) might suggest that further investigation to detect cancer is warranted. Some authorities believe that a particularly raised ESR (i.e. >100 mm/hr) in a patient with cancer is reliable evidence of tumour spread beyond the primary site (metastasis).

The only widely accepted use of the ESR so far as malignant disease is concerned is in the diagnosis of multiple myeloma, a malignant disease of bone marrow in which uncontrolled proliferation of plasma cells within the bone marrow causes bone pain and bone destruction. These malignant plasma cells synthesise huge quantities of abnormal immunoglobulin at the expense of normal immunoglobulin (antibody) production. Since immunoglobulin is one of those proteins which increase rouleaux formation, and thereby the ESR, multiple myeloma is almost always associated with an increase in ESR (often >100 mm/hr). So consistent is this finding that a raised ESR was once among the criteria required for diagnosis of multiple myeloma.

Finally ESR is almost always raised in patients with Hodgkin's disease (malignant tumour of lymph nodes). The ESR is not used to make a diagnosis but is frequently use to monitor disease progress and therapeutic effectiveness.

Other common causes of raised ESR

Myocardial infarction (heart attack) involves tissue injury to heart muscle (myocardium). The consequent inflammatory response to this injury includes increased synthesis of plasma proteins (fibrinogen), which causes increased red cell aggregation and therefore raised ESR. Thus myocardial infarction is a common cause of raised ESR. Typically ESR rises after an infarct, peaking one week later. A gradual return to normal is usual over the next few weeks. A raised ESR is also common in patients suffering renal disease.

Causes of reduced ESR

A reduced ESR is far less common than an increased ESR and actually of little clinical significance. An abnormally high red cell count (polycythaemia) is the most frequent cause. Rare causes include sickle cell anaemia and hereditary spherocytosis; both conditions are associated with abnormally shaped red cells which slow the rate at which they sediment.

C-reactive protein (CRP)

Normal physiology – synthesis and function

C-Reactive protein (CRP) is so called because the first of its properties to be identified at the time of its discovery, in 1930, was its ability to react with (precipitate) C-polysaccharide, a constituent of the wall of streptococcal bacteria. CRP is synthesised in the liver and is one of a number of proteins present in blood plasma that are collectively called the acute phase proteins. Fibrinogen, a protein already discussed for its significance in the ESR test, is another of these acute phase proteins. In health acute phase proteins are present in blood plasma at low concentration. However following any tissue injury, infection or acute inflammation, blood concentration rises. This acute phase reaction, as it is called, is one part of the body's overall complex protective response to tissue injury or microbial attack. The ESR test owes its clinical utility to the acute phase reaction, because it is the increase in plasma concentration of the acute phase protein fibrinogen that accounts for the increased rate of red cell sedimentation associated with disease.

CRP is considered the archetypal acute phase protein. Under the influence of a chemical messenger called interleukin 6 (IL-6) released from macrophages at the site of infection or tissue injury, liver cells are stimulated to increase synthesis of CRP. Within five to six hours of the initial insult, plasma CRP concentration begins to rise rapidly to a maximal peak concentration at around 48 hours. In the case of bacterial infection, concentration can increase up to 10 000 fold[1]. As the stimulus for increased production ceases, plasma CRP concentration falls rapidly to normal concentration; CRP has a half-life in plasma of 19 hours, meaning plasma concentration is halved every 19 hours, once the stimulus for increased production is removed.

The physiological function of CRP is as a contributor to the body's overall innate defences against microbial attack. In this regard it is potent activator of the complement cascade, which leads to phagocytosis and bacterial destruction.

Laboratory measurment

Patient preparation

No particular patient preparation is necessary.

Sample timing

Blood for CRP may be taken at any time of the day, ideally at a time that allows immediate transport to the laboratory. However CRP is stable and samples can be stored at room temperature or in a sample fridge for up to 48 hours before being processed in the laboratory.

Sample requirements

Around 5 ml of blood is required for CRP measurement. Analysis can be performed on either serum or plasma. If local policy is to use serum the blood must be collected into a plain tube (without additives). If local policy is to use plasma blood must be collected into a tube containing the anticoagulant lithium heparin.

Interpretation of results

Approximate reference range

Adults and children	<10 mg/L
Pregnant women	<20 mg/L
Neonates	<4 mg/L (a high sensitivity assay [hs-CRP] is required to reliably distinguish normal and abnormal CRP concentration in neonates)

Causes of increased CRP

General considerations

Increase in both CRP and ESR are due to an acute phase reaction (APR) to tissue injury, infection, inflammation or malignancy. ESR is an indirect measure of APR (because it measures an effect of APR, namely the increased rate of red cell sedimentation) whereas CRP is a more direct measure. Still, in general terms, the conditions that give rise to a raised ESR, also give rise to an increase in CRP; like ESR, CRP is a non-specific indicator of tissue injury, infection, inflammation and malignancy.

CRP has some advantages over ESR. These include:

- Rapidity of response – CRP rises within hours of an insult (e.g. infection); ESR is slower to respond, over a period of days and weeks rather than hours.
- Sensitivity – CRP is generally a more sensitive test of inflammation; minimal inflammation might not be detected if only ESR is measured.
- Specificity – CRP is not affected, as ESR is by abnormality in red cell numbers and shape. So that, for example, CRP remains normal in patients whose sole problem is anaemia. ESR is raised in this condition, giving false evidence of inflammation or infection etc.

Infection

CRP is raised following infection. Bacterial infection is associated with highest concentration (in the range 80–1000 mg/L). The rise is more modest during viral infection (10–20 mg/L). This difference has been utilised clinically, for example, in identifying the cause of meningitis (bacterial versus viral). Measurement of CRP has proven useful for early identification of bacterial infection in a variety of clinical contexts. For example, detection of postoperative infection and infection among patients being cared for in intensive care (a group at particularly high risk of hospital acquired infection).

Inflammation

CRP is a very sensitive indicator of severity of inflammation. Highest concentration (>200 mg/L) indicates acute inflammation, for example, during the active phase of chronic conditions such as rheumatoid arthritis and Crohn's disease. With few exceptions, all conditions with an inflammatory component are associated with increase in CRP concentration; the magnitude of the increase reflecting severity. The test is very helpful in providing objective evidence of the therapeutic effect (or the lack of it) of treatment for inflammatory disease.

Tissue injury

Tissue injury, whatever its cause, is associated with increased CRP concentration. Severity correlates with concentration so that particularly high concentrations (>500 mg/L) might be evident following severe trauma or major surgery. The necrosis of heart muscle associated with myocardial infarction causes increase.

Clinically useful anomalies

As we have seen the normal response to active inflammatory disease is an increase in plasma CRP concentration. For reasons that remain unclear that response is either significantly lower in magnitude or entirely absent in a few inflammatory conditions. This has proven diagnostically useful because there are very few inflammatory conditions in which ESR is significantly raised (reflecting an inflammatory process) but plasma CRP is only slightly raised or even normal. One of these conditions is systemic lupus erythematosus (SLE or lupus), a relatively common chronic autoimmune disease that predominantly affects women of child-bearing age. Joint inflammation similar to that seen in rheumatoid arthritis is a common feature of lupus. When this inflammation occurs in the lupus patient it is accompanied as expected by a marked increase in ESR. However in contrast to most other inflammatory conditions, the plasma CRP remains resolutely normal. The combination of raised ESR and normal CRP is a useful diagnostic feature of SLE.

A similar combination of results (raised ESR and normal or only slightly raised CRP) is typical of the inflammatory bowel disease, ulcerative colitis. This feature distinguishes it from the only other inflammatory bowel disorder Crohn's disease, in which the increase in ESR and CRP are equal. The difference can be diagnostically helpful.

CRP and cardiovascular disease

The development of highly sensitive assays for CRP measurement that are capable of detecting concentration well below 10 mg/L (the limit of original assays used for CRP testing) has revealed that the mean concentration of plasma CRP in apparently healthy individuals is around 0.8 mg/L with a range of 0.01–10 mg/L. Many studies conducted over the past decade have demonstrated that CRP within this normal range predicts future risk of cardiovascular disease. The higher the plasma CRP concentration the greater is the risk of cardiovascular disease[2]. The only blood test currently used to assess an individual's risk of cardiovascular disease is blood cholesterol measurement (see Chapter 8). It seems possible that in the future measurement of plasma CRP might also be used in this way. Indeed at least one authoritative guideline[3] recommends this use of the high-sensitivity CRP test, and states that statin (cholesterol lowering) therapy aimed at reducing an individual's risk of cardiovascular disease should be offered to all those with a CRP >2 mg/L, irrespective of their blood cholesterol level.

Case history 26

Alex Manson was a cheerful healthy five year old until he first became acutely ill just over six months ago. His first complaint was a sore throat. Over the next two weeks he had a spiking fever almost every day and a recurring rash on his trunk. His knee joints became painful making him uncharacteristically tearful. He was often tired and spent long periods just lying on the couch. After a course of antibiotics prescribed by his GP failed to have any effect, and during a particularly severe fever, Alex was admitted for investigation to his local hospital nearly three weeks after the first sign of illness. Among the blood tests performed was an ESR, which was reported as 89 mm/hr. A diagnosis of Still's disease (a form of juvenile chronic arthritis) was eventually made and the intensity of symptoms resolved with administration of the anti-inflammatory drug naprosyn. After three weeks in hospital

Alex was discharged home with prescriptions for naprosyn and methotrexate. At his most recent rheumatology outpatients' clinic, blood was collected from Alex for ESR. The result on this occasion was 18 mm/hr.

Questions

(1) Was Alex's ESR normal at the time of admission to hospital?
(2) Was this ESR result consistent with a diagnosis of Still's disease?
(3) What is the significance of the ESR result at Alex's recent outpatient appointment?
(4) What is meant when ESR is described as a non-specific test?
(5) Would you have expected Alex's plasma CRP concentration to be reduced, normal or raised on admission to hospital.

Discussion of case history 26

(1) No. Alex's ESR was grossly elevated.

(2) Yes. Like many other forms of arthritis, Still's disease is a chronic condition characterised by inflammation of the joints. A raised ESR is almost always a feature of active inflammatory disease.

(3) The most recent ESR shows a marked reduction, reflecting a reduction in disease activity. The result provides objective evidence that the prescribed drug regime (naprosyn and methotrexate) is, for the moment at least, keeping this chronic disease under control.

(4) A non-specific test like ESR is one that is abnormal in a wide range of pathological conditions. By contrast a specific test is one that is abnormal in one or a few related conditions. There are few tests that are absolutely specific for a single disease, but nearly all are more specific than ESR. In the context of this case history the non-specificity of the ESR means that although ESR is usually raised in patients with Still's disease it is not useful to make the diagnosis, there are many other conditions in which a raised ESR is equally likely.

(5) Alex's plasma CRP concentration would have been increased.

References

1. Pepys, M. and Hirshfield, G. (2003) C-reactive protein: a critical update, *J Clin Invest*, 111: 1805–12.
2. The Emerging Risk Factors Collaboration (2010) C-reactive protein concentration and risk of coronary heart disease stroke and mortality: an individual participant meta-analysis, *Lancet*, 375: 132–40.
3. Genest, J., Mcpherson, R., Frolich, J. et al. (2009) Canadian guidelines for the diagnosis and treatment of dyslipidaemia and prevention of cardiovascular disease in the adult: 2009 recommendations, *Can J Cardiol*, 25: 567–79.

Further reading

Batlivala, S. (2009) Focus on diagnosis: The erythrocyte sedimentation rate and the C-reactive protein test, *Pediatrics in Review*, 30: 72–4.
Fincher, R. and Page, M. (1986) Clinical significance of extreme elevation of the erythrocyte sedimentation rate, *Arch Intern Med*, 146: 1581–3.
Windgassen, E., Funtowicz, L. and Lunsford, T. (2011) C-reactive protein and high-sensitivity C-reactive protein: an update for clinicians, *Postgrad Medicine*, 123: 114–19.

PART 4

Blood Transfusion Testing

CHAPTER 20

BLOOD GROUP, ANTIBODY SCREEN AND CROSSMATCH

Key learning topics

- ABO and Rh blood group systems
- Incompatible transfusion reaction
- Other risks of transfusion
- Safe transfusion practice
- Antibody screening during pregnancy
- Haemolytic disease of the newborn

Every year in the UK over 2.5 million units of donated red cells are transfused to hospital patients. Transfusion is such a commonplace procedure that it is perhaps easy to underestimate the dangers involved. Although often of life-saving benefit, red cell transfusion is associated with considerable potential risk to the recipient patient. The two most significant risks are: transmission of serious blood born infection and the potentially fatal haemolytic transfusion reaction that can occur if patients receive incompatible red cells. The risk of infection is virtually eliminated[1] by careful donor selection and rigorous screening of all blood donations for evidence of infection (Table 20.1). In the UK, this screening procedure, which ensures supply of the safest possible blood products to local hospital blood transfusion laboratories, is the responsibility of the four national blood transfusion services. Prevention of the second major risk associated with red cell transfusion, incompatible transfusion reaction, begins with the pre-transfusion tests of donor and recipient blood conducted in local hospital blood transfusion laboratories. Of crucial importance are the three tests that are the subject of this chapter: determination of blood group, antibody screen and crossmatch. In order to understand what is meant by an incompatible red cell transfusion and the significance of these tests for its prevention, a little background immunology is required.

Understanding Laboratory Investigations: A Guide for Nurses, Midwives and Healthcare Professionals, Third Edition. Chris Higgins.
© 2013 John Wiley & Sons, Ltd. Published 2013 by John Wiley & Sons, Ltd.

Table 20.1 Some of the selection criteria for blood donors and mandatory tests on donated blood to prevent transmission of infectious disease.

Blood donors must:
be aged between 17 and 65 years
be in good health
weigh more than 50 kg
have a haemoglobin (Hb) greater than 13.5 g/dl if male and greater than 12.5 g/dl if female

Blood donors must not:
be pregnant or have been pregnant during previous 12 months
have ever suffered from cancer, syphilis or brucellosis
have a recent history of malaria, hepatitis jaundice or glandular fever
be in a high risk group for HIV infection
have received a blood product transfusion since 1980
donate blood more than three times a year

All donated blood is tested for the presence of:
hepatitis B surface antigen
antibody to hepatitis C
hepatitis C nucleic acid
antibody to *Treponema pallidum*

Background immunology

What are antigens and antibodies

Our ability to withstand attack from invading micro-organisms, such as bacteria and viruses, depends in part on antibody produced by plasma cells, derived from white blood cells called B-lymphocytes. Antibodies are immunoglobulin proteins. They bind to and neutralise bacteria and viruses. Each antibody is very specific in its action, so that an antibody that binds and neutralises one sort of bacteria will have no effect on another. This specificity is due to the specific nature of the molecular target on the surface of each sort of bacteria. This molecular target is called the antigen. Recognition by B-lymphocytes of specific bacterial or viral antigens induces specific antibody production.

This ability of the body to produce destructive antibodies to 'foreign' antigens is not confined to those antigens present on the surface of bacteria or viruses. Proteins and other molecular substances present on the surface of any foreign (i.e. non-self) cell are 'seen' as antigens and provoke a similarly destructive specific antibody response. It is, for example, this same antibody response to foreign antigens that accounts in part for the tissue rejection that can occur following organ transplantation.

To summarise then:

An **antigen** is any substance (most commonly a protein, but may be a carbohydrate) that causes production of antibodies by plasma cells (B-lymphocytes). Antigens are found usually, although not exclusively, on the surface of cells.

An **antibody** is a protein (immunoglobulin) which circulates in blood plasma and binds only with the antigen that provoked its production.

When an antibody binds with an antigen present on the surface of a cell, be it a bacteria, virus or tissue cell, a sequence of events follows which invariably leads to that cell's disruption or destruction.

One of the characteristics of the immune system is its ability to remember. On the first occasion lymphocytes 'meet' a foreign antigen, antibody production is low and therefore not very effective. However the immune system is now primed. Specialised lymphocytes (called memory lymphocytes) 'remember' the antigen, so that when it is encountered on subsequent occasions, both speed and intensity of antibody production are greatly increased. This is the basis of the concept of acquired immunity: we have limited protection (immunity) against a particular bacteria or virus until our immune system has been primed by initial exposure.

Clearly it is vital for health that we do not produce antibodies to our own antigens, and the immune system has the means to prevent this occurring. However it is worth mentioning in passing that there are a large group of pathological conditions, collectively known as the autoimmune diseases, in which this ability to distinguish 'self' from 'non-self' antigens is lost. These diseases are characterised by the production of antibodies (autoantibodies) directed at 'self' antigens. Common diseases with an autoimmune component include rheumatoid arthritis, Type 1 diabetes, most thyroid diseases and systemic lupus erythematosus (SLE); there are many others.

Notwithstanding these pathological exceptions, it is important to remember for the discussion here that it is normally not possible to produce antibodies to one's own antigens.

Red cell antigens and blood group

The surface of red cells like all other cells are covered with inherited antigens. These red cell antigens (or the lack of them) determine an individual's blood group. More than 700 different red cell antigens (most very rare) have been identified; these make up the 30 blood group systems so far described. Fortunately, only a tiny minority of these antigens are of significance in transfusion medicine. Of those that do have significance, the antigens of the ABO and Rh blood group systems are of prime importance.

ABO blood group system

We all belong to one of four groups of the ABO blood group system determined by the inheritance or non-inheritance of two red cell antigens, A and B. Those who inherit neither A nor B red cell antigens belong to group O; those who inherit the A red cell antigen belong to group A, those who inherit the B red cell antigen belong to group B and those inherit both the A and the B red cell antigen belong to group AB. Most (88%) of the UK population belong to either group O or group A.

Rh blood group system

The Rh blood group system, so called because early research was conducted on rhesus (Rh) monkeys, is the only other blood group system of major significance to blood transfusion. There are five red cell antigens in the Rh system – C, c, D, E and e – but only the D antigen is of major significance. Around 85% of UK population have the D antigen on their red cells and are said to be Rh D positive, the remaining 15% do not have the D antigen and are Rh D negative.

Other less significant red cell antigens

A routine blood group means determination of patient ABO group type and Rh D type (either positive or negative). Of the remaining 400 plus red cell antigens, which may or may not be present on the surface of an individual's red cells, a few have occasional significance for transfusion medicine. Among these are other antigens of the Rh blood group system (i.e. the c, C, E and e antigens) and antigens of the Kell (K), Duffy (Fy), Kidd (Jk), MNS and Lewis (Le) blood group systems. These antigens are rare causes of transfusion reaction either because they are themselves rare or because they are relatively weakly immunogenic.

Antibodies to red cell antigens: incompatible blood transfusion

The significance of red cell antigens for blood transfusion medicine lies in the specific antibodies to these red cell antigens, which may or may not be present in the recipient's plasma. An incompatible transfusion reaction occurs when antibody present in the patient's (recipient) plasma binds to its complementary antigen present on the surface of (donor) transfused red cells. Such antibody–antigen binding can result in the destruction of the donated red cells; this destruction is called haemolysis so that the term immune haemolytic transfusion reaction is used to describe this adverse effect of blood transfusion. So long as the patient's plasma contains no significant antibodies to the antigens present on the red cells of donated blood, the patient and donor blood are said to be compatible and donor blood can be safely transfused.

Production of red cell antibodies

It was stated above that antibodies are only produced when B-lymphocytes come into contact with the relevant 'foreign' antigen. There are two situations in which an individual's antibody producing lymphocytes may come into contact with 'foreign' red cell antigens. The first of course is blood transfusion, and the second is pregnancy. During labour of pregnancy, and sometimes earlier in pregnancy, foetal blood leaks to maternal circulation. The volume of this so called fetomaternal haemorrhage is usually <0.1 ml but can, in a small minority of pregnancies, be as much as 30 ml. If foetal red blood cells bear antigens inherited from the father, which are not present on the mother's red cells, they are 'seen' as foreign by the mother's lymphocytes, which then proceed to manufacture antibody.

As with any other immune response, initial antibody production during the first immunising blood transfusion or pregnancy is low and usually has no effect. But the immune system is now primed to synthesise large quantities of antibody, the next time the 'foreign' red cell antigen is encountered. Antibodies produced in this way are called immune red cell antibodies. The clinically most significant immune red cell antibody is anti-D, the antibody to the Rh D antigen. Of course only those who lack the Rh D antigen (i.e. the 15% of the population who are Rh D negative) can be immunised to produce anti-D in this way. In fact around 1% of the population have anti-D in their plasma, all the result of previous immunising transfusion

Table 20.2 The ABO blood group system and RhD type.

ABO blood group	Antigen present on red cells	Naturally occurring antibody in plasma	Frequency in UK population
O	Neither A nor B	anti-A and anti-B	47%
A	A	anti-B	42%
B	B	anti-A	8%
AB	A and B	None	3%

Note: RhD antigen present on the red cells of 85% of UK population; these individuals are RhD POSITIVE. RhD antigen is not present on red cells of the remaining 15%; these are RhD NEGATIVE.
Routine blood grouping: ABO group and RhD type (positive or negative) is determined.

or pregnancy. If such people were transfused with Rh D positive blood, the anti-D in their plasma would bind to the D antigen on the surface of donated red cells, resulting in a haemolytic transfusion reaction.

If immune red cell antibodies were the only red cell antibodies present in plasma, then only those who have a history of previous blood transfusion or pregnancy would be at risk of incompatible blood transfusion; this is not the case.

The overriding clinical significance of the ABO blood group system lies in the fact that antibodies to ABO antigens are naturally occurring, that is they do not arise as a result of immunisation by 'foreign' red cells. All of us have antibodies to the A or B antigen that we lack. Thus all those who belong to group O and lack both the A and B antigen have antibodies to both antigens (i.e. anti-A and anti-B) in their plasma; all those who belong to group A and have the A antigen on their red cells have antibodies to the B antigen (i.e. anti-B) in their plasma and all those of group B have the antibody to the A antigen (i.e. anti-A) in their plasma. Only the 3% of the UK population belonging to group AB, who have both the A and B antigen on their red cells, have no naturally occurring anti-A or anti-B in their plasma. The antigens and antibodies associated with the four groups of the ABO blood group system are summarised in Table 20.2.

It is the relative ubiquity and potency of naturally occurring anti-A and anti-B that determines the prime clinical importance of the ABO blood group system. Like anti-D, practically all other clinically significant red cell antibodies are immune antibodies so they cannot be present in the plasma of a person who has not been immunised by a previous transfusion or pregnancy. Thus the only significant red cell antibodies present in an individual who has never received a blood transfusion or been pregnant is naturally occurring anti-A or anti-B. It has been estimated that if only ABO compatibility were ensured and no other tests were performed red cell transfusion would be immunologically safe in 97% of cases.

Immune haemolytic transfusion reaction – ABO incompatibility

The consequences of transfusing ABO incompatible blood are described in Figure 20.1. Such a reaction can occur after only a few millilitres of blood have been transfused, such is the potency of anti-A and anti-B. In this example, blood

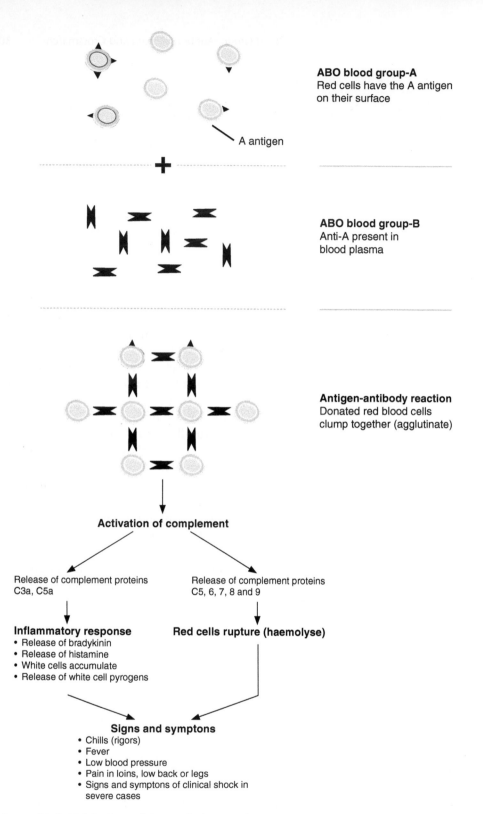

ABO blood group-A
Red cells have the A antigen on their surface

A antigen

ABO blood group-B
Anti-A present in blood plasma

Antigen-antibody reaction
Donated red blood cells clump together (agglutinate)

Activation of complement

Release of complement proteins C3a, C5a

Release of complement proteins C5, 6, 7, 8 and 9

Inflammatory response
• Release of bradykinin
• Release of histamine
• White cells accumulate
• Release of white cell pyrogens

Red cells rupture (haemolyse)

Signs and symptons
• Chills (rigors)
• Fever
• Low blood pressure
• Pain in loins, low back or legs
• Signs and symptons of clinical shock in severe cases

Figure 20.1 ABO incompatible transfusion reaction.

from a donor who is blood group A is transfused to a patient who is blood group B. Anti-A present in the patient's plasma binds to the A antigen on the surface of donated red cells. The red cells clump together (agglutinate). Antigen-antibody binding activates the so called complement pathway; it is the complement proteins (by convention denoted by the letter C followed by a number), produced as a result of this activation, which accounts for many of the signs and symptoms of a haemolytic transfusion reaction. Complement proteins C5, C6, C7, C8 and C9 are all involved in the process of red cell destruction (haemolysis), in which holes are made through the red cell membrane. By this complement mediated haemolysis, all donated red cells are destroyed in the most severe cases of ABO incompatibility. Complement proteins C3a and C5a initiate an inflammatory response that includes release from activated mast cells of various potent chemicals (e.g. histamine, bradykinin) that causes a sudden fall in blood pressure (hypotension) and other very visible symptoms. The fall in blood pressure leads to symptoms of clinical shock and reduced flow of blood to the kidneys with the onset of acute kidney disease (renal failure) in the most severe cases. Other complications of severe haemolytic transfusion reaction include disseminated intravascular coagulation, a condition discussed briefly in Chapter 17. The excess Hb released from damaged red cells is metabolised to bilirubin, causing jaundice.

Other immune haemolytic transfusion reactions

Even if donated blood is ABO compatible with recipients blood, there remains a risk of immune haemolytic transfusion reaction if there are other significant red cell antibodies present in the patients plasma. Since these are all immune antibodies, they can only be present in the plasma of those patients who have been immunised by previous blood transfusion or pregnancy. The most important of these is anti-D. Others include anti-C, anti-c, anti-E and anti-e (i.e. remaining antibodies to Rh blood group antigens); anti-K (antibody to the Kell (K) blood group antigen); anti-Fy^a and anti-Fy^b (antibodies to two of the Duffy (Fy) blood group antigens); and anti-Jk^a and anti-Jk^b (antibodies to two of the Kidd (Jk) blood group antigens). Symptoms of haemolytic transfusion reaction which result from these antibodies are generally speaking less severe than those associated with ABO incompatibility. The reaction may be delayed for up to ten days after the transfusion, when chills and fever develop. Red cell destruction may cause anaemia and mild jaundice.

Laboratory testing: blood group, antibody screen and crossmatch

Sample collection

When a patient requires a blood transfusion, 7.5 ml of venous blood must be collected into a plain tube containing no additives, or a bottle containing the anticoagulant EDTA, depending on local policy. Blood transfusion laboratories supply designated tubes (usually pink top) that are to be used only for these tests.

Because of the potentially fatal consequences of giving donated blood product to the 'wrong' patient, scrupulous attention to the detail of patient identification and documentation is vital when collecting blood for all of these tests. Before taking blood ensure beyond any doubt the identification of the patient, by asking the patient his or her name and cross-checking with his or her identification armband.

The following minimum information must be written legibly on the sample label and accompanying request card:

- Patient's first and last name (taken from the patient's armband).
- Hospital number (taken from the patient's armband).
- Patient's ward or department.
- Date and time of collection.
- Initials of person taking the blood.

The request card should include the following additional details:

- The nature of donated blood required (whole blood, packed red cells etc.).
- Number of donated units required.
- When the blood is required – level of urgency.
- Why the blood is required (acute blood loss, chronic anaemia, elective surgery etc.).
- ABO and rhesus blood group (if known).
- Any relevant transfusion or obstetric history (if known).
- Signature of the medical officer making the request.

These are guidelines only; healthcare workers involved in the collection of blood for pre-transfusion testing must adhere scrupulously to protocol contained in the local blood transfusion policy document, which should reflect best practice as defined by the British Committee for Standards in Haematology (BSCH) in collaboration with the Royal College of Nursing and the Royal College of Surgeons[2,3].

Principles of the three tests

The purpose of the three tests is to prevent immune haemolytic transfusion reaction by issuing only donated red cells that are immunologically compatible with the blood of the patient who is to receive the transfusion. In essence this means first determining which antibodies to red cell antigens are present in the patient's plasma and then selecting donated blood (red cells) that contain none of the relevant red cell antigens. The only significant antibodies that can be expected with certainty to be present in patient's plasma are the naturally occurring antibodies to the red cell antigens of the ABO group system, so that determination of the patient's ABO blood group is the prime test. At the same time as the ABO group is determined the Rh D status (either negative or positive) is also determined. Together these are the routinely determined 'blood group' or 'blood type'.

The binding of red cell antibody to its complementary antigen results in agglutination (clumping together) of cells. This visible phenomenon is exploited in all

	Patient 1	Patient 2	Patient 3	Patient 4
Anti-A				
Anti-B				
Result	No agglutination when either anti-A or anti-D is added	Agglutination only when anti-A added	Agglutination only when anti-B added	Agglutination when both anti-A and anti-B are added
Interpretation of result	**Group O**	**Group A**	**Group B**	**Group AB**
Per cent frequency in UK population	47	42	8	3

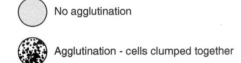

No agglutination

Agglutination - cells clumped together

Figure 20.2 Determination of ABO blood group

blood banking tests and is reflected in the alternative name for red cell antibodies and antigens. In many texts red cell antibodies are referred to as agglutinins and antigens as agglutinogens.

Blood grouping

Patient's ABO blood group is determined by simply mixing a sample of patient's red cells with sera containing anti-A and sera containing anti-B. The red cells either agglutinate or stay separate in suspension (Figure 20.2). As an additional check a reverse group is performed in which the patient's serum is added to red cells of known ABO group. Rh D type is determined by mixing patient's cell with a solution of anti-D. Agglutination indicates the presence of the D antigen on patient's cells (Rh D positive). No agglutination indicates the patient's blood is Rh D negative.

Antibody screen

By performing an ABO blood group we know that patient's plasma contains either anti-A or anti-B, both of these, or neither of these. In around 97% of cases no further antibody is present. With a few very rare exceptions all other significant red cell antibodies, including antibody to the Rh D antigen, are present in the patient's plasma only as a result of previous immunising blood transfusion or pregnancy. However since the presence of some of these red cell immune antibodies may provoke a haemolytic reaction if red cells to be transfused bear the relevant antigen, a search for the presence of any significant atypical antibodies (i.e. not anti-A or anti-B) is performed on the serum of all patients who are to receive donated blood. This is the antibody screening test.

Essentially, the antibody screening test is performed by adding a drop of patient's plasma to a panel of different group O red cells, each bearing a different and known combination of the most common red cell antigens known to cause immune haemolytic reactions. Since group O red cells do not have the A or B antigen on their surface, any agglutination when the patient's plasma is added to this panel of red cells must be due to the presence of an atypical antibody in the patient's plasma. No agglutination indicates no atypical antibodies and the result 'antibody screen negative' is reported. The antibodies tested for in the antibody screening test usually include at least all of the following:

- Anti-D, anti-C, anti-c, anti-E and anti-e (antibodies to Rh blood group antigens).
- Anti-K and anti-k (antibodies to Kell (K) blood group antigens).
- Anti-Fy^a and anti-Fy^b (antibodies to two of the Duffy (Fy) blood group antigens).
- Anti-Jk^a and anti-Jk^b (antibodies to two of the Kidd (Jk) blood group antigens).
- Anti-S, anti-s, anti-M and anti-N (antibodies to four of the MNS blood group antigens).

If the screen is positive, the identity of the antibody or antibodies causing the positive result can usually be deduced from the pattern of reactions displayed by the panel of O red cells.

Selection of donor blood

Having established what significant red cell antibodies are present in the patient's plasma, the next step is selection of a suitable red cell donor unit. What is required is blood whose red cells do not bear any of the antigens that react with any significant antibodies present in the patient's (recipient) serum. For those patients whose antibody screen is negative (the vast majority), the only consideration is ABO and Rh D compatibility. In most instances this simply means selecting blood (packed red cells) that has the same ABO and Rh D type as the patient. Recommended policy[4] is that whenever possible all patients should receive donated red cells of the same ABO and Rh D type as their own. However if ABO/Rh D identical blood is not available, there is some room for manoeuvre:

- Those people whose ABO blood type is AB have no ABO antibodies in their plasma, so they can safely receive donated blood product of any ABO group. In fact it is recommended[4] that to preserve group O stocks, only group A and group B red cells be given to group AB recipient patients, in the event that group AB blood is not available.

- The red cells of blood group O have no A or B antigens on their surface so can be safely transfused to patients of any ABO group. A donor of blood type O Rh D negative has no ABO antigens and no Rh-D antigens. This is the only blood type that can be relatively safely given without crossmatch to a patient whose blood ABO and Rh type are unknown. This is only considered in the rare event of life-threatening haemorrhage, where the clinical need for a blood transfusion is so urgent that it does not allow time for laboratory testing.
- Patients who are Rh D positive cannot have antibodies to the D antigen and can therefore be given blood which is either Rh D positive or negative.
- Patients who are Rh D negative may or may not have antibodies to the D antigen, but whether they do or not transfusion of Rh D positive red cells almost invariably invokes anti-D production, which is best avoided. For this reason only Rh D negative red cells should be selected for transfusion to Rh D negative individuals. This is particularly important for Rh D negative women who could become pregnant (i.e. all pre-menopausal women) because of the risk of haemolytic disease of the newborn associated with having anti-D in their blood (discussed further).
- When giving blood of one ABO type to a recipient patient of another ABO type, consideration must be given to the naturally occurring antibodies (i.e. anti-A and anti-B) present in the plasma of donated blood. There is the potential for a haemolytic reaction caused by binding of these to A and/or B antigens present on the surface of patient's red cells. In practice this is not usually a problem because most of the donors plasma and therefore most of the offending anti-A and/or anti-B is removed in preparing packed red cells for transfusion. However it is a potential problem in the rare event that whole blood (rather than packed red cells) of ABO type O is transfused to patients of group A, B or AB. Only blood labelled 'high titre negative' (which has relatively low amounts of anti-A and anti-B) should be transfused in this circumstance.

Table 20.3 summarises the criteria for selection of donor unit for transfusion, based on the ABO group and Rh D type of the patient.

For those patients whose antibody screen is positive a further step is required. First ABO-Rh D identical or compatible donated blood units are selected as described above. The red cells of these are then tested for the presence of red cell antigens that react with the atypical antibody found in the patient's serum. So, for example, suppose the antibody screen revealed that the patient had the antibody that reacts with the Rh C antigen (i.e. anti-C), the red cells of donated blood must be tested for the presence of the C antigen. Only blood that is negative for the C antigen can be transfused.

Crossmatch

Having selected a unit of donated blood whose red cells have no antigens that could react with clinically significant antibodies present in the patient's plasma, one final checking test must be performed to ensure compatibility. This is the crossmatch in which transfusion is simulated in a test tube. Essentially a sample of

Table 20.3 Selection of donor red cell units for transfusion.

Donor blood group	Recipient (patient) blood group							
	O RhD Pos	O RhD Neg	A RhD Pos	A RhD Neg	B RhD Pos	B RhD Neg	AB RhD Pos	AB RhD Neg
O RhD Pos	✓	✗	✓	✗	✓	✗	✓	✗
O RhD Neg	✓	✓	✓	✓	✓	✓	✓	✓
A RhD Pos	✗	✗	✓	✗	✗	✗	✓	✗
A RhD Neg	✗	✗	✓	✓	✗	✗	✓	✓
B RhD Pos	✗	✗	✗	✗	✓	✗	✓	✗
B RhD Neg	✗	✗	✗	✗	✓	✓	✓	✓
AB RhD Pos	✗	✗	✗	✗	✗	✗	✓	✗
AB RhD Neg	✗	✗	✗	✗	✗	✗	✓	✓

✓ ABO compatible. No risk of Rh sensitisation. Safe to transfuse if patient antibody screen is negative.
✗ ABO incompatible or risk of Rh sensitisation. Not safe to transfuse.

donor red cells is mixed with a sample of patient's (recipient) serum and inspected for agglutination. No agglutination indicates there is no red cell antigen/antibody reaction and that the donor red cells are compatible with patient's plasma, and can be safely transfused.

Pre-transfusion checks on the ward

Severe acute haemolytic reactions are rare events but when they do occur the cause is usually transfusion of blood to the 'wrong' patient due to clerical error or error in patient identification. The commonest single error is failure to check at the bedside that the right blood is being given to the right patient.

Adherence to the agreed protocol for pre-transfusion checks, contained in the local blood transfusion policy document, is vital. Local protocols must reflect best practice as defined by the British Committee for Standards in Haematology (BSCH) in collaboration with the Royal College of Nursing and the Royal College of Surgeons[2,3].

Pre-transfusion checks, which ideally should be made by two nurses one of whom is state registered should include:

- Confirmation of patient's identity, by asking the patient and cross-checking with their identity armband.
- Confirmation that the patient details on the blood compatibility report match in every detail the identity of the patient to be given blood.
- Confirmation that the identifying unit number printed on the unit of blood to be transfused matches the unit number on the compatibility report.
- Confirmation that the ABO blood group and Rh D type printed on the blood unit is the same as, or compatible with, the patient's ABO and Rh D blood group.
- Confirmation that the unit of blood to be transfused has not passed its expiry date, and that no more than 30 minutes have elapsed since the unit was removed from the blood bank refrigerator.
- Baseline measurement of patient's blood pressure, temperature, pulse and respiration rate must be recorded immediately before the start of blood transfusion.

Other transfusion reactions

The laboratory tests discussed in this chapter are designed solely to prevent immune haemolytic transfusion reactions, but these are not the only adverse reactions that a patient can suffer during a blood transfusion.

Febrile reactions

Patients who have received previous blood transfusions may have developed antibodies to antigens present on the surface of white cells. If blood with white cells that bear these antigens is transfused to such patients then a febrile reaction, characterised by shivering and fever, may develop. The symptoms are due to potent chemicals (cytokines) released from damaged white cells. Although quite common among patients who have previously received multiple transfusions, febrile reactions are usually mild and self-limiting.

Allergic reaction

Mild allergic reactions to a variety of donated plasma constituents are common, occurring in 1–2% of all transfusions. They are manifest as a red itchy skin rash (hives) within an hour of starting transfusion; anti-histamine treatment is effective in such cases. Rarely, potentially fatal systemic allergic (anaphylactic) reactions occur; patients with IgA deficiency are particularly vulnerable. Dramatic effect may be seen after transfusion of just a few millilitres. Signs and symptoms include flushing of the skin, hypotension, nausea, abdominal pain, respiratory distress and cyanosis. Rapid treatment response is vital for survival in these extreme, but rare, allergy cases.

Transfusion related acute lung injury (TRALI)

This is a serious condition with a mortality rate of around 10%. It is caused by the presence of antibodies in donor plasma directed at antigens present on recipient patient's white cells. Agglutinated white cells, sequestered in the microvasculature of the lungs, release a range of toxic products that damage the endothelial lining of these vessels, allowing fluid to leak to air sacs of the lungs (pulmonary oedema). The resulting severe acute respiratory distress can be rapidly fatal or resolve without long-term effect within a few days to a week. Signs and symptoms, which usually appear within an hour or so of transfusion and by definition within six hours of transfusion, include breathlessness, coughing, hypotension, rigors (sudden chills and shivering) and fever. Severe hypoxaemia is usual and many affected patients require mechanical ventilation for a short period. The critically ill represent a patient group who are at greater than normal risk of TRALI.

Transfusion associated circulatory overload (TACO)

This condition, which disproportionately affects the very young and elderly, shares many of the features of TRALI. Positive fluid balance consequent on transfusion leads to (hydrostatic) pulmonary oedema and respiratory distress. Like TRALI, symptoms develop usually within an hour or two of transfusion and always within six hours. They include breathlessness, cough, headache and hypertension. There is an associated risk of convulsions and cerebral haemorrhage. The condition has a reported mortality rate of 5–15%. Transfusing blood of inappropriately large volume (i.e. too many units) or transfusing inappropriately rapidly can precipitate TACO.

Bacterial infection

Scrupulous aseptic technique during donor blood collection and care that donated blood is stored at a temperature (+4°C) that minimises bacterial growth ensure that donated blood is free from significant numbers of bacteria at the time of transfusion. Additional safeguards include pre-transfusion visual check of red cell pack for evidence of bacterial infection, the disposal of blood products that have passed their expiry date, and protocols which ensure that donated blood is not left at room temperature for longer than four hours before transfusion is complete. Although rare, reactions due to transfusion of bacterially contaminated blood can occur. Depending on the nature of the contaminating bacteria, symptoms vary. In the most severe cases symptoms can develop within a few minutes of starting the transfusion. These include fever, rigors, nausea and vomiting. Sudden fall in blood pressure can herald severe sepsis and risk of multi-organ failure. Transfusion of bacterially contaminated blood is potentially fatal.

Patient monitoring during transfusion

The vast majority of blood transfusions are uneventful, but because of the potentially serious adverse effects, careful observation of the patient is necessary during blood transfusion. Locally agreed protocol for the monitoring and management of patients receiving a blood transfusion must reflect best practice as defined by the BCSH in collaboration with the Royal College of Nursing and the Royal College of Surgeons[2,3]. Some general points are made here. Monitoring is particularly important during the early stages when most severe haemolytic reactions develop. Temperature, pulse, respiration and blood pressure should be checked at 15 minute intervals during the first hour and at hourly intervals thereafter. Patients should be observed for signs and symptoms of all adverse reactions. In the event of a suspected reaction, the transfusion should be stopped immediately and medical staff summoned. The management of a patient suffering a transfusion reaction depends on its cause and severity. Mild febrile reactions may require only the administration of an anti-pyretic drug (e.g. aspirin) to control temperature. The transfusion can be restarted, only at a slower rate. Mild allergic reactions may be treated with antihistamine drugs. For severe acute reactions such as immune haemolytic reactions, severe allergic reactions and those caused by bacterial infection, the principle first objective is to maintain blood pressure in order to preserve blood flow to the kidneys. Adrenalin and steroids may be administered to control allergy and shock. Diuretics may be administered to increase urine flow. In the case of suspected bacterial infection, broad-spectrum antibiotics are administered.

Chest X-ray, arterial blood gas analysis and assisted ventilation might be considered if respiratory distress caused by TRALI and TACO is suspected. Since both of these potentially fatal reactions can occur up to six hours after the transfusion, observation for signs of respiratory distress should continue after the transfusion has finished.

Laboratory investigation of transfusion reaction

In all cases of severe reaction, the laboratory must be informed as soon as possible, so that the cause of the reaction can be investigated. A fresh sample of patient's blood collected into a plain tube, along with the donor blood pack, must be sent to the laboratory for this purpose. Blood group, antibody screen and crossmatch will be repeated. Because of the risk of disseminated intravascular coagulation (DIC) and resulting excessive bleeding, associated with severe immune haemolytic reaction and reaction due to transfusion of bacterially contaminated blood, a sample of blood for Hb estimation and a further sample of blood for coagulation studies should also be sent to the laboratory. Finally blood from the donor pack and blood from the patient must be cultured for the detection of bacteria.

Post transfusion reactions

For the vast majority of patients, blood transfusion passes uneventfully. There remains a small risk of a delayed immune haemolytic reaction (usually mild) during the days that follow a blood transfusion. Sudden onset of chills, rise in temperature, anaemia and jaundice at any time during the ten day period following a transfusion may signal such a reaction.

Incidence of serious adverse events – how safe is transfusion?

Transfusion transmitted infection

Measures taken to minimise the risk of HBV, HCV, HIV and HTLV infection during transfusion have been highly successful. The blood supply has never been safer and the theoretical risk of contracting these viral infections during red cell transfusion is now vanishingly small. The chance that a unit of donated blood that is infected with HIV might enter the UK blood supply is currently estimated at 0.16 per million donated units[1]. The relevant figures for HCV, HBV and HTLV are respectively 0.014, 0.94 and 0.13. Around 2.5 million blood donations are made annually in the UK so that it is expected that a single HIV infected donation is released to the UK blood supply every two to three years. The relevant figures for HCV, HBV and HTLV are: one every 29 years; two every year; and one every three years.

Incidents of blood transfusion adverse events in the UK are collated in an annual Serious Hazards of Transfusion (SHOT) report. For the five year period 1999–2004 SHOT identified 24 cases of probable transfusion transmitted infection for all blood products, of which six were viral (two HBV, two HIV, one HTLV and one case of hepatitis E). There was one case of malarial transmission and the remaining 16 were bacterial (15 during platelet transfusion and just one during red cell transfusion). During the succeeding six years (2005–2010) there were no cases of virus (HIV, HBV, HCV, HTLV) or malaria transmitted infection and 15 cases of bacteria transmitted infection (12 during platelet transfusion and three during red cell transfusion).

It is now clear that the prion agent that causes the inevitably fatal, variant Creutzfeldt-Jacob disease (vCJD) (the human equivalent of bovine spongiform encephalitis or 'mad cow disease') is transmissible during transfusion, and a prototype blood test that might be suitable for testing all donated blood for the presence of this prion agent has recently been developed[5]. A number of measures have already been adopted to reduce the risk of transmitting vCJD during transfusion, and as of June 2012 there have only been five cases of possible or probable transfusion transmitted vCJD since the early 1990s, when vCJD was first described.

ABO incompatibility

The transfusion of ABO incompatible red cells is entirely avoidable and each case represents a system failure, invariably involving human error. Initiatives aimed at greater vigilance and awareness of the risk of transfusion among healthcare workers involved in the transfusion process have had the desired effect of reducing the number of ABO incompatible transfusions. For the period 1996–2004 there were on average 25 cases of ABO incompatible transfusion each year in the UK. That has been reduced to just 11 cases on average per year for the period 2005–2010; there were just four cases in 2010[6]. Most cases of ABO incompatible red transfusion result in minor or no ill effects, but in up to third of cases patients suffer serious morbidity requiring admission to intensive care and very rarely nowadays patients die as a direct result of receiving ABO incompatible red cells[7].

TRALI and TACO

Over the past five to ten years TRALI and TACO have emerged as significant causes of transfusion related morbidity and mortality; these now eclipse those due to ABO incompatibility. There are around 15–20 TRALI cases each year in the UK; they almost always result in major morbidity. TRALI accounts for one to two transfusion related deaths each year. Forty cases of TACO were identified by SHOT in 2010; these resulted in major morbidity requiring admission to intensive care for 15 patients, six of whom died.

Haemolytic disease of the new born (HDN)

Both determination of blood group and the antibody screening test are important not only for the prevention of haemolytic transfusion reactions but also for prevention and diagnosis of haemolytic disease of the newborn (HDN). As part of all pregnant womens' antenatal care a sample of blood is taken, usually at their first antenatal appointment, for blood group determination and antibody screen in case a blood transfusion is required either during pregnancy or in the post partum period. Another purpose of this testing is to identify those women whose developing baby is at risk of HDN, a condition which, at best, threatens the well being of the baby during the first weeks of life and, at worst, threatens survival of the developing foetus.

What is HDN?

Some red cell antibodies can pass from the mother's blood across the placenta to the foetal circulation. If the baby has inherited red cell antigens from the father that these maternal antibodies react with, an immune haemolytic reaction occurs and foetal red cells are destroyed.

Pregnancies most at risk are those in which the mother is Rh D negative and the father is group Rh D positive. There is a one in four chance that the baby of such a union will be Rh D positive. If the baby is in fact Rh D positive then when foetal red cells, as they do in all pregnancies, pass from foetal circulation to the mother's blood, the mother's lymphocytes 'sees' the D antigen present on the baby's red cells as foreign and produces anti-D.

During the first such pregnancy the titre (amount) of anti-D in the mother's plasma is usually insufficient to have any effect. But the mother's immune system is now primed to produce massive quantities of anti-D the next time it encounters Rh D positive red cells. In subsequent pregnancies, if the baby is once again Rh D positive, large amounts of anti-D pass from the mother to foetal circulation, bind to the D antigen on foetal red cells, provoking a massive haemolytic reaction, with destruction of the developing baby's red cells.

The effects of Rh D HDN are variable; some babies are unaffected but in the most severe cases, the severe anaemia that results from red cell destruction can lead to anaemia sufficiently severe to cause death *in utero*. More often babies are born anaemic and jaundiced. The jaundice is due to increased production of bilirubin from Hb released from haemolysed (destroyed) red cells. If haemolysis is particularly marked and serum bilirubin concentration rises very high, there is a risk of permanent brain damage caused by the deposition of bilirubin in the cells of the brain, a condition called kernicterus. Affected babies may need exchange transfusion, in which O Rh D negative blood (which because it lacks the Rh D antigen cannot be destroyed by any anti-D present) is transfused, as the babies' O Rh D positive blood, containing the damaging antibody and bilirubin, is removed. This transfusion corrects the anaemia and prevents further red cell damage; the severe jaundice resolves. If the developing foetus is severely affected, consideration may be given to intrauterine transfusion from as early as 18 weeks into the pregnancy.

Prevention of Rh D HDN

To prevent HDN caused by Rh D incompatibility, all Rh D negative women who have not been previously immunised to produce anti-D are offered an injection of anti-D at 28 and 34 weeks of pregnancy and immediately after birth, if the baby is confirmed to be Rh D positive. This administered anti-D binds to and destroys any foetal Rh D positive red cells present as a result of feto-maternal haemorrhage before the mother can mount an effective immune response, thereby preventing maternal production of anti-D that could jeopardise subsequent pregnancies. This anti-D treatment is also given to Rh D negative women immediately after any obstetric complication or investigation that might be associated with a potentially sensitising feto-maternal haemorrhage; these include miscarriage, abortion, intrapartum haemorrhage, ectopic pregnancy, chorionic villus sampling and amniocentesis. It is of course not necessary to give prophylactic anti-D if it is known with certainty that the developing foetus is Rh D negative.

HDN can be caused by other red cell antibodies

Although Rh D incompatibility between mother and baby is the cause of the most severe presentation of HDN, other red cell antibodies that may or may not be present in the mother's serum can cause HDN. For example, HDN can arise if there is

ABO blood group incompatibility between mother and baby due to the cross-placental passage of anti-A and anti-B from mother (group O) to baby (group A or group B). The anti-A and anti-B antibodies bind to foetal red cells, resulting in their destruction. For a number of reasons, HDN caused by ABO incompatibility is usually mild and of much less clinical significance than that due to Rh D incompatibility. However it can, unlike Rh D related HDN, occur during the first pregnancy because it does not depend on sensitisation of mother's immune system; anti-A and anti-B are naturally occurring antibodies already present in mother's blood.

Other immune antibodies of significance for possible HDN are antibodies to other Rh blood group antigens (i.e. anti-C, anti-c, anti-E and anti-e), anti-K (antibody to Kell blood group antigens), anti-Jk^a (antibody to Kidd blood group antigen) and anti-Dfy (antibody to Duffy blood group antigens). Together, anti-D, anti-K and anti-c are responsible for most cases of severe HDN.

The antibody screening test performed early in pregnancy (8–12 weeks gestation), and again later (at 28 weeks gestation) if initially negative, is designed to detect whether any immune red cell antibodies capable of causing HDN are present in the mother's blood plasma. In the event of a positive antibody screen the pregnancy is carefully monitored to assess the risk of HDN and its likely severity. This would include serial measurement of the amount (titre) of the offending antibody; a low and unchanging titre indicates a less severe outcome than a rising antibody titre.

Case history 27

Mrs Greenwood, a 24 year old mother, attends a surgical outpatient department to have blood taken for various tests prior to surgery scheduled later in the week. Among the blood tests requested is 'group, screen and save'.

Mrs Greenwood's blood group is found to be AB Rh D negative. During surgery Mrs Greenwood suffers a significant haemorrhage and a request for 2 units of cross-matched packed red cells is sent urgently to the laboratory.

During the pre-transfusion checks in the recovery room, prior to administration of the first unit, it is noted that the red cells to be transfused are A Rh D negative.

Questions

(1) What sample is required for 'group, screen and save' test request?
(2) What is the purpose of the test?
(3) In view of the ABO blood group discrepancy between donor and Mrs Greenwood, is it safe to go ahead with the transfusion?
(4) Why is it important that Mrs Greeenwood does not receive Rh D positive red cells?

Discussion of case history 27

(1) A 7.5 ml sample of venous blood collected into either a tube without anticoagulant or a tube containing the anticoagulant EDTA, specially designated for blood transfusion tests. For most laboratories these have pink tops and are labelled 'FOR BLOOD TRANSFUSION TESTING ONLY'.

(2) These tests are performed to reduce delay should Mrs Greenwood require a blood transfusion during surgery. Her ABO group and Rh D type will be determined. The term 'screen' refers to the antibody screening test in which her plasma is tested for the presence of any

atypical red cell antibodies, which may complicate the selection of a suitable donor unit. 'Save' simply means store the sample. Should a blood transfusion become necessary, the only remaining test to be performed is the crossmatch test in which Mrs Greenwood's stored sample of plasma is mixed with the red cells of a selected ABO and Rh compatible donor unit. If Mrs Greenwood were scheduled for major surgery in which excessive bleeding were a routine and expected complication, blood would be crossmatched prior to surgery.

(3) Although the ABO blood group of the donated unit is not identical, it is compatible with Mrs Greenwood's group. The donated red cells bear the A antigen; it is imperative that these are not given to a patient whose serum contains anti-A. Mrs Greenwood is group AB and her serum therefore contains no anti-A or anti-B, so she can be given group A red cells. Only 3% of the population belong, like Mrs Greenwood, to group AB so that a stock of ABO identical blood for such patients is sometimes not available; group A or group B packed red cells is a suitable and safe alternative.

(4) Mrs Greenwood belongs to the 15% of the population whose red cells do not bear the Rh D antigen. She is Rh D negative. If she were given blood whose red cells did bear the antigen (i.e. Rh D positive blood) her body would 'see' these cells as foreign and invoke an immune response with production of anti-D. This would be significant for future transfusions. If in any subsequent transfusion she were again given Rh D positive blood, her primed immune system would produce large quantities of anti-D, which would bind to the D antigen on transfused red cells and initiate an acute immune haemolytic reaction. There is also a risk that if Mrs Greenwood became pregnant any time after being given Rh D positive blood, her pregnancy would be complicated by severe haemolytic disease of the newborn. For this reason it is imperative that Rh D negative women of childbearing potential like Mrs Greenwood do not receive Rh D positive blood.

References

1. Health Protection Agency (2011) Safe supplies: focusing on epidemiology, *Annual Review from the NHS Blood and Transplant/Health Protection Agency Colindale Epidemiology Unit, 2010*, Health Protection Agency.
2. Department of Health (2007) Better blood transfusion – safe and appropriate use of blood, *Health Services Circular 200/9*, Dept of Health.
3. British Committee For Standards in Haematology (2009) Guidelines for the administration of blood and blood components and the management of the transfused patient, available at: http://www.bcshguidelines.com/documents/Admin_blood_components_bcsh_05012010.pdf.
4. Chapman, J., Elliot, C., Knowles, S. et al. (2004) Guidelines for compatibility procedures in blood transfusion laboratories, *Transfusion Medicine*, 14: 59–73.
5. Edgeworth, J., Farmer, M., Sicilia, A. et al. (2011) Detection of prion infection in variant Creutzfeldt-Jakob disease: a blood based assay, *Lancet*, 377: 487–93.
6. SHOT (2011) *Serious Hazards of Transfusion, Steering Group Annual Report 2010*, SHOT office Manchester Blood Centre Manchester, available at http://www.shotuk.org.
7. Janatpour, K., Kalmin, N., Jensen, H. et al. (2008) Clinical outcomes of ABO-incompatible RBC transfusions, *Am J Clin Path*, 129: 276–81.

Further reading

Bell, E. (2008) When to transfuse preterm babies, *Arch Dis Child Fetal Neonatal Ed*, 93: F469–F473.

Contreras, M. (1998) ABC of transfusion. In McClelland, D. (2007) *Handbook of Transfusion Medicine* (4th edn), BMJ Publishing Group, Her Majesty's Sationary Office, Norwich.

Oldham, J., Sinclair, I. and Hendry, S. (2009) Right patient, right blood, right care: safe transfusion practice, *Br J Nursing*, 18: 312–20.

Rauen, C. (2008) Blood transfusions in the intensive care unit, *Critical Care Nurse*, 28: 78–80.

Watson, D. and Hearnshaw, K. (2010) Understanding blood groups and transfusion in nursing practice, *Nursing Standard*, 24: 41–8.

PART 5

Microbiology Testing

URINE MICROSCOPY, CULTURE AND SENSITIVITY (M,C&S)

In this chapter and Chapter 22, attention is focused on the work of the clinical microbiology laboratory. Of all microbiological tests conducted in clinical laboratories, urine microscopy, culture and sensitivity is the most frequently requested. The test is used to help make or exclude a diagnosis of urinary tract infection (UTI) among patients who exhibit signs and symptoms of UTI, and among patients who are asymptomatic, but at high risk of UTI. After the respiratory tract, the urinary tract is the most frequent site of bacterial infection.

Normal physiology

The urinary tract

The urinary system (Figure 21.1) comprises the kidneys and ureters (the upper urinary tract), and bladder and urethra (lower urinary tract). The nephrons in kidneys are the site of urine formation, a topic considered in Chapter 5. Urine flows from nephrons into a system of collecting ducts. These ducts join at the pelvis of the kidney, where urine leaves the kidney.

Understanding Laboratory Investigations: A Guide for Nurses, Midwives and Healthcare Professionals, Third Edition. Chris Higgins.
© 2013 John Wiley & Sons, Ltd. Published 2013 by John Wiley & Sons, Ltd.

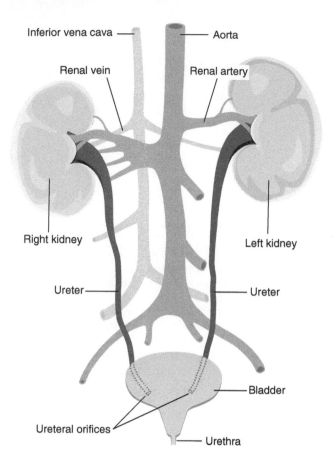

Inferior vena cava — Aorta

Renal vein — Renal artery

Right kidney — Left kidney

Ureter — Ureter

Bladder

Ureteral orifices — Urethra

Figure 21.1 Urinary tract.

Urine is continuously conducted from the pelvis of each kidney to the bladder, via two tubes called ureters. The walls of the ureters contain smooth muscle. Peristaltic contractions of this muscle wall, occurring around three times per minute, propel urine towards the bladder. The ureters are joined obliquely to the bladder at its base, and urine enters the bladder in continuous spurts due to the peristaltic action of the ureters. The oblique entry of ureters to bladder ensures that the opening to the bladder is kept closed, except during peristaltic contraction when urine enters. This effectively prevents urine passing from the bladder in the reverse direction up the ureters.

The bladder is an innervated muscular bag whose function is to store urine prior to urination, and expel all the urine it contains at the time of urination. The volume of the bladder increases as it fills with urine. Between 150 ml and 400 ml of urine are collected in the adult bladder before the conscious need to urinate arises; as accumulated volume increases beyond 400 ml this need becomes increasingly urgent and painful. A sphincter muscle (the external urethral sphincter), situated where the urethra joins the bladder, prevents accumulating urine leaving the bladder. At the time of urination this sphincter is relaxed; the detrusor muscle in the wall of the bladder contracts, forcing urine out of the bladder and urine flows from the bladder down the urethra.

The urethra is the tubular structure through which urine flows on the final part of its journey from the bladder out of the body. In females the opening of the urethra (called the meatus) is above and in front of the vaginal opening, and in the male it is at the tip of the penis. The male urethra is thus significantly longer than the female urethra.

Bacteria in the urinary tract

The urinary tract, from kidney to the final distal third of the urethra, normally contains no bacteria, so that in health the urine present in the bladder is sterile. Bacteria normally present on the skin of the perineum and in faeces can find their way up the urethra, so that bacteria may be present without any untoward effect in the lower third of the urethra. The normal flushing effect of urine as it passes down the urethra and other non-immune and immune defence against bacterial invasion serve to keep this bacterial contamination of urethra under control. In health, normally voided urine is either sterile (contains no bacteria) or contains low numbers of bacteria, flushed from the urethra during urination.

Urinary tract infection

Route of infection

Urinary tract infection (Figure 21.2) most often results from ascending infection by bacteria that constitute part of the normal bacterial flora of either the gastrointestinal tract or skin. Bacteria normally present in the gastrointestinal tract are present in faeces. These bacteria find their way from the perianal region via the perineum to the urethra and up into the bladder. The skin of the perineum is also a source of urinary tract pathogens. Bacteria that are normally present specifically in the female genital tract are a less common cause of UTI.

Infection and resulting inflammation of the bladder is called cystitis. This is the most common form of UTI. In a minority of individuals infection spreads up the urinary tract, infecting the kidney. Although far less common than infection of the lower urinary tract, infection of the kidney (pyelonephritis) is more serious than cystitis. Scarring of kidney tissue can in the long term reduce kidney function. Chronic infection of the kidney may result in renal failure. Pyelonephritis is associated with increased risk of infection spreading to the blood causing septicaemia and sepsis.

Although the ascending route of infection is the most usual, UTI may be caused by septicaemia. In this case bacteria present in blood may initiate descending infection of the urinary tract affecting first the kidneys and then the lower urinary tract.

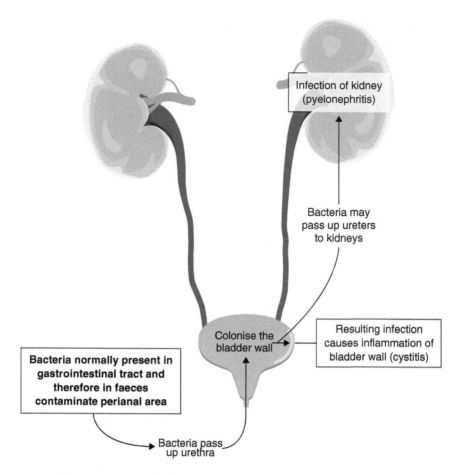

Figure 21.2 Ascending route of urine infection.

Predisposing factors

Gender

The relatively short female urethra is considered the principle reasons for the particular susceptibility of women to ascending UTI. Around a third of all women have a UTI before the age of 26[1], whilst for men under the age of 50 UTI is rare. The incidence of UTI infection among men increases significantly with age past 50 years, so that there is no gender difference in UTI prevalence among elderly patients. Among children, girls are more prone to UTI than boys.

Sexual activity

Women who are sexually active are more likely to suffer UTI than those who are not.

Pregnancy

Changes in the urinary tract from early in pregnancy increase the risk of bacteria present in the bladder spreading up the urinary tract with resulting pyelonephritis. For this reason all pregnant women are screened for the presence of significant numbers of bacteria in urine (bacteriuria) at least once during the first half of pregnancy.

Urine stasis

One of the principle physiological processes that prevents UTI is the flushing effect of sterile bladder urine through the lower urinary tract. Any disease process that inhibits urine flow or complete bladder emptying increases the risk of UTI. Obstruction of the urinary tract by stones (urinary calculi) or tumour, and disease of the prostate, which all impair urine flow, contribute to the increased incidence of UTI in older men, compared with younger men. Constipation is associated with incomplete bladder emptying and resulting predisposition to UTI, particularly among those with chronic constipation.

Immunosuppression

A suppressed immune system reduces host defence against bacterial invasion of the urinary tract. This explains the increased incidence of UTI among HIV patients and those who have been given immunosupressive drug (e.g. transplant patients). Generalised reduced immunity is a feature of advancing years and contributes to pathogenesis of UTI in the elderly.

Diabetes mellitus

Diabetics are more likely to suffer infections than non-diabetics. Urinary tract infection is a particular complication of long-standing diabetes.

Vesicoureteral reflux

Anatomy of the normal urinary tract prevents urine from passing from the bladder back into the ureters. Vesicoureteric reflux is a pathological condition in which reflux of urine from bladder to ureters greatly predisposes to ascending infection with resulting pyelonephritis. This is a particular problem among children and is a major cause of pyelonephritis among this age group. Other congenital abnormalities of the urinary tract cause UTI in babies and young children. If not identified and treated these anomalies, and associated recurrent UTI can lead to renal failure later in life. For this reason, UTI in childhood often warrants intensive urological investigation[2].

Hospitalisation

Illness that necessitates a stay in hospital is quite commonly associated with a temporary state of reduced immune defence against infectious disease. Furthermore the hospital environment is one in which the risk of coming into contact with infectious organisms is high. It is perhaps not surprising then that many patients acquire an infection as a direct result of being admitted to hospital. Around half of all patients in hospital who are suffering an infection, acquired the infection after admission. The principle site of hospital acquired (nosocomial) infection is the urinary tract; around 40% of all nosocomial infections are UTIs[3]. Patients at particularly high risk of nosocomial UTI are those who require urine catheterisation or cystoscopy (endoscopic examination of the urinary tract). Urological surgery is also associated with an increased risk of UTI. All patients who require long-term catheterisation, that is for more than a month, whether in hospital or the community, almost inevitably contract a UTI, though most are asymptomatic (i.e. they have significant bacteriuria, but do not feel unwell).

Signs and symptoms

Lower UTI (cystitis)
The principle signs and symptoms of cystitis are:

- Frequent urge to urinate even when there is not much urine in the bladder (frequency and urgency).
- Burning pain during and immediately after urination (dysuria).
- Supra-pubic pain (i.e. pain in the lower central abdomen).
- Fever may be a feature.

Upper UTI (acute pyelonephritis)
Those with upper UTIs are usually significantly more unwell than those with uncomplicated cystitis. Principle signs and symptoms include:

- Fever and rigors (fits of shivering).
- General malaise with nausea and vomiting.
- Renal (i.e. low back/flank) pain.
- Symptoms of lower UTI may also be present.

Microbiological examination of urine

Specimen collection (MSU)

The sample required is a 'clean catch' mid stream specimen of urine (Table 21.1). It is important that the sample is taken before antibiotics are given, as these can reduce the numbers of any bacteria present, resulting in a falsely negative result. If antibiotics have been given, then this should be stated on the accompanying request card.

Specimen collection (CSU)

The once widely adopted practice of catheterising patients simply to obtain a specimen of bladder urine for microbiological testing was abandoned when it was realised that the process of catheterisation itself increases the risk of UTI. However the collection of a catheter specimen of urine (CSU) is necessary for the investigation of catheterised patients. Any bacteria present in bladder urine will quickly multiply as it stands in a catheter drainage bag. Urine should not therefore be sampled from the drainage bag; it will give a false impression of the bacterial content of bladder

Table 21.1 Collection of 'clean catch' midstream urine (MSU) specimen.

OBJECTIVE

To collect a specimen of bladder urine uncontaminated by bacteria which may be present on:

- skin
- external genital tract
- perianal region or
- in the environment (on worktop surfaces, outside of collection bottle etc.)

PRINCIPLE

Any bacteria present in the urethra are washed away in the first portion of urine voided. This is not collected. All other potential contamination is avoided by thorough cleansing and effective aseptic technique.

PROTOCOL (for women)

1. Wash hands thoroughly with soap and water and dry.
2. With one hand separate the labia.
3. Area around the urinary meatus must be cleansed from front to back with soap and water and dried.
4. Still with labia separated, the patient voids the first 20 ml or so of urine into the toilet bowl, and then collects a portion of the remaining urine passed into a sterile universal container.
5. Screw on cap of urine bottle immediately taking care not to touch either the rim of the bottle of inside of the bottle cap.

PROTOCOL (for men)

1. Wash hands thoroughly with soap and water and dry.
2. Retract foreskin and clean around the urinary meatus with soap and water.
3. Patient must void the first 20 ml or so of urine into the toilet bowl, and then collect a portion of the remaining urine passed into a sterile universal container.
4. Screw on cap of urine bottle immediately taking care not to touch either the rim of the bottle of inside of the bottle cap.

---

urine. Urine should instead be sampled using scrupulous aseptic technique by syringe and needle from the self-sealing sleeve of the drainage tube. Aseptic technique is important for three reasons:

- It reduces the risk of infecting the catheterised patient.
- It reduces the risk of cross-infection from the catheterised patient to staff and other patients.
- It reduces the risk of the specimen being contaminated with bacteria in the environment.

Specimen collection (supra pubic aspiration)

The ideal 'gold standard' urine sample for microbiological examination is one obtained directly from the bladder, because it is free of contaminating bacteria normally present in the distal part of the urethra.

Bladder urine is normally sterile so any bacteria present in such a sample are always pathological. A bladder urine sample is obtained by inserting a sterile needle through the skin above the pubic bone into the bladder and aspirating urine into a sterile syringe. Such a procedure is clearly invasive, potentially hazardous and only rarely considered if collection of a clean catch urine is not possible, for example from babies.

Specimen collection bottle

Urine (either MSU or CSU) must be collected into a sterile bottle. It is not necessary to fill the bottle; 5–10 ml is all that is required.

Transport to the laboratory

Urine is a good medium for bacterial growth. Any bacteria present in the urine at collection will continue to multiply in the specimen bottle, giving falsely positive results. It is important then that the urine is examined within a few hours of collection. The time of sample collection should be recorded on the accompanying request card. If there is to be any delay in transport to the laboratory, urine is best stored in a designated refrigerator, as low temperature slows bacterial growth. Some laboratories provide sterile universal bottles that contain boric acid, a chemical that inhibits bacterial growth. The dip-slide culture method is designed for immediate culture of urine the moment the sample is voided. The slide, which is covered with a culture medium, is dipped into freshly voided urine, drained and then sent to the laboratory.

In the laboratory

As with any specimen submitted for microbiological examination, urine is:

- Examined macroscopically.
- Examined microscopically.
- Cultured to detect and identify any bacteria present.
- Any potential pathogenic bacteria discovered are tested for sensitivity or resistance to a range of anti-microbial drugs.

Macroscopic examination

Normal urine is a clear straw/yellow coloured fluid. Although by no means diagnostic, the appearance of urine can sometimes provide suggestive evidence of UTI. Like any other bacterial infection, UTI is associated with recruitment of phagocytic white blood cells (WBC) to the site of infection. Dead and dying white cells are removed from the site of any infection in an inflammatory exudate called pus. Pus in urine (pyuria) turns clear urine turbid (cloudy). The absence of cloudiness however does not rule out an infection and turbid urine does not necessarily mean the urine is infected; there are other benign causes of urine turbidity. Infection with some bacteria can make urine foul smelling.

Microscopical examination

A measured volume of urine is examined under the microscope principally for the presence of white and red blood cells. Urine normally contains a few white and red blood cells but a significant increase in white cell numbers particularly is strong evidence of an infective process. However an increased white cell count is occasionally seen in urine which when cultured is found to contain no bacteria. Conversely, a small minority of urines from patients suffering UTI contain normal numbers of white cells. Infection is sometimes associated with an increase in red cell numbers (haematuria). There are other pathological causes (mostly renal disease) for an increase in urine red cell numbers[4]. Epithelial (skin) cells naturally shed from the surface of the female genital tract may be seen in urine; these have no pathological significance but rather indicate that the urine was not collected properly and may contain contaminating bacteria from the genital tract. Bacteria if present in large enough numbers may be seen during microscopical examination of urine.

Culture

The only sure way of confirming the presence or absence of bacteria and identifying the species is to culture the urine. Culture in this context means grow. A measured volume of urine is placed on a sterile solid culture medium in a petri dish. The culture medium contains all the nutrients necessary for bacterial growth. The petri dish is then covered and placed in an incubator at 37°C (optimum temperature for bacterial growth) and left for 24 hours. Any bacterial growth is seen as visible colonies on the surface of the solid medium. Each colony contains many thousands of bacteria, all derived from a single bacterium present in the urine sample. The number of these visible colonies is directly related to the number of organisms in the urine sample. If the urine were sterile (i.e. contained no bacteria) there would be no visible colonies, the culture medium would appear unchanged.

As previously stated, it is quite normal for urine to contain small numbers of bacteria, mostly derived from the distal third of the urethra, so that the mere presence of bacteria in urine (bacteruria) is not sufficient to make a diagnosis of UTI. The term 'significant bacteruria' was first used by Kass in 1956[5] to diagnose UTI. He determined that, with some provisos, a bacterial count of more than 10^5 (i.e. 100 000) organisms per millilitre of urine was diagnostic of UTI. Although it has been demonstrated since that symptoms of UTI can occasionally occur when bacterial count drops as low as 10^3/ml and that some patients have no symptoms when their bacterial count is above 10^5/ml, Kass's dictum is still widely applied and a bacterial count of $>10^5$/ml remains a working definition of UTI. By counting the number of colonies in culture grown from a known volume of urine, it is possible to deduce the original concentration of bacteria in the urine specimen.

Each colony is the product of division of a single bacterium, so that each colony is pure (i.e. contains only one sort of bacteria). The macroscopic appearance of the colony provides some evidence of the sort of bacteria it contains but further testing is required for positive identification.

Although several types of bacteria are known to cause UTI, the commonest being *E.coli.* (Table 21.2), it is very rare for the infected urinary tract of any one patient

Table 21.2 Most common bacterial species to cause urinary tract infection (UTI).

Bacterial species	Normally present in:	% of UTI acquired in community	% of UTI acquired in hospital
Escherichia coli (*E.coli*)	GI tract, faeces	75–80%	50–60%
Staphylococcus epidermidis (*S. epidermidis*)	Skin, external genital tract	5–10%	<5.0%
Staphylococcus saprophyticus (*S. saprophyticus*)	GI tract, faeces	5–10%	<5.0%
Proteus species	GI tract, faeces hospital environment	<5.0%	10–15%
Klebsiella species	GI tract, faeces, external genital tract	<5.0%	10–15%
Pseudomonas aeruginosa (*P. aeruginosa*)	GI tract, faeces, hospital environment	<5.0%	5–10%
Other (many species)		<5.0%	5–10%

(except catheterised patients) to be colonised by more than one sort of bacteria. Thus the finding of many sorts of bacteria and no single one predominating (called a mixed bacterial growth) tends to indicate, not that the urinary tract is infected, but rather that the urine has been contaminated with the mixture of bacteria normally present in the lower third of the urethra or genito-anal area. In other words, the sample was not collected properly. A pure growth (i.e. growth of one type of bacteria) with a bacterial count of $>10^5$ organisms/ml or urine is virtually diagnostic of urinary tract infection.

Sensitivity

The results of this final test inform the decision about which antibiotic is to be prescribed in cases of bacterial infection. It is therefore a test that would not be performed if the results of urine culture revealed that the urine was sterile or contained insignificant numbers of bacteria. The object of the test is to determine the resistance or sensitivity of the particular strain of bacteria causing the UTI to a range of antibiotics. Bacteria are said to be resistant to an antibiotic if that antibiotic fails to kill the bacteria in culture. If prescribed, that particular antibiotic would not be effective in eradicating the infection. Conversely a strain of bacteria that is sensitive to a particular antibiotic will be killed by that antibiotic.

Essentially, the test is performed by taking colonies of bacteria previously grown by culture of the urine specimen and re-inoculating them on culture medium as before, but this time in the presence of a range of antibiotics. After a period of incubation the culture medium is inspected. If the strain of bacteria is resistant to the antibiotic being tested then no effect on bacterial growth is seen; the culture appears as it would if the antibiotic were not present. If however the bacteria are sensitive to the antibiotic being tested, there is no evidence of bacterial growth; the bacteria are killed and the culture medium appears as if no bacteria had been applied.

Since sensitivity testing involves a further period of incubation, there is an inevitable delay of up to 24 hours before the final report can be issued. If there is strong evidence of UTI at microscopy, that is there is a high white cell count and bacteria are visible, some laboratories perform sensitivity tests on urine directly, without waiting for the bacteria to grow in culture.

Interpretation of results

- Pure growth of bacteria with bacterial count of $>10^5$ organisms/ml urine **indicates UTI.** Increase in number of white cells (i.e. $>10/ml^3$ urine) provides supportive evidence.
- Pure growth of bacteria and bacterial count of 10^3-10^5 organisms/ml urine **indicates equivocal result.** May or may not be UTI. The presence of increased numbers of white cells (i.e. greater than $10/ml^3$ urine) supports a diagnosis of UTI. The higher the white cell count the stronger is the possibility of infection.
- Mixed bacterial growth indicates **probable contamination**, especially if epithelial cells are present. However this mixed growth may be masking urinary tract infection caused by one type of bacteria within the mixed growth, particularly if the bacterial count is high (i.e. $>10^5$ organisms/ml urine.) A carefully collected repeat sample may be indicated. A normal white cell count tends to suggest there is no UTI, whereas a raised white cell count suggests there might be.
- Sterile urine (no bacteria detected) or bacterial count of $<10^3/ml$ urine indicates **no evidence of UTI.** A white cell count of $<10/ml^3$ urine also indicates no evidence of UTI.

Post treatment testing

Symptoms of UTI may disappear within a few days of beginning a course of antibiotic therapy, but the only way of ensuring that a cure has been elicited is microbiological examination of urine. Although often not clinically necessary, an MSU can be examined at around one to four weeks after the course of antibiotics has been completed. If the bacterial species that caused the infection cannot be isolated from urine culture, a cure is proven.

Dipstick testing for UTI

Rapid dipstick tests to screen for UTI are commercially available. The tests are discussed in Chapter 25.

Although extremely convenient, these rapid dipstick methods have limitations. The number of false positive/negative results associated with their use is unacceptably high to make a definitive diagnosis of UTI[6]. In any case without culture of the urine, it is not possible to identify the causative bacteria and perform sensitivity studies.

Urines found to be positive by dipstick testing should be submitted to the laboratory for full urine culture and sensitivity. Recent clinical study[7] and current guidelines[8] suggest that this is not necessary in the case of the typical young non-pregnant woman who exhibits symptoms (dysuria, frequency and urgency) strongly suggestive of uncomplicated upper UTI (cystitis). For these women empirical antibiotic treatment, without urine culture and sensitivity testing, is considered acceptable. It is also not considered necessary to culture urines from elderly patients with asymptomatic bacteriuria (evidenced by positive dipstick test result) because these patients do not benefit from antibiotic therapy.

Some studies have concluded that a negative result using urinalysis dipstick testing is reliable[6,9]. So long as the manufacturers' instructions are followed to the letter, the finding of no bacteria, white cells, blood or protein in urine by dipstick testing is strong evidence that the patient is not suffering a UTI. Unless there is particularly strong clinical evidence suggestive of UTI, most authorities agree that such negative testing urines need not normally be submitted for full microbiological examination.

Case history 28

Hayley Smith is a 24 year old mother of two who is 16 weeks pregnant. At her most recent routine antenatal care appointment she was asked to provide a mid stream urine (MSU) specimen for microscopy, culture and sensitivity (M,C&S).

A few days later the laboratory report of this test is received. The report includes the following results:

WBC $<5/mm^3$
RBC $<5/mm^3$
Urine culture $<10^3$ bacteria/ml 'Mixed coliform growth'

Questions

(1) Why is microbiological examination of MSU a routine part of antenatal care?
(2) Do the results suggest Hayley is suffering a urinary tract infection?

Discussion of case history 28

(1) Pregnancy is normally associated with changes in the gross structure of the urinary tract, in part caused by compression of the growing uterus on the kidneys and lower urinary tract. The ureters are elongated, widen and become more curved. One effect of these changes is a relative urine stasis (urine flow is not as efficient as usual) and resulting higher than normal risk of infection of the lower urinary tract spreading upwards to the kidneys with resulting infection of the kidney (pyelonephritis). An estimated 20–40% of pregnant women with significant bacteriuria early in pregnancy, even if asymptomatic, will go on to develop pyelonephritis later in pregnancy if the bacteria are not quickly eliminated with antibiotic therapy. Pyelonephritis is a serious infection that may lead to renal failure. Babies of mothers suffering pyelonephritis during pregnancy may

be born prematurely or have a low birth weight. To prevent pyelonephritis, all pregnant women are screened for evidence of UTI. Since significant bacteriuria may occur without any symptoms, testing in this context should not be confined to those who have symptomatic UTI.

(2) Despite the finding of bacteria in Hayley's urine, there is no evidence of infection. The numbers of bacteria are not significant and those discovered are a mixed growth of many bacterial species suggesting contamination of the specimen with bacteria normally present in the lower part of urethra or the perianal region. There is also no increase in the number of white blood cells in Hayley's urine, providing further evidence that her urinary tract is not infected.

References

1. Gieson, L., Cousins, G., Dimitrov, B. et al. (2010) Predicting acute uncomplicated UTI in women: a systematic review of the diagnostic accuracy of symptoms and signs, *BMC Family Practice*, 11: 78–92.
2. National Institute for Health and Clinical Excellence (2007) Urinary tract infection in children: diagnosis, treatment and long term management, NICE clinical guideline 54, NICE.
3. Kalsi, J., Arya, M. and Wilson, P. (2003) Hospital-acquired urinary tract infection, *Int J Clin Prac*, 57: 388–91.
4. Cohen, R. and Brown, R. (2003) Clinical practice. Microscopic hematuria, *N Eng J Med*, 348: 2330–8.
5. Kass, E.H. and Finland, M. (1956) Asymptomatic infection of the urinary tract, *Trans Assoc Am Physicians*, 69: 56–64.
6. Patel, H., Livsey, S., Swann, R. et al. (2005) Can urine dipstick testing for urinary tract infection reduce laboratory workload, *J Clin Pathol*, 58: 951–4.
7. Little, P., Moore, M. and Turner, S. (2010) Effectiveness of five different approaches in management of urinary tract infection: randomized controlled trial, *BMJ*, 340: c199.
8. Health Protection Agency (HPA) and British Infection Association (BIA) Diagnosis of UTI: quick reference guide for primary care, available at HPA website: http://www.hpa.org.uk/webc/HPAwebFile/HPAweb_C/1194947404720.
9. Whiting, P., Westwood, M., Watt, I. et al. (2005) Rapid tests and urine sampling techniques for the diagnosis of urinary tract infection (UTI) in children under 5 years: a systematic review, *BMC Pediatrics*, 5: 4–17.

Further reading

Beveridge, L., Davet, P., Phillips, G. et al. (2011) Optimal management of urinary tract infections in older people, *Clinical Interventions in Aging*, 6:173–80.

Dailly, S. (2012) Auditing urinary catheter care, *Nursing Standard*, 26: 35–40.

Gould, D. and Brooker, C. (2008) *Infection Prevention and Control Applied Microbiology for Healthcare* (2nd edn), Palgrave Macmillan.

Hooton, T. (2012) Uncomplicated urinary tract infection, *N Eng J Med*, 366: 1028–37.

Naish, W. and Hallam, M. (2007) Urinary tract infection: diagnosis and management for nurses, *Nursing Standard*, 21: 50–7.

Schmiemann, G., Kniehl, E., Gebhardt, K. et al. (2010) The diagnosis of urinary tract infection, *Dtsch Arztebl Int*, 107: 361–7.

Schnarr, J. and Smaill, F. (2008) Asymptomatic bacteriuria and symptomatic urinary tract infections in pregnancy, *Eur J Clin Invest*, 38: 50–7.

Slater, R. (2011) Preventing infection with long-term indwelling urinary catheters, *Br J Community Nursing*, 16:168–72.

CHAPTER 22

BLOOD CULTURE

Key learning objectives

- Normal defence against blood stream infection
- Factors that increase risk of blood stream infection
- Bacterial species that cause blood stream infection
- Symptoms of blood stream infection
- Defining sepsis, SIRS and septic shock
- Collection of blood for culture
- Interpretation of blood culture report

In this second of two chapters highlighting the work of the clinical microbiology laboratory, attention is focused on blood culture, a test used to confirm the presence of bacteria or fungi in blood (bacteraemia or fungaemia). Blood culture is useful in three broad clinical contexts. The first is among patients who are suspected of suffering sepsis (systemic disease caused by bacterial and, much more rarely, fungal infection). Secondly, there are several infectious diseases, whose pathogenesis involves spread of bacteria via the bloodstream. These diseases include endocarditis (infection of the valves of the heart), osteomyelitis (infection of bone) and infective arthritis (infection of joints). A positive blood culture provides supportive evidence for diagnosis of these conditions. Finally, the third group of patients who are likely to have their blood cultured are those with PUO (pyrexia of unknown origin). This is usually defined as a raised body temperature for more than ten days, with no immediate explanation. The clinical investigation of a patient with PUO routinely includes a blood culture in the search for an infective cause of pyrexia.

Understanding Laboratory Investigations: A Guide for Nurses, Midwives and Healthcare Professionals, Third Edition. Chris Higgins.
© 2013 John Wiley & Sons, Ltd. Published 2013 by John Wiley & Sons, Ltd.

Normal physiology

Blood is normally sterile (contains no bacteria or other microbes). However, normal life is associated with the risk of bacteria coming into contact with circulating blood, and transient bacteraemia may occur from time to time without ill effect. For example, bacteria normally present in the mouth have access to the blood stream during dental surgery; transient bacteraemia invariably follows dental surgery. Even vigorous chewing has been shown to facilitate entry of bacteria, normally present in the mouth, to the blood stream. Likewise a 'dirty' cut allows environmental bacteria, and bacteria normally present on the skin, access to the blood stream. Small numbers of bacteria or fungi may enter the blood stream from an existing infection site (e.g. the urinary tract, the respiratory tract, a wound infection etc.). Despite scrupulous aseptic technique, any surgical procedure may be associated with passage of bacteria from sites (e.g. the skin and bowel), where bacteria are normally present in abundance, to the blood stream.

It is the innate and acquired immune defences of blood that maintain its sterility, and prevent transient bacteraemia – which inevitably occurs from time to time – developing to clinically significant bacteraemia, usually called blood stream infection or septicaemia.

Innate immune defences in blood

Innate immunity is the sum of the protective mechanisms against infection that we are born with. One of the principle functions of skin, for example, is to act as a physical barrier to invading organisms; in this way skin makes a major contribution to the body's innate immune defence. The most significant innate immune defence against bacterial invasion in blood is neutrophils, phagocytic white blood cells. These cells engulf invading bacteria by the process of phagocytosis. Once phagocytosed, bacteria are killed by enzymes and highly reactive 'free radical' chemicals, produced within the neutrophil. The process of phagocytosis is greatly enhanced by the so-called complement proteins, which also make a significant contribution to innate immunity. Production of these blood proteins is activated by some species of invading bacteria. One of the complement proteins, known as C3b binds to the surface of bacteria. Bacteria that are coated with C3b are much more easily phagocytosed by neutrophils. Other complement proteins (C6, C7, C8 and C9) kill or damage some species of bacteria directly by insertion in bacterial membranes, and some (e.g. C5a) act by attracting neutrophils towards bacteria, thus enhancing phagocytosis.

Acquired immune defence in blood

We are not born with this form of immune defence, rather it is acquired as a result of exposure to invading organisms. It is very specific; meaning that exposure to one invading bacterial strain provides immunity (protection) only for that bacterial strain. (By comparison, innate immune mechanisms are non-specific: for example, skin protects against invasion from all bacterial species.)

Acquired immunity depends on the presence of antibodies in blood. Bacterial invasion results in production of specific antibodies (immunoglobulins) to bacteria by plasma cells; these cells are derived from a sub-group of the white blood cell population called B-lymphocytes. Antibody binds to the specific protein (antigen) present on bacterial surface that induced its production by plasma cells. This antibody binding of bacteria has two damaging effects for the bacteria: firstly it enhances neutrophil phagocytosis of bacteria and secondly it enhances the bactericidal effect of complement proteins. Many bacteria produce chemical toxins; specific antibodies bind to these toxins, effectively neutralising them. Finally, antibodies can activate production of the protective complement proteins by an alternative pathway to that induced by bacteria.

Thus by the complex synergistic action of both innate and acquired immune mechanisms, any bacteria present in blood are destroyed and blood remains essentially sterile.

Bacteraemia and fungaemia

Pre-disposing factors

If bacteria (or fungi) invade the bloodstream and the normal (innate and acquired) defences against invasion are overwhelmed, blood stream infection ensues.

Contributory factors include:

- Reduced host defences.
- Existing focus of infection.
- Virulence of invasive organism.
- Hospital procedures that facilitate entry of bacteria to the blood stream.

Reduced host defences

Any condition associated with reduced immune (either innate or acquired) defence against microbial invasion, predisposes to blood stream infection.

So, for example, major burns victims are predisposed to blood stream infection because as a result of their injury they lack the innate immunity provided by an intact covering of skin.

Those with AIDS, and those prescribed cytotoxic drugs, are particularly vulnerable to blood stream infection because of the reduced innate and acquired immunity associated with marked reduction in white blood cell numbers. Such patients are often so severely immunosuppressed that they are vulnerable to so called opportunistic bacteria and fungi (i.e. bacteria or fungi of such low virulence that they never pose a threat for those with a functioning immune system).

Any chronic debilitating illness (e.g. cancer, renal failure, heart failure etc.) or major trauma is associated with some degree of reduction in the normal immune response to infection. Premature babies have an under developed immune system and are particularly prone to infection during the first few months of life. The immune response to infection becomes less effective with advancing years; blood stream infections occur much more commonly among the elderly (>65 years), than among younger adults. Finally diabetic patients are more at risk of some bacterial infections spreading to the bloodstream than non-diabetics.

Existing focus of infection

In most cases of blood stream infection there is a pre-existing infection at some site (called the focus of infection) in the body. Bacteria from this primary site invade the blood. If the organisms are not susceptible to the bactericidal (bacterial killing) action of blood, or the numbers of organisms are overwhelming, bacteria multiply within the blood stream. The most common foci of infection in patients with bacteraemia are the lower respiratory tract and urinary tract, but bacteria may enter blood from any site of infection and, if the conditions are 'right', multiply within the blood stream.

Virulence of invading organism

The vulnerability of bacteria to blood defences varies between species so that, for example, Gram positive bacteria are generally speaking resistant to the bactericidal properties of antibody and complement, although they are vulnerable to phagocytosis. This variation determines that invasions by some species of bacteria (highly virulent bacteria) are more likely to result in significant bacteraemia than others of low virulence. However if there is an established focus of infection in the body and/ or the patient's defences are sufficiently impaired, any bacterial species no matter what its virulence can cause blood stream infection. In fact, although only a few species of bacteria cause most cases, all species of pathogenic (disease causing) bacteria and even some normally non-pathogenic species can cause clinically significant bacteraemia if present in large enough numbers, and host (patient) immune defences are sufficiently debilitated.

Hospital procedures that facilitate entry of bacteria to the blood stream

Around 60% of all patients with blood stream infection have acquired the infection whilst in hospital[1]. Patients at greatest risk of hospital acquired (nosocomial) bacteraemia are those who are subjected to surgical procedures, intravenous or urinary catheterisation, cystoscopy and other operative invasive interventions. An infected intravenous catheter (most commonly a central line) is the focus of infection in around 20% of all patients suffering hospital acquired bacteraemia and most of those patients with hospital acquired bacteraemia whose focus of infection is the urinary tract have been catheterised, or have had their urinary tract investigated using a cystoscope. Surgery of areas that are normally heavily contaminated with bacteria (e.g. the mouth, the colon, genital area) carry the highest risk of post-operative bacteraemia.

Causative bacteria

Usually a single species of bacteria is the cause of blood stream infection, but in around 8% of cases more than one bacterial species is found in blood[1]. All pathogenic (disease causing) bacteria and, more rarely, some usually non-pathogenic (opportunistic) bacteria have been implicated as causative in particular cases of blood stream infection. There are however a few species of bacteria which account for the vast majority of cases.

The two most common causes are the Gram-negative bacterium *Escherichia coli* (*E.coli*) and the Gram-positive bacterium *Staphylococcus aureus* (*S.aureus*)[1,2]. *E.coli* is the causative organism in around 25% of blood stream infections and *S.aureus* is the cause in around 12%, so together these two bacterial species account for close to a little over a third of all cases.

E.coli is present as part of the normal bacterial flora of the gastrointestinal tract, and many cases of blood stream infection associated with this organism result from disease or trauma of the abdominal area and resulting blood invasion of bacteria from the gut. Abdominal surgery, for example, is associated with risk of *E.coli* bacteraemia.

E.coli is responsible for most cases of urinary tract infection so that the focus of infection in many cases of *E.coli* blood stream infection is the urinary tract, particularly the upper urinary tract.

In recent years the incidence of *E.coli* blood stream infection has been steadily increasing. In an effort to understand this increase, and hopefully devise the means to combat it, mandatory reporting of all cases of *E.coli* blood stream was introduced in 2011; the only other blood stream infection that requires mandatory reporting in the UK is that caused by *S.aureus* (mandatory reporting introduced over a decade ago).

S.aureus is present without ill effect in the nose of 20–30% of the population and the skin of 5–10%. It is however also a common pathogen of the skin, being responsible for superficial skin infections such as boils and carbuncles. Surgical and trauma induced wound infections are frequently caused by *S.aureus* and the organism is responsible for most (>80%) cases of bone infection (osteomyelitis) and joint infection (septic arthritis). The most common foci of infection in cases of *S.aureus* blood stream infections are infected wounds and infected intravenous catheters. In around 10% of cases caused by *S.aureus*, the particular strain is resistant to methicillin and related antibiotics – it is an MRSA (methicillin resistant *Staphylococcus aureus*) strain. UK government led initiatives[3] over the past decade aimed at reducing the incidence of hospital acquired infection have been particularly successful in combating blood stream infections caused by MRSA. The annual rate of MRSA blood stream infections has fallen year on year from 7700 in 2003 to 1100 in 2011[4]. As a percentage of total *S.aureus* blood stream infections, those due to MRSA has fallen during that period from 40% to just 10%.

In excess of 150 species of bacteria are the cause in the remaining two thirds of cases. The vast majority of these are rare but the following are relatively common causes of blood stream infection, together accounting for around another third of cases: *Streptococcus pneumoniae, Streptococcus pyogenes,*

Staphylococcus epidermidis, Pseudomonas aeruginosa, enterococcal species, Klebsiella species and Proteus species.

Streptococcus pneumoniae

A Gram-positive cocci, which may be present in the mouth and nose of healthy people, but is the most significant bacterial cause of the common lower respiratory tract infection, pneumonia. It is the causative organism in around 2–5% of cases of bacteraemia; most of these are the result of spread of the organism to blood from infected respiratory tract, in patients suffering pneumococcal pneumonia.

Streptococcus pyogenes

A common pathogen of the upper respiratory tract: responsible for pharyngitis ('strep throat'); skin infections (e.g. impetigo, cellulitis) and serious invasive tissue infection (necrotising fasciitis). *Strep pyogenes* infections are usually community-acquired.

Staphylococcus epidermidis

This is the most significant of a group of staphylococcal bacteria known collectively as cogulase negative staphylococci (CNS). In common with all other species in the group, *Staph epidermidis* is abundantly present on the skin and inside the nose of healthy individuals and this determines that it is a common contaminant of blood cultures. However it can also be a causative organism in cases of blood stream infection, most particularly among immunocompromised patients who have undergone some invasive procedure (e.g. intravenous catheterisation). Blood stream infection caused by this organism is usually hospital acquired.

Pseudomonas aeruginosa

A Gram-negative bacillus (rod shaped), this is a common environmental bacterium that thrives on moist surfaces and can be found contaminating hospital environment, surfaces, equipment etc. Most cases of blood stream infection caused by this organism are related to infected venous or urinary catheters, so is usually hospital acquired.

Enterococcal species

These are Gram-positive cocci (sphere shaped) normally present in the gastrointestinal tract. Clinically, the most significant species are *Enterococcus faecium* and *Enterococcus faecalis,* which can be the causative organism in cases of abdominal infections (e.g. peritonitis) and urinary tract infection. Spread from these sites of infection to blood can occur in severely debilitated patients.

Klebsiella and Proteus species

These are a relatively common cause of urinary tract infection and much more rarely, lower respiratory tract infection (pneumonia). The urinary tract or infected wounds is usually the focus of infection among those with bacteraemia associated with these organisms.

Causative fungi

Fungi are the cause in fewer than 2% of cases of blood stream infection[3]. Almost all of these occur in patients who are severely immunosuppressed. The causative organism in almost all cases of fungaemia is *Candida albicans*, a fungus that is present in low numbers on the skin of healthy individuals. It is the cause of common superficial skin and nail infections and vaginal candidosis, a superficial infection of the vagina.

Consequences of bacteraemia/fungaemia

The symptomatic and potentially life threatening consequences of bacteraemia and fungaemia are due in large part, not to the invading organism, but to dysregulation of the body's normal physiological response to infection, which has already been very briefly outlined. The detail of the dysregulation is complex, only partially understood and the object of intensive current research[5,6]. It is manifest clinically as sepsis, which can quickly progress to severe sepsis, septic shock and death. An outline understanding of the clinical significance of blood stream infection depends crucially on defining the following terms:

- Systemic inflammatory response syndrome (SIRS).
- Sepsis.
- Severe sepsis.
- Septic shock.

Systemic inflammatory response syndrome (SIRS)

Inflammation is the normally protective response to any injury that ensures limitation and resolution of injury (healing). In health the inflammatory response is limited to the site of injury and is exquisitely controlled by an opposing anti-inflammatory process. SIRS is defined as an abnormal (dysregulated) inflammatory response that has effect in organs or sites removed from the site of injury. It is thus inappropriate and harmful. SIRS can be caused by any major insult to the body, for example, severe trauma and major surgery; burns; diseases like acute pancreatitis that are associated with extensive tissue damage; and infection. A diagnosis of SIRS is made if patients exhibit at least two of the following abnormal signs of systemic inflammation:

- High or low body temperature $< 36°C$ or $> 38°C$.
- Tachycardia   heart rate greater than 90 beats/minute.
- Hyperventilation   respiratory rate > 20 breaths/minute or $PaCO2$ < 4.2kPa.
- High or low white cell count $> 12.0 \times 10^9/L$ or $< 4.0 \times 10^9/L$.

Sepsis

Sepsis is defined as infection in the presence of SIRS. Thus the finding of bacteraemia in a patient exhibiting two or more of the qualifying SIRS signs allows a diagnosis of sepsis. Since bacteraemia is a systemic infection, eliciting a blood-borne systemic inflammatory response, sepsis is usual in those with bacteraemia. However bacteraemia is not necessary for a diagnosis of sepsis; focal infection at any site can elicit SIRS, so that a diagnosis of sepsis can be made even if blood is sterile, so long as there is evidence of infection somewhere in the body in association with systemic inflammation. The term septicaemia (infection of blood) is often used as a synonym for sepsis, but since sepsis can occur in the absence of blood infection they are not synonyms. Experts now argue that because of this confusion, use of the term septicaemia should be discouraged in favour of the term blood stream infection.

Severe sepsis

The dysregulated response to infection that sepsis represents is associated with inappropriate release of a host of potent chemicals (cytokines) to blood from a range of cells involved in the immune process. Unchecked, pro-inflammatory cytokines cause damage to the endothelial cells that line the microvasculature making capillaries leaky with loss of fluid to the interstitial space, hypovolaemaia and fall in blood pressure (hypotension). Inappropriate inflammation and damaged endothelium activates the clotting cascade as well as platelets, and a pro-coagulant state ensues in which micro-thrombi (small blood clots) form inappropriately within capillaries. The damaging cascade continues as the reduced blood pressure, presence of micro-thrombi and endothelial damage combine to reduce blood flow through the microvasculature. This leaves tissues deficient of the oxygen required for cells to survive and ischaemic tissue damage progresses to organ dysfunction; it is this organ dysfunction that defines severe sepsis

Progression to severe sepsis occurs unpredictably in around a third of sepsis cases, but may be prevented by early recognition and prompt antibiotic therapy. It is defined as sepsis with evidence of organ dysfunction, hypotension or poor tissue perfusion. The damaging effects on the microvasculature are widespread so any or all organ systems can be affected.

Septic shock

The most severe presentation of sepsis is septic shock, characterised by acute circulatory failure and persistent hypotension (systolic pressure <90 mmHg), despite adequate fluid resuscitation. Reduced tissue perfusion can lead to multiple organ failure and death.

Sepsis, severe sepsis and septic shock are not separate conditions but rather represent a continuum of severity of the same condition, namely an abnormal systemic response to microbial (usually bacterial) infection. Patients with blood stream infection may present at any stage. Severity is reflected in mortality rates: sepsis is associated with around 25% mortality, severe sepsis with 40% mortality and septic shock with 60% mortality[7]. Sepsis and its sequalae remains the most common cause of death among patients being cared for in intensive care units, and currently accounts for an estimated 37 000 deaths in the UK every year.

Following the collaborative effort of critical care expertise from around the world, the now influential Surviving Sepsis Campaign (http://www.survingsepsis.org) was launched in 2004. The campaign has allowed preparation of internationally agreed clinical guidelines[8] aimed at significantly reducing sepsis related mortality. The so called 'care bundles' (which include the use of blood culture and other laboratory tests) promoted by these guidelines are now being applied by nursing[9] and medical staff in emergency and intensive care units at hospitals around the world.

Summary of the general symptomatic effects of bacteraemia

Infection caused by particular bacterial species may be associated with specific symptoms. The most common general symptoms are:

- Fever (body temperature >38 °C).
- Rigors (shivering chills).
- Tachycardia (heart rate >95 beats/minute).
- Increased respiratory rate.
- Alteration of mental state (confusion, apprehension).
- Hypotension (reduced blood pressure).

Signs and symptoms associated with organ dysfunction in severe sepsis include:

- Jaundice (liver).
- Increased tendency to bleed (coagulation defects).
- Reduced urine output (kidney).
- Respiratory distress, breathlessness – reduced PaO2 (respiratory system).

Principles of microbiological examination of blood

The primary objective of the laboratory is to determine if the patient's blood contains bacteria (or fungi). It is not possible to confirm or exclude the presence of bacteria in blood by merely examining a sample under the microscope: there simply are not sufficient numbers present. Instead bacteria must first be grown (cultured) in a liquid (called the culture medium) that contains the nutrients necessary for bacteria to multiply. The culture medium containing the blood sample is incubated at 37°C the optimum temperature for bacterial growth, until there is evidence of bacterial growth. This usually takes 6–18 hours, but may take days for particularly slow growing species. In practice, if there is no evidence of bacterial growth after three days of incubation it is highly unlikely that the culture (and therefore the blood sample added to the culture medium) contains any bacteria. However the culture may continue to be monitored for longer to allow for the possibility that rare, slow growing species were present in the blood sample.

As soon as there is evidence of bacterial growth, a sample of the culture, now rich in bacteria, is stained and examined under the microscope. This provides the first evidence of the identity of the species of bacteria present (e.g. whether Gram positive or Gram negative, cocci or baccilli etc.). More precise identification may require that the liquid culture be further grown (sub-cultured) on a solid culture medium in a petri dish. This allows the growth of visible, pure colonies of bacteria, each colony being the product of multiplication of a single bacterium. A sample of the visible colony is then subjected to a range of chemical tests that finally determine the identity of the bacteria it contains.

Having isolated and identified the bacteria present in the culture, the final step is sensitivity testing. This involves testing the bacteria isolated in culture for reaction with a range of antibiotics, to establish which antibiotic is likely to be most effective in combating this particular infection.

Bacteraemia and fungaemia are potentially life-threatening conditions which demand immediate antibiotic treatment. It is often not practicable therefore to wait for the results of laboratory tests before starting treatment, and initial antibiotic therapy must be based on the clinical history, which provides important clues as to the likely nature of the invading bacterial species. However when the results of laboratory tests, particularly sensitivity testing, become available (usually within a day or two) antibiotic therapy can be altered if necessary.

Sample collection

Objective

To introduce a sample of patient's blood into culture bottles without **any** bacterial contamination (e.g. from environment, operators or patient's skin etc.).

Timing of sampling

Blood for culture should be sampled before administration of antibiotic therapy as antibiotics may delay or prevent bacterial growth, causing falsely negative results. For patients with intermittent fever, blood should ideally be taken while temperature is rising, or as soon after the spike of temperature as is possible, when the bacteria are present in blood at highest concentration. Most laboratories recommend taking a second or third sample, not less than one hour after the first to increase the chances of recovering bacteria and to distinguish true bacteraemia (which would be present in all culture sets) from bacterial contamination.

Blood culture bottles

Blood must be collected into specially designated blood culture bottles. There are several commercially available blood culture systems, but they all contain a sterile liquid mixture of nutrients (called the culture medium) necessary for bacterial growth. Most laboratories supply two blood culture bottles per blood culture set. The first has oxygen in the space above the culture medium to allow growth of those species of bacteria that require oxygen. The second bottle has a mixture of gases without oxygen. This bottle is required for culture of anaerobic bacteria (i.e. bacteria which only grow best in an oxygen-free environment). A sample of blood must be introduced into both bottles.

Volume of blood required

In a patient with bacteraemia there may be as few as one bacterium per millilitre of blood, so that a falsely negative result can occur if insufficient blood is introduced into the culture bottle. Paradoxically, a false negative result can also occur if too much blood is introduced. This is because blood continues to have bactericidal effect in culture. This effect is diluted out in the liquid culture medium. A compromise must be sought between too small a volume of blood, which might well contain insufficient bacteria and too large a volume, which would remove the dilution effect of the culture medium on bactericidal property of blood. An approximate 1:10 dilution of blood in culture medium is optimal but the actual volume required (usually 5–10 ml) depends on the blood culture system being used. It is vital that no less than the local laboratory recommended minimum volume of blood be sampled for each culture bottle.

Technique

Aseptic technique is essential throughout to ensure that no bacterial contamination of the culture occurs. If successful, only bacteria present in the patient's blood will be transferred to the culture bottle.

- Blood should be sampled from a peripheral vein, not via an indwelling catheter, which might itself be contaminated with bacteria.
- With sterile gloved hands, the venipuncture site must be cleansed with 2% tincture of iodine, or some other suitable disinfectant. The iodine should be removed after a minute or two with 70% alcohol, ensuring that the site is dry. The top of both blood culture bottles, through which the sample is introduced, must be similarly disinfected.
- Taking care not to touch the venipuncture site, blood is collected using sterile syringe and needle.
- Blood is inoculated into the blood culture bottle via the rubber septum in the blood culture top. Never remove the top of a blood culture bottle. This would expose the culture to environmental bacteria.
- If blood is being collected for other tests, always inoculate blood culture bottles first, to prevent bacteria present on other specimen bottles being transferred to the culture.
- Blood culture bottles must be carefully labelled with patient details and sent along with the appropriate request card to the laboratory without delay. If blood is collected out of normal laboratory hours, blood cultures must be placed in a specially designated 37°C incubator to facilitate bacterial growth.

It is important to record on the request card outline clinical details and any antibiotic therapy if given before blood sampling.

Blood culture reports

Interim reports of progress in examination of a blood culture are issued daily. A final report will include the identity of any bacteria recovered from the culture, along with a report of the sensitivity or resistance of that particular strain to a range of antibiotics.

Results of blood culture fall into one of three main groups:

- Blood culture negative – no bacterial growth.
- Blood culture positive – pure growth.
- Blood culture positive – mixed bacterial growth.

Blood culture negative – no bacterial growth

This is a normal result, that is one which would be obtained from a person whose blood was sterile (contained no bacteria). Before a negative culture result is interpreted in this way, it is important to consider the possibility that the result is falsely negative, that is the patient has bacteraemia but the test has failed to detect it. Causes of false negative results include:

- Insufficient blood added to culture bottle.
- Antibiotic therapy administered before blood sampled.
- Incubation period insufficient for growth of rare, slow growing organisms.

Blood culture positive – pure growth

This means that a pure growth of a single identified species of bacteria (e.g. *E.coli*, *Strep pneumoniae*, *Staph aureus* etc.) was isolated from the culture. This is the result that would be expected from a patient with blood stream infection. However, in around 10–20% of positive blood cultures, the bacteria isolated and identified is derived not from the patient's blood but is present as a result of bacterial contamination of the culture due most often to poor aseptic technique at the time of sample collection. Since all species of bacteria have been implicated in bacteraemia, and as a cause of sepsis at one time or another, it is sometimes difficult to decide whether a positive blood culture is due to contamination (false positive) or reflects bacteraemia and possible sepsis (true positive).

To illustrate this, suppose a blood culture yields a pure growth of the organism *Staph epidermidis*. This organism, which is normally present in abundance on the skin of us all, could be transferred from the skin of patient or staff to the blood culture during the process of blood collection. In fact it is one of the most common organisms to contaminate blood cultures. However, *Staph epidermidis* is also a quite common cause of sepsis among debilitated patients whose focus of infection is an infected catheter. It is also the most significant cause of endocarditis among patients who have received heart surgery. The finding may reflect contamination, but in some circumstances can be of clinical significance.

It is the bacteria, like *Staph epidermidis*, that are part of the normal resident flora of skin that usually contaminate blood cultures. A pure growth of any organism in blood culture is more likely to be due to bacteraemia than contamination, if:

- The same organism has been isolated from the same patient at some other infected site.
- The same organism is isolated from repeated blood cultures.

Blood culture positive – mixed bacterial growth

This result indicates that more than one species of bacteria was isolated from the blood culture. It is rare for blood to be infected by more than one species of bacteria, although it may occur. A mixed growth of bacteria suggests that the culture was contaminated, particularly if the bacterial species isolated are common contaminants. Interpretation may be difficult and frequently requires the expert help of a clinical microbiologist.

Case history 29

Until the evening prior to hospital admission, 18 year old Kevin Thomas was a fit and healthy student. On that evening he went to bed early complaining of a headache; he was also feverish. Early the next morning his mother, a nurse, went to check on him. He was clearly very ill, moaning quietly, with a very high temperature. He had vomited during the night. Mrs Thomas was so alarmed by Kevin's condition that she took him straight to the local A&E department where she worked, believing that he may be suffering from meningitis. On admission Kevin's temperature was 40°C, his heart rate was 126 and he was becoming increasingly drowsy. A rash was noted on Kevin's legs. Blood was sampled for among other tests, blood culture. In view of his rapidly deteriorating condition Kevin was given a broad-spectrum antibiotic intravenously and admitted to the intensive care unit. Later that day the laboratory reported the presence of Gram-negative diplococci bacteria in the culture of Kevin's blood, which was subsequently identified as *Neisseria meningitidis*.

Questions

(1) What was the diagnosis?
(2) What other serious infectious disease is caused by the bacteria isolated from Kevin's blood?
(3) Is it possible to isolate the bacteria causing Kevin's illness from normally healthy individuals?

Discussion of case history 29

(1) Kevin was suffering meningococcal sepsis, a life threatening infection of the bloodstream caused by the bacteria, *Neisseria meningitidis*. A diagnosis of sepsis depends on two elements: infection and systemic inflammation. Raised body temperature and heart rate provided sufficient evidence of systemic inflammation and the positive blood culture (bacteraemia) was evidence of infection.

(2) The same bacteria strain is one of two main causes of bacterial meningitis; the other is *Streptococcus pneumoniae*. When the causative bacteria strain is *N. meningitidis* the condition is known as meningococcal meningitis. Usually meningococcal meningitis and meningococcal infection of the blood coexist in the same patient, but in recent years there has been an increase in the number of patients whose infection is confined to blood and have, like Kevin, no infection of the meninges.

(3) Yes. *Neisseria meningitidis* is present in the nose and throat of around 10–20% of the healthy population.

References

1. Luzzaro, F., Ortisi, G., Larosa, M. et al. (2011) Prevalence and epidemiology of microbial pathogens causing blood stream infections: results of the OASIS mulitcenter study, *Diagnostic Microbiology and Infectious Disease*, 69: 363–9.
2. Health Protection Agency (2012) Polymicrobial bacteraemias and fungaemias in England, Wales and Northern Ireland: 2010, available at: http://www.hpa.org.uk/webc/HPAwebFile/HPAweb_C/1317132423063.
3. Department of Health (2010) The Health and Social Care Act 2008 Code of Practice on the prevention and control of infections and related guidance, Dept of Health, available at: http://www.dh.gov.uk/prod_consum_dh/groups/dh_digitalassets/documents/digitalasset/dh_123923.pdf.
4. Health Protection Agency (2012) Quarterly Analysis: Mandatory MRSA, MSSA and *E.coli* bacteraemia and CDI in England (up to October–December 2011), Health Protection Agency, available at: http://www.hpa.org.uk/webc/HPAwebFile/HPAweb_C/13171331482973.
5. Fry, D. (2012) Sepsis, systemic inflammatory response, and multiple organ dysfunction: the mystery continues, *The American Surgeon*, 78: 1–8.
6. Vincent, J., Martinez, E. and Silva, E. (2009) Evolving concepts in sepsis, *Crit Care Clin*, 25: 665–75.
7. Alberti, C., Brun-Busisson, C., Sergey, V. et al. (2003) Influence of systemic inflammatory response syndrome and sepsis on outcome of critically infected patients, *Am J Crit Care Med*, 168: 77–84.
8. Dellinger, R., Levy, M., Carlet, J. et al. (2008) Surviving Sepsis Campaign: international guidelines for management of severe sepsis and septic shock, *Crit Care Med*, 36: 296–327.
9. Aitken, L., Williams, G., Harvey, M. et al. (2011) Nursing considerations to complement the Surviving Sepsis Campaign guidelines, *Crit Care Med*, 39: 1800–18.

Further reading

Gould, D. and Brooker, C. (2008) *Infection Prevention and Control Applied Microbiology for Healthcare* (2nd edn), Palgrave Macmillan.

Nelson, D., LeMaster, T., Plost, G. et al. (2009) Recognizing sepsis in the adult patient, *Am J Nursing*, 109: 40–5.

Oakley, C. and Chowdhury, C. (2010) Benefits of a network approach to managing neutropaenic sepsis, *Cancer Nursing Practice*, 9: 17–21.

Pomeroy, M. (2009) A patient with sepsis: an evaluation of care, *Emergency Nurse*, 17: 12–17.

Royal College of Obstetricians and Gynaecologists (2012) Bacterial sepsis in pregnancy (Green-top guideline No. 64a), RCOG, available at: http://www.rcog.org.uk/files/rcog-corp/25.4.12GTG64a.pdf.

Sriskandan, S. (2011) Severe peripartum sepsis, *J R Coll Physicians Edin*, 41: 339–46.

Steen, C. (2009) Developments in the management of patients with sepsis, *Nursing Standard*, 23: 48–55.

Williams, E. (2006) Taking blood for culture, *Br J Hosp Med*, 67(2): M22–23.

PART 6

Screening Tests

PART 6

CHAPTER 23

NEWBORN SCREENING BLOOD TESTS

Key learning topics

- Screening for disease – general consideration
- Aims and organisation of the newborn bloodspot programme
- Collection of bloodspot sample
- Laboratory role in the newborn bloodspot programme

As part of their early routine health assessment, all babies born in the UK are, with parental agreement, submitted for the blood tests that are the subject of this chapter. So of all laboratory blood tests, these are the most universally applied. The tests, collectively known as the newborn bloodspot screening test (formerly called the Guthrie test), require a single heel-prick blood sample collected, usually by the midwife or health care visitor, when babies are five to eight days old. The blood is collected directly onto a newborn bloodspot card (a special filter paper, formerly called a Guthrie card), which is sent by post to one of 20 specialist laboratories located throughout the UK. The object of this nationally co-ordinated blood testing is to identify those babies who are at high risk of suffering any one of five rare but serious congenital conditions that have lifelong health significance. Early diagnosis and treatment reduces the severity of all five conditions and may be life saving. The five conditions are: phenylketonuria (PKU), congenital hypothyroidism (CH), cystic fibrosis (CF), medium-chain acyl CoA dehydrogenase deficiency (MCADD) and sickle cell disease (SCD).

In this chapter we consider each of these conditions in turn and the specific blood tests used to screen for them, but first there follows a brief general discussion about screening for disease and nationally co-ordinated screening programmes to place the one under discussion here in a wider context.

Understanding Laboratory Investigations: A Guide for Nurses, Midwives and Healthcare Professionals, Third Edition. Chris Higgins.
© 2013 John Wiley & Sons, Ltd. Published 2013 by John Wiley & Sons, Ltd.

Table 23.1 UK Nationwide screening programmes.

Screening Programme	Who is screened (frequency)	Condition(s) being screened for	Method of screening
NHS Newborn Bloodspot Screening Programme	All newborns at age 5–8 days (once only)	• PKU • CH • CF • MCADD • SCD	Blood testing
NHS Newborn Hearing Screening Programme	All newborns within 2 weeks of birth (once only)	Hearing deficit	Audio Automated Otoacoustic Emission (AOAE) hearing test
NHS Newborn and Infant Physical Examination	All newborns within 72 hours of birth and again at 6–8 weeks	• Congenital heart disease • Development dysplasia of the hips • Cataracts • Undescended testes	'Top to toe' systematic physical examination
NHS Down's and Foetal Anomaly Screening Programme	All pregnant women 1st–2nd trimester	• Down's syndrome • Foetal anomalies	Blood testing and ultrasound scan
NHS Infectious Disease in Pregnancy Screening	All pregnant women at first antenatal appointment (once only)	• Hepatitis B infection • HIV infection • Syphilis infection • Rubella immunisation status	Blood testing
NHS Antenatal Sickle Cell and Thalassaemia Screening Programme	All pregnant women by 10th week of pregnancy and, if necessary, their partners (once only)	• Sickle cell trait • Thalassaemia trait	Blood testing
NHS Diabetic Eye Screening Programme	All diabetics aged 12yrs or over (every year)	Diabetic retinopathy	Digital imaging of retina
NHS Abdominal Aortic Aneurysm Screening Programme	All men at age 65yrs (once only)	Abdominal aortic aneurysm	Abdominal ultrasound scan
NHS Breast Screening Programme	All women aged 50–70yrs (every 3 years)	Breast cancer	Digital mammography (low dose X-ray exam)
NHS Bowel Cancer Screening Programme	All men and women aged 60–69yrs (every 2 years)	Bowel (colorectal) cancer	Test for presence of blood in faeces (occult blood)
NHS Cervical Cancer Screening Programmes	All women aged 25–65yrs (every 3yrs for those aged 25–49 and every 5 years for those aged 50–65)	Cervical cancer	Cervical smear test (discussed in Chapter 24)

Screening tests and national screening programmes

Screening tests are those that are offered to apparently healthy people in order to identify those who may be at high risk of a particular disease or condition. These tests are not intended to identify those with a particular disease or condition – that is the object of the diagnostic process, which is invariably more expensive and in one way or another less easily applied to large numbers of people. The value of the effective screening test is that it relatively easily and cheaply eliminates the vast majority who are not at risk of the disease or condition being screened for, so that only a very small number need be submitted for the usually more expensive, complex diagnostic testing and clinical assessment that either confirms or excludes the disease.

It is only considered justifiable to screen for a disease if early identification of that disease before symptoms develop leads to a better outcome. If there is no effective treatment or early treatment has no benefit there is arguably limited value in knowing you have the disease, indeed the knowledge may, on balance, have harmful effect.

The screening process has an ethical dimension because it exposes those who do not have the disease – the vast majority – to a process from which they gain no tangible health benefit. Indeed if such people screen positive they often have to undergo extra tests and investigations and be caused the anxiety associated with knowing they *might* have the disease, again without any benefit. For any proposed screening process the benefit gained by those who have the disease must be rigorously weighed against the potential harm that the screening process might cause those who do not have the disease.

Finally, no screening procedure is entirely reliable. For a number of reasons, some avoidable and some unavoidable, a small minority of those with the disease will be given a negative screen result, and a small minority of those without the disease will be given a positive screen result. Either scenario may have devastating consequence for the, thankfully few, individuals concerned and national screening programmes are constantly updated in the light of new research that reveals ways in which the number of false positive and false negative screening results can be minimised.

The limitations and cost of screening determine that national screening programmes are only used to screen for a small number of diseases/conditions, although it is true that the number has increased in recent years and the appropriateness of extending screening programmes is under constant review. Table 23.1 lists the 11 national screening programmes currently operational within the UK.

The screening process does not necessarily involve laboratory testing but clinical laboratories have a role in six of the 11 programmes, including two that are discussed in this book: the cervical cancer screening programme (Chapter 24) and the newborn bloodspot screening programme.

Newborn bloodspot programme – sample collection

As with all other UK nationally co-ordinated screening programmes, the effectiveness of the newborn bloodspot programme depends on the cooperative effort of several groups of healthcare workers, all working to well defined standards of

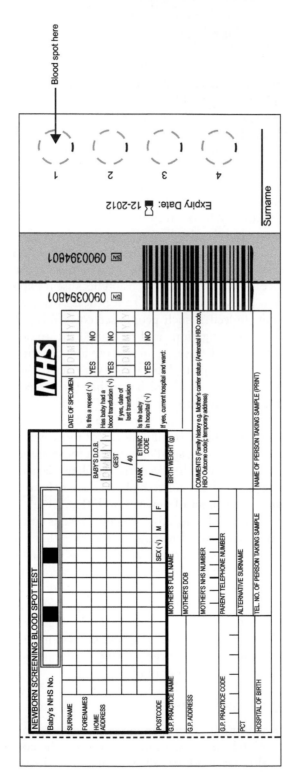

Figure 23.1 The newborn bloodspot card.

quality and timeliness at each step of what is a quite complex process. The standards of the programme, for example, demand that laboratory staff complete all screening tests, including where necessary repeat analysis, within four days of receiving the bloodspot sample. On the same day that a positive screening result is identified, the defined local clinical liaison team (CLT) must be informed by telephone. On that day the CLT are required to arrange an urgent (ideally next day) follow up clinic appointment for diagnostic blood testing/clinical assessment of the baby, and parental counselling. Diagnosis should be confirmed within a few days of that appointment, using a clearly defined protocol. When all standards are observed, babies found to be affected by one of the conditions being screened for start appropriate treatment within two to four weeks of birth. Delay beyond this may have lifelong deleterious effect.

The first step in the process, usually the responsibility of midwife or health visitor, is collection of the bloodspot sample, after gaining informed consent of parents. The detail of standards for bloodspot sample collection is contained in published guidelines[1] from which the following bullet points are derived:

- The bloodspot sample should be taken on day five, but in exceptional circumstances between days five and eight (day zero is taken as day of birth).
- Details must be entered on the bloodspot card (Figure 23.1) at the time of blood sampling. It is mandatory to include the baby's identifying NHS number; the sample cannot be processed in the laboratory if this is absent or other details are undecipherable. Bar coded labels, that contain all essential details relating to the baby, are preferred.
- The baby's heel from which blood is sampled must be clean and dry – it is essential that there is absolutely no trace of faecal matter because faeces contains large amounts of trypsin, a substance measured in blood to screen for cystic fibrosis. Failure to clean the heel sufficiently could lead to faecal contamination of the blood sample and a falsely positive screening result.
- An automated incision device that penetrates no more than 2 mm should be used to obtain the sample – manual lancets should not be used. The bottom (fleshy) surface of the heel should be punctured, not the back of the heel where the heel bone (calcaneus) can be felt.
- The aim is to fill each circle on the bloodspot card using a single drop of blood. Allow blood to form a drop on the heel. It is important that blood flows freely without the need to squeeze the foot. Allow one spot of blood to drop onto each of the circles. Do not allow the card to make contact with the heel. There should be sufficient blood for it to seep naturally through to the other side of the card and evenly saturate the whole of each circle. Insufficient sample, evident as multiple small spots of blood within the circle, will be rejected by the laboratory and a repeat requested. Too much blood caused by layering of blood drops on top of each other can cause erroneous results.
- Allow the bloodspots to air dry before placing in the glassine envelope and place the bloodspot card in the prepaid addressed envelope and post (first class) on the day the sample is collected. Standards demand that bloodspot cards are received by the laboratory within three days of sample collection.

- Blood transfusion prior to bloodspot sampling can adversely affect screening tests for SCD. This is of course only usually an issue for sick or premature babies admitted to neonatal care units. All these babies should have a bloodspot sample on admission in case they have a blood transfusion before day five. This is stored labelled as 'pre-transfusion sample' and must be sent with the normally timed sample if they have a blood transfusion in the interim. It can be discarded if no blood transfusion is given by day five. It is important to record any transfusion history on the bloodspot card.

Conditions screened for with the bloodspot test

Phenylketonuria (PKU)

This is an inherited disturbance of amino acid metabolism, specifically the amino acid phenylalanine [2]. It affects around 1 in 10 000 babies; so, as the current annual UK birth rate is around 800 000, close to 80 PKU affected babies are born every year in the UK.

The principle biological significance of all amino acids (there are 23 in total) is as the building blocks of all proteins. Some amino acids, including phenylalanine, cannot be synthesised in the body and must be provided for in the diet; they are called the 'essential' amino acids. We obtain all the phenylalanine we need to synthesise proteins only by eating protein-containing foods. Tyrosine is an example of an amino acid that *can* be synthesised in the body; it is a 'non-essential' amino acid. In the body tyrosine is made from phenylalanine; the two are structurally very closely related.

The conversion of phenylalanine to tyrosine, which occurs principally in the cells of the liver, is a metabolic process that depends on the enzyme phenylalanine hydroxylase (PAH). Those with phenylketonuria have one of many possible inherited defects (mutations) in the gene that codes for synthesis of PAH. This results in absent or reduced activity of PAH (depending on the particular mutation), and therefore absent or reduced conversion of phenylalanine to tyrosine.

The condition is inherited in an autosomally recessive mode, meaning that it is necessary to inherit two copies of the mutated PAH gene, one from each parent. Those who inherit just one copy are unaffected 'carriers' of the condition. There is a one in four chance that a baby born to parents who are both healthy 'carriers' will be affected by PKU.

As a consequence of the inherited genetic defect, phenylalanine accumulates in blood and tissues. Some is metabolised to a group of substances known collectively as phenylketones, which are excreted in urine. The presence of phenylketones in urine is called phenylketonuria, which gives the condition its name, and once provided the only diagnostic signal of PKU. However, the most significant clinical consequence of PKU stems from the toxic effect of accumulating phenylalanine on brain function. Without early treatment very soon after birth, PKU in its most severe 'classical' form results in permanent brain damage and profound mental disability manifest as progressive intellectual impairment, accompanied by a range of symptoms that may include seizures and autism. Late in childhood or adolescence behavioural and psychiatric problems may emerge.

Since accumulating phenylalanine is the problem, and all phenylalanine is derived from food, treatment of PKU is based on simply restricting phenylalanine intake. Introduction of a phenylalanine-restricted diet soon after birth prevents brain damage and nearly all of the PKU associated neuro-psychological problems. The diet, which is essentially a very low protein diet almost devoid of phenylalanine, must be continued certainly until adolescence and ideally for life; efficacy must be monitored by regular blood phenylalanine measurement.

The PKU screening test

Screening for PKU is based on measurement of phenylalanine (and if necessary tyrosine) concentration in the blood spot sample by an automated technique known as tandem mass spectrometry. This technique allows phenylalanine/tyrosine measurement in a few minutes and the ability to process up to 600 bloodspot samples every day. The technique is suited for simultaneous measurement of all amino acids and many intermediary metabolites from a single sample, and so is a potential screening tool for many other congenital metabolic defects, including MCADD (explained further).

A healthy newborn baby has a blood phenylalanine in the approximate reference range 50–110 µmol/L. Severe 'classical' untreated PKU is typically associated with blood concentration in excess of 1000 µmol/L, but levels are lower than this in less severe forms. PKU is not the only cause of mildly increased blood phenylalanine concentration.

A negative screen (PKU not suspected) is reported if blood phenylalanine is less than 200 µmol/L on initial testing. This eliminates the vast majority of samples. The remaining samples with phenylalanine >200 µmol/L are analysed again but this time both phenylalanine and tyrosine are measured. For this second round of testing a negative screen (PKU not suspected) is reported if phenylalanine is <240 µmol/L, irrespective of the tyrosine result. A positive screen (PKU suspected) is reported if phenylalanine is >240 µmol/L *and* tyrosine is <240 µmol/L (i.e. not increased). The finding of increased phenylalanine *and* increased tyrosine is not consistent with PKU and is thus reported as 'PKU not suspected'.

Cystic fibrosis

Cystic fibrosis (CF) is one of the most common serious inherited diseases, affecting 1 in 2500 births. Based on annual UK birth rate of 800 000, then, close to 300 CF affected babies are born every year in the UK. The inherited defect is one of many possible mutations in the gene that codes for production of a protein called cystic fibrosis transmembrane conductance regulator (CFTR). It is necessary to inherit a mutant copy of the CFTR gene from both parents for a baby to have CF. Inheritance of one normal and one abnormal CFTR gene confers healthy 'carrier' status; around 1 in 25 of the UK (Caucasion) population are CF 'carriers'. The genetic defect is much less common in those of other racial descent. There is a one in four chance that the offspring of parents who are both healthy CF 'carriers' will be born with CF.

Mutations in the CFTR gene give rise to absent or dysfunctional CFTR protein, and to understand cystic fibrosis it is useful to have some understanding of normal

CFTR function. CFTR is located in the membrane of epithelial cells that line the surface of secretory glands throughout the body. Its function is to regulate the passage of ions (sodium, chloride etc.) and water across these epithelial cell membranes. This function is important for optimum constitution of glandular secretions. For example, the volume and viscosity of the protective mucous secretion that lines the respiratory tract depends on CFTR function in epithelial cells of the respiratory tract.

Glandular secretions of those with CF are abnormally thick (viscous), and it is this feature that can account for the principle effects of CF in the intestine, pancreas and lungs.

The only early sign or symptom of CF is a condition called meconium ileus, which is evident in a minority (around 10–20%) of CF affected neonates. Meconium is the dark green tar-like substance that is usually expelled from the baby's intestine during the first bowel movement in the hours after birth. In CF affected babies, meconium is unusually thick, and may form a plug in the ileus (the lower part of the small intestine). This intestinal obstruction, which causes vomiting and the possible need for urgent surgical intervention, is called meconium ileus.

Failure to thrive and achieve normal growth targets during the first months and years of life is common in babies and infants with CF. This results from failure of the pancreas to deliver the digestive enzymes to the intestines that are necessary for food to be absorbed. This effective malnutrition is due to unusually 'thick' pancreatic juice and resulting blockage of pancreatic ducts.

The abnormally thick mucus secretion in the lungs of CF affected individuals hampers effective elimination of inhaled bacteria. This predisposes to recurrent respiratory infection and eventually to progressive irreversible inflammatory lung damage. Declining lung function is the principle cause of serious illness and premature death among adult CF patients.

The sweat of CF affected neonates is abnormally concentrated (salty). Although this has no great clinical effect, it has proved to be of great diagnostic significance; indeed measurement of the concentration of sodium or chloride in sweat provides the only widely available reliable means for confirming CF.

Although CF remains incurable, improved understanding of the condition and resulting more effective treatment regimes have greatly improved the health of CF sufferers and had a remarkable impact on life expectancy. When the condition was first described in 1938 most affected babies died before their first birthday. By the mid 1990's the average age of death was 31 years, and babies born today are expected to survive their fiftieth birthday. Early diagnosis and treatment (within a few weeks of birth) has proved a significant contributory factor towards both improved quality of life and life expectancy.

The CF screening test

Screening for CF is based on measurement of trypsin in bloodspot samples and, if necessary, DNA analysis of the bloodspot sample. Trypsin is an intestinal digestive enzyme derived from pancreatic trypsinogen. Pancreatic involvement in the pathogenesis of CF determines that blood concentration of trypsin is temporarily increased in neonates with CF. (As the disease progresses beyond the neonatal period blood trypsin levels fall below normal.) The test is called immunoreative trypsin (IRT); immunoreactive here merely defines the method of measurement (it is an immunoassay that employs antibodies that only react with trypsin).

Median IRT in healthy neonates is around 20 ng/ml, whereas IRT of CF affected neonates usually exceeds 100 ng/ml and is commonly considerably higher. CF is not the only condition that is associated with increased IRT, so DNA analysis to detect CF mutations is an essential part of the screening process for samples with increased IRT.

Initially blood spot samples are submitted for IRT analysis. A negative screen, reported as 'CF not suspected', is given to all those with IRT <60 ng/ml. This eliminates the great majority. The remaining samples whose IRT is >60 ng/ml are retested again twice. On this round of testing a negative screen, reported as 'CF not suspected', is applied to all those samples in which the mean of the two IRT results is <70 ng/ml. Samples with IRT >70 ng/ml are submitted for DNA analysis. This involves testing for the presence of the 30 most common CFTR mutations, which together account for 90–95% of all CF cases. (It is impractical to test for all CFTR mutations – there are in excess of 1600.) A positive screen result – CF suspected – is reported if two mutations (one from each parent) are identified. If only one mutation is detected this most likely indicates healthy carrier status but it could mean that the individual has CF, the second unidentified mutation being one of those rare mutations not tested for. In order to discriminate these two possibilities the screening protocol uses the IRT measurement. If IRT is <120 ng/ml the report is 'probable carrier' and if the IRT is >120 ng/ml the report is 'CF suspected'. The same IRT criterion is applied to those samples whose DNA analyses reveal no mutations, on the basis that no mutation could mean either CF (two unidentified rare mutations) or, most likely, normal healthy status (no CF mutations).

Congenital hypothyroidism (CH)

[Note: The thyroid gland, thyroid hormones and adult hypothyroidism are discussed in Chapter 10.]

This condition[3], which affects approximately 1 in 3500 births, is defined simply as deficiency of thyroid hormones at birth. Around 230 CH affected babies are born annually in the UK.

CH has two principle causes: abnormal development of the thyroid gland (around 80–85% of all cases); and inherited genetic defect that results in reduced synthesis of thyroid hormones (around 10–15% of all cases). Abnormal development of the thyroid gland includes complete absence of thyroid gland (thyroid agnesis), a thyroid of reduced size (thyroid hypoplasia) or a thyroid of reduced size that is located in an abnormal position (thyroid ectopy). These conditions are not inherited – they occur sporadically during embryonic/foetal development; it remains largely unclear why.

A number of inherited single gene defects result in reduced synthesis of thyroid hormone. The most common is in the gene that codes for the enzyme thyroid peroxidase (TPO), which is required for the first step in thyroid synthesis, the iodination of tyrosine (see Chapter 10, Figure 10.2). The genetic defect results in reduced activity of TPO and thereby reduced thyroid hormone synthesis.

Very rarely CH is due *not* to abnormality in the thyroid gland or defect in thyroid hormone synthesis within a normally developed thyroid gland, but to a defect in the pituitary gland that results in reduced production of the pituitary hormone, thyroid stimulating hormone (TSH). As its name suggests TSH is required for normal production of thyroid hormone by the thyroid gland. For reasons that will become clear, the screening process does not readily identify that very small minority whose CH is due to reduced TSH (i.e. defect in the pituitary).

All the abnormalities that give rise to CH discussed thus far are permanent and therefore require lifelong treatment. Occasionally CH is transitory, meaning it is due to a condition that resolves with time during the first months or years of life. Transitory CH can be a feature of moderate to severe prematurity. The screening process detects transitory as well as permanent CH.

Thyroid hormone is essential for early growth and brain development both *in utero* and postnatally. To a significant extent the effects of any thyroid hormone deficiency during foetal development are mitigated by the transplacental passage of maternal thyroid hormones, but from birth continuing growth and brain development depends on the baby's ability to produce adequate amounts of thyroid hormone. Irrespective of its cause, untreated CH leads to permanent physical and mental disability. The longer treatment is delayed the more significant is the disability.

There are usually no early clinical signs and symptoms of CH. Those that occur in the minority of newborns with particularly severe CH are non-specific and include prolongation of jaundice, feeding difficulty, lethargy and constipation.

Early treatment with thyroid hormone replacement therapy starting within the first two to three weeks of birth ensures normal growth and intellectual development. Given the lack of specific early clinical signs and symptoms, CH could hardly ever be diagnosed within this time frame without the benefit of screening during the first week of life. Since a sufficiency of thyroid hormones is essential for good health throughout life, replacement therapy is a life-long requirement in most cases.

The CH screening test

Screening for congenital hypothyroidism is based on measuring the concentration of thyroid stimulating hormone (TSH) in the bloodspot sample. TSH is a pituitary hormone required for normal regulation of thyroid hormone production (see Chapter 10, Figure 10.3). This role determines that primary hypothyroidism, which includes almost all cases of CH, is associated with increased TSH.

Although there is a surge of TSH release at the time of birth, blood concentration quickly falls over the first few days of life so that the TSH of a healthy full term neonate aged five to eight days old <5 mU/L. Typically CH is associated with TSH levels >20 mU/L, although in mild cases it can be 10–20 mU/ml.

A negative screen result reported as 'CH not suspected' is applied to all those with bloodspot TSH <8 mU/L. This eliminates the vast majority. For those remaining in the screening process whose initial blood spot TSH is >8 mU/L, TSH assay is repeated in duplicate. On this second round of testing a negative test result reported as 'CH not suspected' is applied to all those whose mean of three TSH results is <10 mU/L. A positive screen result reported as 'CH suspected' is applied to those whose mean of three TSH results is >20 mU/L. Finally an equivocal screening test result, reported as 'CH borderline', is applied to those whose mean of three TSH results is 10–20 mU/L. The screening process demands that all babies with 'CH borderline' result on initial screening have a second bloodspot sample taken within seven days of the first. If on testing this second bloodspot sample TSH is <10 mU/L a negative screen 'CH not suspected' is reported; and if it is >10 mU/L then a positive screen 'CH suspected' is reported.

Babies born very prematurely (<32 weeks of gestation) must have a second bloodspot sample taken for CH screening only. That sample should be taken 28 days after birth or on the day of discharge, whichever is the sooner. The same TSH cut-off (10 mu/L) is used to distinguish positive from negative screening result.

Medium chain acyl-CoA dehydrogenase deficiency (MCADD)

This condition affects 1 in 10 000 births[4], so around 80 MCADD affected babies are born each year in the UK. It is a disturbance of fatty acid oxidation, a metabolic process that allows our fat reserves to provide energy during periods of fasting or stress. Medium chain acyl-CoA dehydrogenase is one of several enzymes required for this metabolic process. Those with MCADD have an inherited defect (mutation) in the gene that codes for synthesis of this key enzyme. The mutation results in deficiency of the enzyme, which in turn inhibits the metabolic pathway leading to abnormal accumulation of fatty acids and their metabolites. This accumulation can result in a potentially lethal acute metabolic disturbance.

Like PKU and CF, MCADD is inherited in an autosomal recessive manner so that the abnormal gene must be inherited from both parents. Inheritance of one abnormal and one normal MCAD gene confers carrier status. Carriers are unaffected but if both parents are carriers there is a one in four chance that their offspring will inherit MCADD.

Since this metabolic pathway is only operational during periods of fasting or stress, MCADD is only significant in these situations. Indeed, an estimated third of those with MCADD remain apparently unaffected by the condition. However during a period of fasting or stress caused, for example, by feeding difficulties or inter-current illness/infection, MCADD can become manifest as a serious acute illness. The hallmark of this illness is abnormally reduced ketones (the products of fatty acid oxidation) and reduced blood glucose (hypoglycaemia). This abnormal metabolic state, called hypoketotic hypoglycaemia may be accompanied by metabolic acidosis and accumulation of toxic ammonia. Seizures, brain damage and coma may ensue. The metabolic disturbance is rapidly fatal in around 25% of cases and may leave those who survive with permanent neurological deficit.

Treatment of MCADD is dietary based. It is important that MCADD affected individuals do not go without food for too long and that they take special precautions to maintain carbohydrate intake when unwell. This may necessitate hospital admission for IV feeding. A very few foods (containing medium chain triglycerides) should be avoided.

Before newborn screening, MCADD was only usually diagnosed when affected individuals suffered the severe metabolic disturbance already described. Early diagnosis through screening, coupled with effective dietary advice can prevent such potentially fatal crises.

The MCADD screening test

Screening for MCADD is based on measuring the blood concentration of two fatty acid metabolites, octoylcarnitine and decanoylcarnitine, in the bloodspot sample. The method of measurement is tandem mass spectrometry, the same as that used for the PKU screening test.

Octoanoylcarnitine is derived from the eight carbon chain (C8) fatty acid, octanoic acid, and decanoylcarnitine is derived from the ten carbon chain (C10) fatty acid, decanoic aid. So the two measured metabolites are commonly referred to as C8 and C10.

A negative screening result reported as 'MCADD not suspected' is initially applied to all bloodspot samples whose C8 is <0.4 µmol/L. This eliminates the majority of samples. The remaining samples with C8 ≥0.4 µmol/L are analysed again this time in duplicate for both C8 and C10. In this second round of testing a negative screen, reported as 'MCADD not suspected', is applied to all those whose mean of three C8 results is <0.5 µmol/L. For all those whose mean of C8 results is ≥0.5 µmol/L, the ratio of C8:C10 concentration is calculated. If the ratio is <1 the screen result is negative 'MCADD not suspected' and if the ratio is >1 the screen result is positive; this is reported as 'MCADD suspected'.

Sickle cell disorders (SCD)

SCD[5] are the most common of a large group of inherited conditions, collectively called the haemoglobinopathies, that are characterised by defect either in the structure or the synthesis of haemoglobin (Hb). Hb is the oxygen carrying protein present in red blood cells. Around 1 in 2000 UK births are affected by a SCD, so close to 400 SCD affected babies are born annually in the UK. SCD predominantly affects those of African, Asian or Mediterranean descent; it is rare among those of Northern European descent (Caucasians).

An understanding of SCD, which are all defects in Hb structure, requires some knowledge of normal Hb structure. This was dealt with in Chapter 15 but the relevant section is reproduced here.

The Hb molecule (see Chapter 15, Figure 15.3) comprises four folded chains of amino acids. These together form the protein or *globin* portion of the molecule. Each of the four globin sub-units has a much smaller *haem* group attached, and at the centre of each haem group is an atom of iron in the ferrous state (Fe^{2+}). Whilst the structure of the haem group is always the same, the exact sequence of amino acids in the globin sub-units varies slightly, giving rise to four possible globin chains: alpha (α), beta (β), gamma (γ) and delta (δ). Around 97% of total Hb is haemoglobin A (HbA) which contains 2 α and 2 δ globin sub-units. The remaining 3% is HbA2 (2 α and 2 δ globins). In the developing foetus, and for the first three to six months after birth, foetal haemoglobin (HbF) is the principle Hb produced.

HbF is composed of 2 α and 2 γ globin sub-units. Slowly over the first six months of life HbF production declines as HbA production increases so that at the end of this period and throughout life, HbF normally constitutes <0.5% of total haemoglobin. At five to eight days of age when bloodspot tests are performed, around 75% of Hb is HbF; just 25% is HbA.

Synthesis of globin chains (α, β, γ, δ) are coded for by separate genes and it is inherited defects (mutations) in these genes that give rise to haemoglobinopathies such as SCD.

SCD is an inherited defect in the gene that codes for the β globin chain. Like all proteins, β globin is composed of amino-acids joined in a very precise sequence. The sixth amino acid in β globin is valine. The genetic defect in those with SCD results in production of β globin with the amino-acid glutamine instead of valine at position 6. This single amino substitution results in production of the abnormal sickle haemogloblin (HbS), which is composed of 2 normal α globin sub-units and 2 abnormal β globin sub-units. If the abnormal sickle cell gene is inherited from just one parent, around half the Hb produced is abnormal HbS and half is normal HbA. This essentially benign heterozygous state is known as 'sickle trait' or 'sickle carrier' status. Around one in seven black Africans and one in eight black Caribbeans are sickle cell carriers, this compared with 1 in 500 among those of northern European descent. All pregnant women are offered a blood test to screen for sickle cell trait during first trimester, and if they test positive the test is offered to their partners.

If a copy of the sickle gene is inherited from both parents all Hb produced is abnormal HbS; this is sickle cell anaemia, by far the most common SCD, accounting for around 80% of all cases in the UK. Less common forms result from inheritance of the sickle gene from one parent and inheritance of a different, rarer β globin gene defect from the other. Those affected produce two kinds of abnormal Hb, HbS and another. Like those with sickle cell anaemia, these individuals produce no normal Hb (HbA).

In its deoxygenated state, HbS polymerises causing structural changes to the red cell membrane, which becomes rigid. The red cells deform into the familiar sickle (crescent) shape that gives the condition its name. These deformed red cells are fragile and haemolyse (breakdown) easily. Normally red cells survive on average for 120 days whereas red cells that contain HbS survive on average for just 15 days. The resulting chronic (haemolytic) anaemia is a hallmark of the disease.

SCD only becomes manifest after the switch from HbF (which of course does not contain β globin) to HbS production at around three to six months of age. There is considerable variability in expression of the disease, a minority are only mildly affected, but for most the disease is characterised by periods of relatively good health, apart from chronic anaemia of variable severity, punctuated by extremely painful sickle cells crises.

These crises may be precipitated by a variety of environmental factors including infection, extreme exercise, emotional stress, extreme cold, dehydration etc. Sickle cell crises are associated with increased haemolysis along with sequestration of sickled red cells in the microvasculature of various organs (spleen, bone, lungs and brain); it is this sequestration that accounts for many of the serious complications of SCD. Microvasculature blocked by sickled cells prevents normal blood flow to tissue cells. Deprived of oxygen, these cells are irreversibly damaged. If the microvasculature of the brain is affected, patients may suffer stroke due to cerebral infarction. Occlusion of vessels in the eye causes visual impairment. Infarcts in growing bone tissue early in childhood may leave single fingers or toes permanently shorter than the rest.

SCD is associated with increased risk of infection, due partly to splenic damage. Overwhelming pneumococcal sepsis was once a significant cause of death in infancy, before daily prophylactic penicillin and pneumococcal vaccination was introduced to routine care.

Early diagnosis, monitoring and prophylactic treatment before symptoms develop has been shown to reduce the complications and premature deaths associated with SCD.

The SCD screening test

Screening for sickle cell disease involves one of two techniques that allow separation and identification of the kinds of haemoglobin present in the bloodspot sample. The two techniques are high performance liquid chromatography (HPLC) and isoelectric focusing (IEF), and the separation reflects the slight differences in Hb structure. These techniques allow separation of HbA, HbA2 and HbF (the haemoglobins that are normally present in a neonatal blood sample) as well as HbS (the abnormal haemoglobin present in a neonate with SCD). Screening by this method allows distinction between sickle cell carriers and those with sickle cell anaemia, because in the first case blood contains predominantly HbF, but also equal amounts of HbA and HbS; and in the second it contains only HbF and HbS, there is no HbA.

- A report of HbFA indicates unaffected by SCD.
- A report of HbFAS is consistent with sickle carrier status.
- A report of HbFS is consistent with sickle cell disease (sickle cell anaemia).

The screening technique also allows detection of abnormal haemoglobins (other than HbS) that are associated with sickle cell disorders, other than sickle cell anaemia. These are: HbC, HbE, HbD[Punjab] and HbO[arab].

Thus a report of HbFSC, for example, is consistent with sickle cell disease (specifically sickle C disease, not sickle cell anaemia).

The screening protocol demands that when an abnormality is found it is confirmed by the alternative technique (HPLC or IEF) before reporting.

References

1. UK Newborn Screening Programme (2012) *Guidelines for Newborn Blood Spot Sampling*, UK National Screening committee, available for download at: http://newbornbloodspot. screening.nhs.uk/bloodspotsampling

2. Blau, N., van Spronsen, F. and Levy, H. (2010) Phenylketonuria, *Lancet*, 376: 1417–27.
3. Rastogi, M. and LaFranchi, S. (2010) Congenital hypothyroidism, *Orphanet J of Rare Diseases*, 5: 17.
4. Oerton, J., Khalid, J., Dalton, R. et al. (2011) Newborn screening for medium chain acyl-CoA dehydrogenase deficiency in England: prevalence, predictive value and test validity based on 1.5 million screened babies, *J Med Screen*, 18: 173–81.
5. McCavit, T. (2012) Sickle cell disease, *Paediatrics in Review*, 33: 195–204.

Further reading

http://newbornbloodspot.screening.nhs.uk

This is the website of the NHS newborn bloodspot programme. It contains a wealth of very accessible information about conditions screened for, organisation and standards of the programme, including those relating to laboratory testing.

CHAPTER 24

CERVICAL SCREENING TEST

Key learning topics

- Gross and micro anatomy of the cervix
- Cervical cancer
- Human papilloma virus (HPV) infection and cervical cancer
- History and organisation of cervical cancer screening
- Defining cervical intraepithelial neoplasia (CIN)
- Defining dyskaryosis
- Collecting a cervical sample
- Colposcopy

The purpose of most clinical laboratory testing is to aid clinical diagnosis and monitor the progress of disease or effectiveness of therapy. By contrast, the purpose of the test that is the subject of this chapter is to *prevent* disease. The cervical screening test (sometimes referred to as the cervical smear or 'Pap' test) involves the microscopical examination of cells recovered by scraping the surface of the cervix. Abnormal changes in the appearance of these cells occur up to 10–15 years before cancer of the cervix develops. Since early treatment of these changes prevents cervical cancer developing, women are actively encouraged to have the test at regular intervals. In the UK around 4.5 million cervical samples are examined in clinical laboratories every year[1,2,3]. This work accounts for a significant proportion of the total workload of cytopathology departments.

The cervix

Anatomy

The cervix (from the Greek meaning neck or neck like) is part of the female genital tract. It is a tubular structure around 3 cm in length that forms the lower part or

Understanding Laboratory Investigations: A Guide for Nurses, Midwives and Healthcare Professionals, Third Edition. Chris Higgins.
© 2013 John Wiley & Sons, Ltd. Published 2013 by John Wiley & Sons, Ltd.

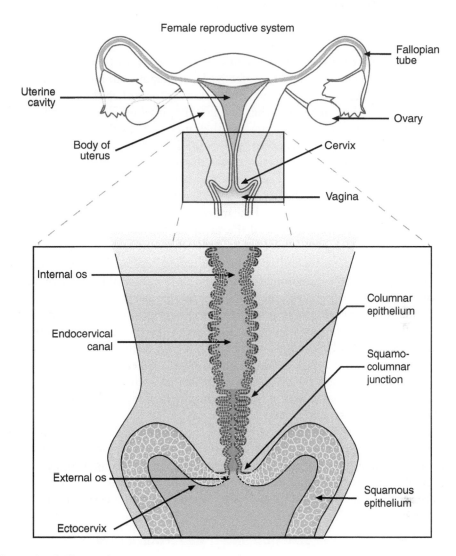

Figure 24.1 The cervix.

neck of the uterus, connecting the uterus to the vagina. Four main anatomical features can be identified (Figure 24.1). The ectocervix is the lower part of the cervix, which extends into the vaginal canal. At the centre of the ectocervix is the external os, the tiny opening to the endocervical canal, which is circular in women who have never been pregnant but otherwise slit-like. The endocervical canal is the tubular structure of the cervix, which opens at the internal os to the uterus.

As the connection between uterus and vagina, the cervical canal is the first part of the birth canal. Late in pregnancy, the normally tough and fibrous cervix softens or 'ripens', allowing the cervical canal to dilate to several times its normal diameter, for passage of the developed foetus from uterus to vagina, during birth.

Cervical epithelium

The surface of the cervix is covered with a protective layer of epithelium. It is the epithelial cells, which make up this protective layer that are sampled for the cervical screening test. In the case of the cervix, there are two sorts of epithelium: squamous epithelium covers the ectocervix, whilst columnar epithelium lines the endocervical canal. Four distinct layers of squamous epithelium can be distinguished on the surface of the ectocervix. The deepest of these is the basal layer, which comprises one row of immature squamous (basal) epithelial cells. Above this is the parabasal layer: two rows of immature squamous (parabasal) cells, which are constantly dividing to maintain the epithelium above. The intermediate layer comprises four to six rows of more mature cells, and the most mature squamous epithelial cells are those within the five to eight rows of the superficial layer. Cells in this superficial layer become increasingly less attached to each other and are continuously cast off from the surface of the ectocervix by a process called desquamation or exfoliation. Constant regeneration of squamous epithelial cells in the basal layers is required to replace those that are lost from the surface of the ectocervix by exfoliation. Most of the squamous epithelial cells recovered for the cervical screening test are from the superficial and intermediate layers. Cells from the parabasal layer constitute only around 5% of all squamous epithelial cells in a normal sample from young women. The cells in a cervical sample from older women contain slightly more parabasal cells, and disease of the cervix is associated with a significant increase in the number of parabasal cells in a cervical sample. Because of their relative depth, basal cells are rarely seen in cervical samples.

The mucous secreting columnar epithelium of the endocervical canal is composed simply of one row of columnar epithelial cells; some are mucous secreting and others have cilia on their surface. The mucous and cilia are thought to facilitate the passage of spermatozoa through the endocervical canal. When columnar epithelial cells are seen in a cervical sample, they are referred to as endocervical cells.

The squamo-columnar junction and transformation zone

The point where the squamous epithelium of the ectocervix meets the columnar epithelium of the endocervical canal is called the squamo-columnar junction (Figure 24.1). This junction is of great pathological significance because it is in this area that most cases of cervical cancer originate. Before puberty the junction lies at the external os, (Figure 24.2) but in response to the normal hormonal changes that occur at puberty, the lower end of the endocervix everts somewhat, so that the junction moves outwards from external os onto the ectocervix. A second important physiological change occurs as a result of this eversion of the endocervix. The columnar epithelium that covers the everted part of the endocervix is now exposed to the acidic vaginal environment and this environmental change, in combination with other factors, induces the exposed columnar epithelial cells to undergo transformation to squamous epithelial cells, a process called metaplasia. The area around the external os of the ectocervix where this transformation of columnar to

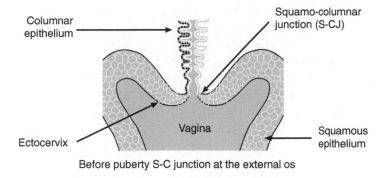

Columnar epithelium

Squamo-columnar junction (S-CJ)

Vagina

Ectocervix

Squamous epithelium

Before puberty S-C junction at the external os

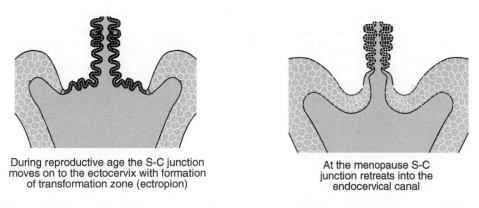

During reproductive age the S-C junction moves on to the ectocervix with formation of transformation zone (ectropion)

At the menopause S-C junction retreats into the endocervical canal

Figure 24.2 Location of the squamo-columnar junction at different stages of a woman's life.

squamous epithelium occurs is called the transformation zone. Epithelial cells undergoing transformation are called squamous metaplastic cells. As the transformation occurs, throughout a woman's reproductive years, the squamo-columnar junction moves back towards the external os. After the menopause the junction usually retreats into the endocervical canal.

Cancer of the cervix

Almost all (85–90%) cervical cancers originate in the squamous epithelial cells of the transformation zone on the ectocervix. This is known technically as cervical squamous cell carcinoma. The rest originate in the columnar epithelial cells of the endocervix; this is known as cervical adenocarcinoma. Generally speaking the second of these two kinds of cervical cancer is considered to have the worst prognosis.

With an annual incidence of around 2 900 in the UK, cervical cancer is currently the twelfth most common cancer to affect women of all ages, and the second most common cancer to affect young women under the age of 35 years[4]. It can affect women of any age but is most often diagnosed between the ages of 25 and 50 years. Younger women, so long as they are of reproductive age, are also at risk; around 2% of cases occur before the age of 25[5].

There are often no symptoms during the early stages of cervical cancer. The only common symptoms are abnormal vaginal bleeding and discomfort during sexual intercourse. Post-coital bleeding is fairly common.

The prognosis for a woman with invasive cancer of the cervix depends, as with most other cancers, on the extent of cancer spread at the time of diagnosis. So long as the cancer is confined to the cervix, the prognosis is good; treatment can effect a cure. Untreated, invasive cervical cancer spreads from the cervix first to the upper part of the vagina, then to the ureters and lower part of the vagina. In the most advanced cases, invasion of the bladder wall and rectum may be evident at diagnosis. Such advanced disease is associated with a poor prognosis; only 15–20% of patients with the most advanced disease survive more than five years. The annual UK death toll due to cervical cancer is currently close to 950[4]. There is now overwhelming evidence that infection with the human papilloma virus (HPV) is the cause of cervical cancer.

HPV and cervical cancer

Early epidemiological studies suggested that a sexually transmitted agent might have a role in cervical cancer. By the end of the 1970s human papilloma virus (HPV) had emerged as the most likely of several candidate sexually transmitted agents. The more recent observation that HPV is present in all cervical cancers and that infection predates cancer development has allowed the now established view that HPV is a necessary, but not sufficient, cause for cervical cancer[6]. Thus only those who have been infected with HPV develop cervical cancer. (It is worth mentioning in passing that since the link between HPV and cervical cancer was first established it has become apparent that some other cancers are caused by HPV infection; these include almost all anal cancers, and some vaginal, vulvar, penile and mouth/throat cancers.)

Cervical cancer is by no means an inevitable consequence of HPV infection. Up to 75% of sexually active women become infected with HPV at some point in their life[7]. The vast majority eradiacte the virus without even knowing they have been infected. It remains unclear why in a small proportion of infected women HPV is not eradicated but persists for many years, eventually causing cervical cancer. Some risk factors have been identified; they include cigarette smoking, the use of oral contraceptives and immune suppression (e.g. co-infection with the human immunodeficiency virus (HIV) that causes AIDS).

There are around 100 different HPV types, which have been broadly categorised to those that infect skin (the cutaneous types) and those that infect the mucosal surface of the mouth and genital tract (mucosotropic types). The cutaneous HPV types are responsible for common, invariably benign, wart infection of hands and feet. The mucosotropic group includes 40 different HPV types that, following transmission by sexual contact, infect the genital tract. These are divided into low risk types that can cause benign genital warts and high-risk types that can, after many years of clinical latency, cause cervical cancer. Seventeen high-risk types have been identified but just five types (HPV 16, 18, 31, 33 and 45) account for 95% of all cervical cancers. The two most common high-risk types, HPV 16 and HPV 18, account for an estimated 70–75% of cases.

The notion that prevention of HPV infection prevents cervical cancer provided the rationale for universal HPV vaccination of girls before they become sexually active, and thereby at risk of HPV infection.

The UK HPV vaccination programme, introduced in 2008, offers vaccination (delivered in three doses) to all girls aged 12–13 years. Initially, the vaccine used was Cervarix, which provides protection against HPV types 16 and 18. Since 2012 an alternative vaccine, Gardisil, has been used. This provides the same level of protection against HPV types 16 and 18, but also provides protection against HPV types 6 and 11 that together cause almost all cases of genital warts. If vaccination achieves 80% coverage it is estimated that by 2025 there will be a 63% reduction in the incidence of cervical cancer; most recent data[8] indicate that 83% of girls are being vaccinated. Since vaccination provides full protection only against HPV types 16 and 18 infection, and other HPV types can cause cervical cancer, it is important that vaccinated women continue to participate in the screening process.

The malignant (cancerous) potential of HPV depends on its DNA being incorporated into the DNA of normal healthy cervical cells. All pre-cancerous and cancerous cervical cells contain HPV DNA. The notion that HPV DNA testing of cervical samples would be of value in screening for cervical cancer has, after many years of research, been established, and this test was introduced to the screening process in 2011. Just how this testing is applied will be discussed further.

Natural history of cervical cancer

The preventative value of the cervical screening test is due to the usually long natural history of cervical cancer. Identifiable pre-cancerous changes occur up to 10–15 years before invasive cancer develops. If these are identified and treated, cervical cancer can be prevented.

Many years before cervical cancer develops, microscopical changes to the squamous epithelial cells in the transformation zone occur. These changes are known technically as cervical intra-epithelial neoplasia (CIN). CIN is a potentially progressive lesion, caused by HPV infection, which may if not treated ultimately lead to cervical cancer. Three grades of severity of CIN have been identified. If the cellular changes which characterise CIN are confined to the lowest third of epithelium, a diagnosis of CIN I is made, if such changes are seen in the lower two thirds, CIN II is diagnosed. The most severe form of CIN, CIN III, is diagnosed when abnormal cells are seen throughout the full thickness of the epithelium; this is also called carcinoma *in situ*. The level of CIN determines the risk of invasive cervical cancer developing. For example, patients with CIN I have a relatively low risk of cancer developing; in around 50% of cases the abnormality resolves spontaneously. However CIN I may persist without any untoward effects; or for an unpredictable small minority of patients may progress through CIN II to CIN III. Around 30% of patients with CIN III if left untreated would progress to invasive cancer within ten years. At the present time there is no way of predicting with any certainty which patients with CIN will progress to invasive cancer, or how speedy that progression will be. All that can be said is that there is an increased risk of cervical cancer for women with CIN and that the risk is highest in those with CIN III. Treatment of CIN prevents cancer developing in nearly all cases. The definitive diagnosis of CIN depends on microscopical examination of a piece of cervical tissue (a biopsy). However the microscopical appearance of cells scraped from the surface of the cervix reflect the abnormalities that constitute CIN. This is the rationale for the cervical smear test as a screening test for prevention of cervical cancer.

Cervical screening

History

The cervical screening test is often referred to as the 'Pap' smear test. This alternative name celebrates the research of George Papanicolaou, a Greek physician who worked in the United States. In the 1920s Papanicolaou first observed that cancerous cervical cells could be found in vaginal smears. To enhance the appearance of these cells he developed a staining technique using the Papanicolaou stain, which is used to this day to stain cervical samples. In the late 1940s, Ayre demonstrated that scraping the surface of the cervix was a more reliable means of recovering cancerous cervical cells. He developed the Ayre's spatula for this purpose. At around this time, the concept of pre-cancerous disease of the cervix was introduced, allowing the rationale for the use of the cervical smear test to screen for early evidence of cervical cancer.

A screening programme using the cervical smear test was first introduced in the UK during 1964. However the organisation of the scheme was not nationally co-ordinated and evolved in an *ad hoc* fashion. The result was that the scheme had much less impact in reducing the incidence of cervical cancer than expected. Experience of cervical screening in other European countries, particularly Denmark, Sweden and Finland, had demonstrated that a well organised scheme in which all women at risk are regularly given a cervical smear test can be successful. In these countries there had been huge steady reduction in the incidence of cervical cancer from the time screening was introduced in the 1960s. In recognition of the relative failure of the *ad hoc* screening programme then in operation in the UK, a nationally co-ordinated cervical screening programme was introduced in 1988. Although there have been changes over the intervening years, the scheme introduced in 1988 remains substantially the same.

Probably the most significant change to the scheme came during the period 2005–2008 when the switch from conventional cervical smear test to liquid based cytology (LBC) occurred in stages across the country. Instead of smearing the sample on a glass slide and sending this to the laboratory, the LBC technique involves collection of the cervical sample into a liquid fixative solution that is sent to the laboratory. This apparently simple change has made the screening process far more efficient and cost effective, principally because the LBC method is associated with a much lower proportion of samples being reported as inadequate, and having to be repeated. Prior to introduction of LBC around 10% of cervical screening tests had to be repeated because of inadequate sampling; now only around 2.5% of tests need repeating[9].

LBC has also allowed much speedier reporting of results. Recent data shows that results of all cervical screening tests are now available within one to two weeks of the sample being taken[10]. Prior to implementation of LBC women had to wait 4–12 weeks for their result, and sometimes even longer. The conventional smear technique only allowed cytological examination of cervical samples, whereas the LBC technique allows both cytological examination and HPV DNA testing. Introduction of selective HPV DNA testing in 2011–2012 represents the most recent improving change to the cervical screening programme.

Organisation and success of cervical screening

The aim of the UK programme is to reduce the incidence of cervical cancer and deaths due to cervical cancer by performing regular cervical screening tests on every woman between the ages 25 and 65 years. Current national policy in England and Northern Ireland is that all women between the ages 25 and 49 should be screened every three years, and those between the ages 50 and 65 every five years. Screening after the age of 65 is reserved for those who have not been screened since the age of 50 and those who have had recent abnormal results. In Scotland and Wales the policy is to screen all women between the ages 20 and 65 (60 in Scotland) every three years, but there is now consultation on the proposal to change this to that which currently pertains in England and Northern Ireland; a decision is expected by 2013.

The responsibility for cervical screening falls largely on the primary healthcare team. A computerised call and recall system implemented by primary care workers (GPs, practice nurses and practice managers) ensures that every woman in the target population of each GP practice is offered a cervical screening test appointment at the prescribed intervals.

Before 1987 only around 40% of women in the then target age range 20–65 years were being screened. With the introduction of the national screening programme in 1988, coverage increased quickly. By 1994, 85% of the target population was being screened; this level of coverage has been maintained broadly ever since, although there is concern that coverage has reduced in recent years, particularly among young women when offered their first screening appointment. In 2010 78.6% of the total target population attended for cervical screening[10].

Notwithstanding this recent concern, there is much evidence that the increased level of cervical screening since 1987 has had a significant effect on incidence of cervical cancer[11]. In England, between 1971 and 1987 the annual incidence stayed fairly steady, fluctuating between 14 and 16 per 100 000 women (i.e. on average

3900 cases a year). Between 1990 and 2003 however, annual incidence fell steadily year on year; by 1995 the incidence was 10 per 100 000 women or 2900 new cases, and in 2003 just 2312 new cases were registered[12]. Since 2003 annual incidence in England has remained fairly static at around 2300.

The screening programme since 1987 has also had an effect on the number of deaths attributed to cervical cancer. From 1950 to 1987 mortality due to cervical cancer fell steadily at the rate of 1.5% every year. Since 1987 this rate of fall has trebled. In 1987, 1800 deaths in England were attributed to cervical cancer; in 2008 this number had fallen to 759. An analysis[13] of trends in mortality before screening was introduced suggests that cervical screening prevents the death of 5000 women in the UK every year.

The cervical screening test

Around 80% of cervical samples are collected in a primary care setting, most often by practice nurses.

Patient preparation

The best time to take a cervical sample is mid cycle to avoid contamination with menstrual blood. It is preferable to delay the test for a few months following child-birth. The patient should be advised to avoid the use of vaginal creams and refrain from sexual intercourse for 24 hours before the test. Many women will be anxious, especially on the first occasion they attend, so that a calm reassuring manner is important. A brief explanation of the test emphasising the points in Table 24.1 will help to allay fears. Any effort made to reduce the tension or anxiety a woman might experience at the time of sampling, will increase the chance of obtaining a suitable sample. Furthermore there is evidence to suggest that women who are dealt with in a sympathetic manner are more likely to re-attend for future testing or further investigation, if an abnormality is discovered.

Cervical sampling technique

The practical detail of collecting an adequate cervical sample is beyond the scope of this chapter. Some general points are made here.

The cervix must first be visualised by passing a vaginal speculum. The cervix must be well illuminated. The object is to sample epithelial cells from the transformation zone and squamo-columnar junction, so that squamous epithelial cells as well as some endocervical cells are recovered. Since the position of the squamo-columnar junction varies with age and parity, sampling technique must take account of these factors.

A disposable sampling instrument called a Cervex-brush is used, the business end of which is a soft flexible plastic brush. The shape of the brush with longest bristles at the centre reflects the contours of the ectocervix and endocervix, allowing the brush to come into contact with all areas of the transformation zone, including

Table 24.1 Topics for discussion with patient prior to cervical smear test.

Why have the test?
- Cervical screening is recommended for all women between the ages of 25 and 65.
- Cervical screening is not a test for diagnosing cervical cancer but to confirm that the cervix (the lower part of the womb) is healthy.
- In over 90% of cases the test confirms a healthy cervix.
- Less than 10% of women have changes to the cervix, which in the vast majority of cases revert to normal over time; a small fraction of these women however have changes that might lead to cancer in the long term.
- Simple out-patient treatment of these pre-cancerous changes prevents cancer.

About the test
- You will be asked to undress from the waist down, but if you wear a full skirt you will not have to remove it.
- The test is performed with you lying on a couch. A small instrument called a speculum is gently placed into you vagina to hold it open so that the cervix can be viewed.
- A small 'brush like' instrument is used to gently wipe some cells from the surface of the cervix.
- The cells are placed in a small container of preservative liquid and sent for examination under the microscope. The liquid might also be tested for the presence of the virus (HPV) that causes cervical cancer.
- The test takes just a few minutes; you might feel some discomfort. Take deep breaths to relax as it may hurt more if you are tense but tell the nurse (or doctor) if you experience pain.

After the test
- The nurse or doctor will tell you when and how you will receive the result of the test.
- There is no reason to be alarmed if you are asked for a repeat test; around 1 in 50 tests have to be repeated because an insufficient number of cells have been collected.

the squamo-columnar junction. The full circumference of the transformation zone must be sampled by applying slight pressure on the cervix with the Cervex-brush and rotating it clockwise through 360° several times. Cervical cells adhere to the brush.

A differently designed brush that allows sampling within the endocervical canal is necessary in the case of post-menopausal women because the transformation zone retreats within the endocervical canal at the menopause.

The brush, whatever its design, is immediately transferred to a glass vial containing fluid fixative, and the sampled cellular material is rinsed from the brush by a swirling motion. Alternatively the head of the brush is removed, placed in the liquid fixative vial and the vial is shaken vigorously to release cellular material. The vial is transported to the laboratory.

In the laboratory cervical cells are separated from other debris in the cervical liquid sample and these cells are transferred in an even distribution to a glass slide, prior to staining and microscopical examination by a cytoscreener.

Results of cervical screening test

Around 93–94% of adequately collected cervical samples are found on microscopical examination to be entirely normal[9] and no further investigation, save recall in three or five years is necessary. The remaining 6–7% have some degree of abnormality ranging from the benign (the vast majority), through entirely curable pre-malignant disease (CIN) to invasive cancer.

The main object of microscopical examination of cervical cells is to search for the abnormal changes associated with the pre-cancerous condition, CIN. These abnormal changes, which are known collectively as dyskaryosis (literally, abnormal nucleus), include an increase in the size of the nucleus compared with surrounding cytoplasm, along with irregularity in the shape and staining characteristics of the cell nucleus. There are three recognised grades of severity of dyskaryosis: mild, moderate and severe. In some cases only slight changes to the nucleus are present which may not be sufficient to warrant a report of even mild dyskaryosis; these are reported as 'borderline nuclear abnormalities'. The severity of dyskaryosis correlates to some degree with the level of CIN that might be expected if a cervical tissue biopsy were examined, so that a report of a smear result from a patient with dyskaryosis implies a prediction of the level of CIN. In broad terms CIN I would be expected if mild dyskaryosis were present; CIN II or CIN III would be expected if moderate dyskaryosis were present and CIN III would be expected if severe dyskaryosis were present. It is not possible to make a definitive diagnosis of CIN or invasive cervical cancer from examination of a cervical smear.

Follow up of abnormal samples – HPV testing

The cytological examination of cervical cells described above is only a screening test; its value lies in its ability to exclude the approximate 93% of women whose cervical cells appear normal. The severity of dyskaryosis found in an abnormal sample merely determines the next step in the diagnostic process. The vast majority (around 90%) of abnormal samples show only the mildest of abnormality, reported as either 'borderline nuclear abnormalities' or 'mild dyskaryosis'. There is a strong likelihood that these mild changes will spontaneously regress to normal. However there remains a risk that over time a pre-malignant lesion might develop. Prior to introduction of HPV testing, those with these mild abnormalities would have been advised to attend for repeat testing at three or six monthly intervals until the abnormality had resolved. Now, their samples are recovered and tested for the presence of HPV DNA. If the test is negative (i.e. cervical cells contain no HPV DNA) there is no risk of pre-malignancy and patients are able to return to routine screening every three or five years. Those with mild cell abnormality (i.e. 'borderline nuclear abnormalities' or 'mild dyskaryosis') and a *positive* HPV DNA result however are referred for colposcopy, as are all patients whose smear show signs of 'moderate' or 'severe' dyskaryosis.

Colposcopy

Colposcopy is a usually pain free, outpatient diagnostic procedure in which the cervix is viewed directly through a specially modified microscope, called a colposcope. A vaginal speculum is passed as for a cervical smear, and the cervix is 'painted' with acetic acid and a stain which both help to visualise abnormal tissue. This is biopsied to determine the level of CIN or confirm the presence of micro-invasive or invasive cancer. The results of colposcopy and cervical tissue biopsy determine the treatment that may be offered. In the absence of invasive cancer, CIN can be treated in an outpatient setting using a colposcope, by a variety of techniques which all involve the destruction (ablation) of abnormal tissue by extremes of heat (e.g. laser vaporisation, cryotherapy, loop diathermy). Surgical excision (cone biopsy) may be necessary, and rarely, in the absence of invasive disease, hysterectomy might be recommended. All patients who have been treated for CIN must be monitored for recurrence of disease. Instead of the normal three or five year interval between cervical screening test, such patients may be recalled every year for up to ten years. HPV testing is used in this follow up – a negative result on both cytological examination and HPV testing is evidence of cure, and an indication to return to normal interval cervical screening.

Case history 30

In 2005 Sally Turnbull, a 25 year old mother of three, had her first cervical smear test at her primary care surgery. The report of the test arrived at the surgery six weeks later and read 'borderline nuclear abnormalities'; it included the advice to repeat the test in six months time. As soon as she received the appointment for the repeat test some seven weeks after her smear was taken, Sally began to worry. She telephoned the surgery for a much earlier smear test booking, insisting 'If I have cancer I want to know now, not wait for six months'.

Questions

(1) What do you understand the laboratory report to mean?
(2) What could you have said to Sally to allay her fears?
(3) Consider the changes to the cervical screening programme since 2005 and how they have helped to lessen the anxieties surrounding cervical screening that Sally experienced.

Discussion of case history 30

(1) The principle object of examining a cervical sample (smear) is to discover if the epithelial cells it contains shows any signs of dyskaryosis (literally, abnormal nucleus). The nucleus of a dyskaryotic cell is typically larger than normal, occupying an increased volume of the cytoplasm. It is irregular in shape and staining characteristics. Dyskaryosis is a signal that the cervical epithelial tissue from which the cells have been sampled has CIN, a condition that may progress to cervical cancer. There are three grades of severity of dyskaryosis: mild, moderate and severe, which broadly correspond to the severity of CIN. If there are only very slight abnormal changes to the nucleus of epithelial cells, insufficient in magnitude to warrant them being labelled even mildly dyskaryotic, a report of 'borderline nuclear changes' is made.

(2) You could have assured Sally that she did not have cancer. Whilst not normal the changes seen in her smear are not uncommon; around 1 in 20 smears have such slight changes. You could have said that in the majority of such cases the changes revert to normal over a period of months and that by the time of her next appointment, it is highly likely that her smear would be entirely normal. However she needed to know that there was a chance that the abnormality might persist

and could, if ignored, progress slowly over many years to cancer. She could have been told that if the abnormality did persist, cancer can be prevented and a 'cure' achieved by a simple outpatient procedure. It is important that women presenting for routine cervical smear realise that the test is not to detect cancer, but to detect a curable condition (CIN) which if left untreated might, though not necessarily, progress to cervical cancer over a number of years.

(3) The two principle changes to the screening programme since 2005 are the introduction of liquid-based cytology and selective HPV testing of cervical samples. The first of these innovations has meant far fewer 'inadequate' samples (itself a source of anxiety for the women who have to re-attend), and much greater efficiency in processing adequately collected samples. Women now only have to wait one to two weeks for their screening test result, compared with the seven weeks that Sally had to wait. Nowadays Sally's sample would be automatically sent for HPV testing because of the mild abnormality found on cytological examination. Supposing the HPV test were negative (the most likely result), Sally would be sent a report stating in essence that all was well and that she should re-attend for scheduled screening in three years time; all this within one to two weeks of her sample being taken.

References

1. NHS Health and Social Care Information Centre (2011) *Cervical Screening Programme, England: 2010–11*, available at: www.ic.nhs.uk.
2. Cervical Screening Wales (2011) *Statistical Report 2010–2011*, available at: http://www. screeningservices.org.uk/csw/prof/reports/KC53-61-65_10-11.pdf.
3. Scottish Health Statistics *No of screening tests processed 2010–2011*, available at: http://www.isdscotland.org/Health-Topics/Cancer/Cervical-Screening/.
4. Cancer Research UK (2012) Cervical cancer statistics UK (2009/10), available at: www. cancerresearchuk.org.
5. NHS Cancer Screening Programme (2011) NHSCSP audit of invasive cervical cancer – national report 2007–2010.
6. Bosch, F. and Iftner, T. (2005) The aetiology of cervical cancer, *NHSCSP publication No 22 NHS*, Cancer Screening programme: Sheffield, available at: http://www. cancerscreening.nhs.uk/cervical/publications/nhscsp22.pdf.
7. Koutsky, L. (1997) Epidemiology of genital human papilloma virus infection, *Am J Med*, 102: 3–8.
8. Department of Health (2012) Annual HPV vaccine coverage in England 2010/2011, available at: http://www.wp.dh.gov.uk/immunisation/files/2012/04/120319_HPV_ UptakeReport2010-11-revised_acc.pdf.
9. NHS Information Centre (2011) *Cervical Screening Programme England 2010–11*, NHS information centre for health and social care.
10. NHS Cancer Screening Programme (2011) *Annual Review 2011* NHS Cancer Screening Programme: Sheffield.
11. Quinn, M., Babb, P. et al. (1999) Effect of screening on incidence and mortality from cancer of cervix in England: evaluation based on routinely collected statistics, *BMJ*, 318: 904–7.

12. National Statistics (2005) *Cancer Statistics. Registrations of cancer diagnosed in 2003, England*, Office for National Statistics.
13. Peto, J., Gilham, C., Fletcher, O. and Matthews, F. (2004) The cervical cancer epidemic that screening has prevented in the UK, *Lancet*, 364: 249–56.

Further reading

Bryant, E. (2012) The impact of policy and screening on cervical screening in England, *Br J Nursing*, 21 (Suppl 4): S4–10.

Gibb, R. and Martens, M. (2011) The impact of liquid-based cytology in decreasing the incidence of cervical cancer, *Obstet Gynecol*, 4 (suppl 1): S2–11.

Hardy, J. (2007) How to take a sample for cervical screening, *Nursing Standard*, 21: 40–4.

Henderson, L., Clements, A., Damary, S. et al. (2011) 'A false sense of security'? Understanding the role of the HPV vaccine on future cervical screening behaviour: a qualitative study of UK parents and girls of vaccination age, *J Med Screen*, 18: 41–5.

Hughes, C. (2009) Cervical cancer: prevention, diagnosis, treatment and nursing care, *Nursing Standard*, 23: 48–56.

National Health Service Cancer Screening Programme (2010) *Colposcopy and Programme Management – Guidelines for NHS Cervical Screening Programme NHSCP Publication No 20*, NHSCP: Sheffield, available at: http://www.cancerscreening.org.uk/cervical/publications/nhscsp20.pdf.

Stanley, M. (2010) Pathology and epidemiology of HPV infection in females, *Gynecol Oncol*, 117 (Suppl 2): S5–10.

Waller, J., Jackowska, M., Marlow, L. et al. (2012) Exploring age differences in reasons for nonattendance for cervical screening: a qualitative study, *BJOG*, 119: 26–32.

http://www.cancerscreening.nhs.uk/cervical/index.html. A full list of NHSCSP publications relating to cervical cancer screening.

CHAPTER 25

DIPSTICK TESTING OF URINE

Key learning topics

- What can be learned from physical inspection of urine
- Principles of performing dipstick testing of urine
- Significance of abnormal urine dipstick test results

Urinalysis is the generic term for all those clinical tests that involve physical, microscopical, chemical or microbiological examination of urine. Microbiological examination of urine is the subject of Chapter 21. Another aspect of urinalysis, dipstick testing of urine, is the focus of this final chapter. In contrast to all other tests considered in this book, dipstick testing of urine is almost always performed outside the laboratory, in clinics, on hospital wards and primary care surgeries by non-laboratory staff, usually nurses; it is a 'point of care test'.

The value of the urine dipstick test lies in its simplicity and potential to screen for serious renal, urological and liver disease as well as metabolic disorders, such as diabetes. A positive result on dipstick testing is never sufficient to make a definitive diagnosis, though it may provide supportive evidence of one. More often a positive result is used to inform what the next step in the diagnostic process should be.

After a general consideration of sample collection and what can be learned from a physical examination of urine, attention will turn to the dipstick test itself. Each of the urine constituents tested for will be considered in turn, highlighting the most common pathological and non-pathological causes of abnormal results.

Urine sample collection

The ideal urine sample for urinalysis, including dipstick testing, is a sample of uncontaminated bladder urine. The 'clean catch' mid stream urine collection

Understanding Laboratory Investigations: A Guide for Nurses, Midwives and Healthcare Professionals, Third Edition. Chris Higgins.
© 2013 John Wiley & Sons, Ltd. Published 2013 by John Wiley & Sons, Ltd.

Table 25.1 Changes that occur in urine after voiding.

Physical
Colour darkens
Odour strengthens
Turbidity increases

Chemical
pH changes (may increase or decrease)
Glucose concentration decreases
Bilirubin concentration deceases
Urobilinogen concentration decreases
Protein concentration changes (may increase or decrease)
Nitrite concentration increases
Ascorbic acid concentration decreases

Cellular changes evident by microscopy
Red and white blood cells lyse (degrade); numbers decrease

If a delay in testing is unavoidable, the sample should be kept in a refrigerator, as reduced temperature slows the rate of these changes.

technique (Table 21.1) was designed for collection of such an ideal specimen. In practice initial screening can be performed on a midstream urine sample collected without the exacting requirements of a 'clean catch' technique, although a chemically clean and sterile container is essential. The manner of sample collection is less important than its freshness. Urine should be dipstick tested within a few hours of voiding, because many urine constituents are unstable. The major changes in urine composition that occur after voiding are summarised in Table 25.1.

Physical inspection of urine

Inspection of urine should focus on: colour, clarity and odour. In health, freshly voided urine is usually a clear, pale yellow/straw coloured fluid, with only slight, if any, odour. Urine appearance and odour can change if left to stand for more than a few hours so that it is important that freshly voided urine is used for physical inspection.

Colour

The pale yellow colour of urine is due to the presence of the pigment urobilin, a product of bilirubin metabolism. In health the variability in intensity of this yellow reflects varying urine concentration; the more concentrated the urine, the darker is the shade of yellow. The main physiological determinant of urine concentration is fluid intake. Overnight urine reflects a prolonged period without any fluid intake, so that the urine passed first thing in the morning is usually the most concentrated and therefore the strongest coloured. Dehydration, whatever its cause, is associated with production of a concentrated urine, that is consequently relatively dark in colour. After heavy fluid intake (particularly alcohol, which has diuretic property), a dilute urine is passed, which may be almost colourless.

Quite apart from these normal physiological changes in colour, urine may be abnormally coloured due to the presence of abnormal urine constituents[1,2]. These may be endogenous, in which case the abnormal colour reflects a pathological condition (e.g. bilirubin turns urine dark yellow, blood and Hb turns urine pink/red) or they may be exogenous in origin, simply reflecting ingestion of certain foods (e.g. acidic urine may be red after eating beetroot) or more frequently, prescribed drugs.

Clarity/turbidity

Freshly voided urine is usually clear, but urine from healthy subjects may become cloudy if left for more than a few hours due to precipitation of phosphates as urine becomes more alkaline, or precipitation of uric acid if urine is acidic. The most common pathological cause of increased urine turbidity is urinary tract infection (UTI). In such cases turbidity is due principally to the presence in urine of the causative bacteria and white cells (leucocytes), recruited to fight the infection.

Odour

Ingestion of certain foods (e.g. asparagus, aromatic spices) can affect the odour of urine. Bacterially infected urine often smells characteristically fishy, particularly if left to stand for more than a few hours. Certain species of bacteria (Proteus, Klebsiella and Pseudomonas) elaborate an enzyme, urease, that acts on urea present in urine to produce ammonia. Urine infected with these bacteria has a strong ammoniacal odour. A few metabolic disorders are associated with urinary excretion of odorous chemicals. The most significant of these is acetone excreted in the urine of diabetics suffering diabetic ketoacidosis.

Dipstick testing

Technical considerations

Commercially available reagent strips for urine dipstick testing consist of an inert plastic strip on which is mounted paper pads impregnated with chemical reagents. Each pad contains the chemicals needed for detection of a particular constituent of urine. The urine constituents that can be tested for using commercial dipsticks varies according to the particular product being used. Urine constituents detectable by commercial dipstick testing are:

- Glucose
- Bilirubin
- Ketones
- Blood
- Leucocyte esterase
- Nitrite
- Protein
- Albumin
- Creatinine
- Trypsinogen
- pH
- Specific gravity

When the dipstick is dipped in urine, the reagents in each pad dissolve, initiating a chemical reaction that results in a colour change. After a set period of time (usually in the range 20–60 seconds) the colour change of each pad is compared with a colour chart provided by the manufacturer, and the result read. In the case of some urine constituents the test is semi-quantitative, in that the more intense the colour change, the higher is the concentration of the particular urine constituent. If a semi-quantitative result is possible, results are typically reported as either trace (lowest detectable concentration) or 1+, 2+, 3+ or 4+ (very high concentration). If a semi-quantitative result is not possible then the report is either positive (the substance is present in urine) or negative (the substance is not present in urine).

Each manufacturer of test strips provides detail of the test procedure that must be followed for accurate results, but some general points are made here:

- The chemical reagents contained on the strip pads have a limited shelf life governed by the expiry date on the container. Always check expiry date before use. Dipsticks should not be used if the expiry date has passed.
- The stability of the chemical reagents depend on the desiccant (which absorbs any moisture) provided either in a sachet or in the lid of the container. To maintain chemical stability it is important that dipsticks are stored in the container provided and that the lid is replaced immediately after use. Only remove enough dipsticks for immediate use.
- The chemicals on dipstick pads dissolve if left in urine long enough. The dipstick must be dipped in urine so that all reagent pads are immersed and then immediately removed.
- It is important that the chemicals from one pad do not contaminate the next. To avoid this, excess urine must be removed as the strip is withdrawn from the urine sample, by dragging the edge of the strip against the urine container and then immediately blotting the side of the strip on an absorbent paper towel.
- Good lighting is essential for accurate reading of colour change.

- Ability to accurately differentiate sometimes subtle colour change is essential. It may be inappropriate for staff with colour blindness to perform dipstick testing.
- The timing of the reaction is vital for accurate results; always observe manufacturers' timing instructions.
- Urine is a biological fluid which must be treated as a potential source of pathogens, with risk to patient and staff of cross-infection. All staff performing dipstick testing must be familiar with local health and safety policy regarding work with body fluids (e.g. the need for protective gloves and apron, what to do in the event of a urine spillage etc.).
- Results must be recorded on a worksheet and in patients' notes.
- The quality of results using dipsticks should be regularly assessed by a local laboratory quality control scheme[3].

Interpretation of results

Glucose

Although in health urine may contain very slight amounts of glucose, concentration is too low to give a positive result using urine dipsticks and a negative result is normal. A positive result only occurs when blood glucose concentration rises above the renal threshold. For most people the renal threshold for glucose, that is the blood concentration above which glucose appears in urine, is around 10.0 mmol/L. A positive urine glucose result (termed glycosuria) then indicates that at some time since the bladder was last emptied, blood glucose concentration was in excess of around 10 mmol/L. The dipstick test is semi-quantitative, allowing an indication of the extent of the increase in blood glucose concentration beyond the renal threshold.

The most common and significant cause of an abnormal rise in blood glucose, sufficient for glucose to be detected in urine, is diabetes mellitus. Other rarer endocrine disorders which result in raised blood glucose and resulting glycosuria include Cushing's syndrome (excess cortisol), acromegaly (excess growth hormone), phaeochromocytoma (excess adrenalin) and hyperthyroidism (excess thyroid hormones). Occasionally a positive glucose urine dipstick may be found in an individual whose blood glucose concentration is not increased. This lowering of the renal threshold for glucose most often occurs during pregnancy. It is also the defining feature of a rare and entirely benign defect of kidney function, known as renal glycosuria. Advancing age is associated with increasing renal threshold so that blood glucose is often well in excess of 10 mmol/L before glycosuria occurs in the elderly.

A positive urine glucose result raises the suspicion of diabetes, but this can only be confirmed or excluded by measurement of blood glucose concentration.

Once diabetes has been confirmed, the principle aim of treatment is to maintain near normal blood glucose concentration. Dipstick urine testing for the presence of glucose is sometimes used by diabetic patients to monitor blood glucose control.

A positive result of course indicates raised blood glucose (at least above the patient's renal threshold) and therefore increasingly poor control. A negative result indicates either normal or reduced blood glucose concentration (hypoglycaemia). Only by measuring blood glucose concentration can hypoglycaemia be distinguished from normoglycaemia. Since the urine test is unable to distinguish hypoglycaemia from normoglycaemia, it is a less satisfactory way of monitoring diabetes than measuring blood glucose concentration directly.

Ingestion of large amounts of vitamin C (ascorbic acid) can cause a falsely negative glucose result.

Bilirubin and urobilinogen

Bilirubin and urobilinogen are waste products of haemoglobin catabolism. Haemoglobin is the oxygen carrying protein contained in red blood cells (erythrocytes). At the end of their 120 day life, red cells are removed from blood and degraded in the reticuloendothelial system, principally the spleen. Here the Hb, contained within them, is broken to its constituent parts: haem and globin. Haem is converted to bilirubin. As a waste product of metabolism, bilirubin must be removed from the body. It is first transported in blood to the liver, where it is conjugated (joined) with glucuronic acid to form so called 'conjugated' bilirubin. Conjugation renders bilirubin water soluble, a necessary state for its elimination from the body. Conjugated bilirubin is excreted from liver cells to the bile canniculi of the liver and out from the liver via the common bile duct, in bile, to the small intestine.

During passage through the intestine bilirubin is converted (oxidised) by gut bacteria to urobilinogen. Most of this urobilinogen is excreted in faeces but some is absorbed into blood. The urobilinogen that is reabsorbed into blood has two possible fates: some of it is taken up by liver cells and excreted in bile, thereby reappearing in the gastrointestinal tract, and some is excreted in urine.

In health then, all bilirubin is excreted via the liver in bile and none is excreted in urine. A negative dipstick result for bilirubin is normal. The presence of bilirubin in urine is always pathological. By contrast normal urine contains a small amount (trace) of urobilinogen, and a negative urobilinogen dipstick result is pathological as is a result indicating more than trace amounts (1+ 2+ etc.).

A positive urine bilirubin result (termed bilirubinuria) indicates abnormal accumulation of conjugated bilirubin in blood. This can only usually occur if the normal excretory route (liver and biliary tract) is impaired. A positive urine bilirubin result thus indicates significant liver or biliary tract disease, and requires further investigation; initially blood should be sampled for liver function tests. A falsely negative result can occur if urine contains large amounts of ascorbic acid (vitamin C).

Normal urine contains a trace of urobilinogen. A negative result is thus pathological and indicates that urobilinogen is not being formed in the intestine, which in turn indicates that conjugated bilirubin is not being excreted in bile to the intestine. Such a negative finding can be expected if the biliary tract is obstructed (e.g. gall stones, cancer of the head of pancreas). An abnormally high concentration of urobilinogen in urine (i.e. greater than 'trace' on dipstick testing) occurs if the portion of urobilinogen normally reabsorbed from intestine cannot be excreted in bile, due to liver disease (hepatitis, cirrhosis etc.).

Increased excretion of urobilinogen in urine also occurs if increased bilirubin is excreted in bile secondarily to increased bilirubin production. Since bilirubin is derived from the Hb in red cells, increased bilirubin production/excretion, and therefore increased excretion of urobilinogen in urine, occurs in the context of increased red cell destruction (haemolysis). A dipstick result indicating abnormally raised urobilinogen thus provides supportive evidence of the haemolytic process associated with haemolytic jaundice and haemolytic anaemia.

To summarise: a positive bilirubin dipstick test result suggests liver disease; a negative urobilinogen dipstick test result suggests biliary obstruction; and a strongly positive urobilinogen dipstick test result suggests either liver disease or increased red cell destruction (i.e. a haemolytic process).

Ketones

Ketones (sometimes called ketone bodies) is the collective name for three chemical substances present in the body. Two are keto-acids (β-hydroxybutyric acid and acetoacetic acid) and the third is acetone. All three are produced during the oxidation of fatty acids, the metabolic process by which the energy contained in fat is released. Normally ketones are rapidly metabolised. However if fat metabolism is abnormally increased, the rate at which ketones are produced exceeds the rate at which they are metabolised (removed). The result is accumulation of ketones in blood (ketonaemia) and excretion of ketones in urine (ketonuria). This abnormal metabolic state is known as ketosis. If the accumulation of keto-acids in blood is sufficient to overwhelm the homeostatic mechanisms that maintain normal blood pH, blood becomes abnormally acidic; this pathological, potentially fatal, state is called ketoacidosis.

The principal causes of increased fat metabolism and resulting positive test for urine ketones are diabetes and starvation. In both of these conditions there is a deficiency of glucose within cells to provide energy. In the case of the diabetic patient, the problem is a deficiency of insulin, the hormone required for entry of glucose into cells. In the case of the patient who is suffering from starvation the deficiency of glucose is simply due to lack of dietary carbohydrate. In both instances stored fat is metabolised to fill the 'energy gap' caused by glucose deficiency within cells.

The ketosis associated with starvation is usually mild and therefore very rarely associated with acidosis. By contrast ketosis in diabetes can be severe giving rise to the acute life threatening complication of diabetes, known as diabetic ketoacidosis. If a diabetic patient is unwell, the finding of a positive urine ketone test is suggestive of diabetic ketoacidosis and the need for emergency medical care.

A positive urine ketone test may occur in normal pregnancy around the time of delivery and in those who are severely dehydrated. A positive ketone test is also a feature of a condition called alcoholic ketoacidosis that can affect chronic alcoholics who fail to eat immediately before or after an episode of binge drinking.

Nitrite

This is a screening test for UTI, a condition discussed in Chapter 21. Normally urine contains no nitrite. However many species of bacteria can convert dietary nitrate, which *is* present in normal urine, to nitrite. A positive result for nitrite indicates that the urine contains bacteria. The test is reasonably sensitive, that is there are few false positive results. In a typical study[4] only 6% of urines with a positive nitrite test did not contain significant numbers of bacteria. However falsely negative results are a limitation of the test. In around 50% (range 45–65%) of urines containing significant numbers of bacteria, the urine nitrite test is negative[4,5]. The reasons for the false negative results are twofold. Firstly there are some species of bacteria (mostly Gram-positive) which can cause urinary tract infection, but which do not have the enzyme necessary for conversion of nitrate to nitrite. Secondly urine must be present in the bladder for around four hours for complete bacterial conversion of nitrate to nitrite. Samples taken during the day may not have been in the bladder for a sufficient time. An early morning specimen, which has been in the bladder overnight, is more likely to result in a positive nitrite test than one taken during the day.

The presence of abnormally high amounts of vitamin C (ascorbic acid) and urobilinogen in urine can affect nitrite detection resulting in falsely negative results.

Leucocyte esterase (white blood cells)

Like the nitrite dipstick test, this is a screening test for UTI. The test detects the presence of the enzyme leucocyte esterase, which is an enzyme present only in phagocytic white blood cells (leucocytes) called neutrophils. The test thus detects the presence of neutrophils in urine. Normally the test is negative; urine from a healthy individual does not contain sufficient neutrophils to produce a positive result. The presence of significant numbers of leucocytes (including neutrophils) in urine is called pyuria. The body's normal response to any bacterial infection is recruitment of neutrophils to the site of infection, where they engulf (phagocytose) and destroy bacteria. Pyuria, and the resulting positive leucocyte esterase urine dipstick test, is thus an indication of bacterial infection of the urinary tract. In around 75–85% of UTI infections the test is positive.

Pyuria, and therefore a positive result, can occur in the absence of bacterial infection of the urinary tract; this is termed 'sterile pyuria'. Conditions associated with sterile pyuria include tuberculosis and inflammatory disease of the kidneys and urinary tract (e.g. chronic pyelonephritis, urethral syndrome). Although the most likely explanation, a positive result clearly does not necessarily indicate urinary tract infection. If nitrite and leucocyte esterase tests are both negative, urinary tract infection is unlikely. A positive result in either or both is suggestive of urinary tract infection but not sufficiently reliable to definitively make the diagnosis.

Blood

The presence of blood in urine is called haematuria. A distinction is made between macroscopic haematuria, the visible presence of blood in urine (this turns urine a reddish brown colour) and microscopic haematuria, the presence of blood in urine that is not obvious to the naked eye, and can only be detected by dipstick testing or examination of urine under the microscope. The number of red blood cells provides an index of the quantity of blood. Normal urine contains small numbers of red blood cells (< 5000/ml)[6]. The sensitivity of the dipstick test is such that only those urines whose red blood cell concentration is greater than normal will give a positive result.

For women of reproductive age, a positive blood dipstick result may simply indicate that the specimen is contaminated with menstrual blood. If urine is very concentrated, the dipstick test may be positive despite the fact that a normal number of red cells are being excreted. Other causes of a false positive result include raised levels of ascorbic acid (vitamin C) in urine. Finally, since the dipstick test is detecting the haem part of haemoglobin, not red cells directly, rare conditions in which there is excessive urine excretion of free Hb and myoglobin (which also contains the haem group) result in a positive result despite no increased excretion of red blood cells (i.e. no haematuria).

Although the dipstick test may be used to confirm the presence of visible blood in urine (macroscopic haematuria), its principle value is detection of microscopic haematuria.

Depending on the age of the population studied, 0.2–22% of apparently well individuals test positive for microscopic haematuria[7]. A positive result is most likely to have a benign cause; for example, exercise can result in transient microscopic haematuria. More rarely it can be the first objective sign of serious urological or renal disease. The most common pathological cause of positive blood dipstick for blood is urinary tract infection. Less common causes include inflammatory disease of the kidney (e.g. glomerular nephritis) and early bladder or renal cancer. A representative study[8] demonstrates just how rare it is for a positive dipstick to be associated with serious pathology. Of 368 patients with positive dipstick result, 40% did not even have significant haematuria when urine was examined in the laboratory. Of the remaining 225 in whom microscopic haematuria was confirmed, just 48 (13% of those with a positive dipstick result) were suffering any sort of pathology; just six were found to be suffering early malignant disease (all bladder tumours). A positive result should not be ignored but confirmed by microscopical examination of urine before intensive urological (or renal) investigation[9].

Protein

The first step in urine production is filtration of blood at the glomerulus. The pores in the glomerular membrane are too small to allow proteins to pass, so that normally urine contains no protein. In health urine dipstick protein result is negative. The presence of protein in urine is called proteinuria. Proteinuria, particularly mild proteinuria (trace/1+), is most often transient, benign and of no particular clinical significance. However it can be the first sign of serious renal disease and, among pregnant women, the first sign of pre-eclampsia, a serious disease of pregnancy that can threaten both the life of the mother and health of her unborn child.

Fever, urinary tract infection and strenuous exercise may all be associated with transient mild proteinuria, which resolves with time (days or weeks) and has no long-term consequences. Orthostatic proteinuria is a relatively common, entirely benign condition with particular prevalence among older children and adolescents. It is characterised by proteinuria in the standing position only and may be associated with positive dipstick result if urine is collected during the day. A morning specimen collected on rising is always negative. The condition usually disappears during adulthood.

Persistent proteinuria, that is positive dipstick results on three occasions separated by intervals of at least a week in an otherwise well patient without orthostatic proteinuria, is indication of possible renal disease and/or hypertension which warrants further investigation, including measurement of blood pressure, 24 hour urine protein estimation to quantify the protein loss and serum creatinine.

All pregnant women have urine tested at first booking for the presence of protein to identify those at risk of pre-eclampsia, a condition characterised by the triad of hypertension, oedema and significant proteinuria (>300 mg/24 hrs).

pH

In contrast to the tight control of blood pH, which is maintained at 7.35–7.45, urine pH may range from 4 to 8, although it is usually within the range 5.5–6.5. Extremes of urine pH can be due to diet. A vegetarian diet, for example, is generally speaking associated with an alkaline pH >6.5. Pathological conditions associated with disturbance of acid-base balance and abnormal blood pH are reflected in urine so that, for example, patients in diabetic ketoacidosis would tend to have an acidic urine pH <5.0, whereas those with systemic alkalosis have an alkalotic urine (pH >6.0).

Urine infections due to some bacterial species (Proteus, Klebsiella, Pseudomonas) are associated with alkaline urine because they elaborate an enzyme, urease, that splits the urea present in urine to carbon dioxide and ammonia.

The pH of urine has little clinical significance except in two conditions – renal tubular acidosis and renal stone disease. Renal tubular acidosis is a defect of renal tubule cells characterised by failure of the kidneys to excrete hydrogen ions effectively. The consequent accumulation of hydrogen ions in blood results in reduced blood pH (acidosis) and inappropriately alkaline urine. Kidney stones are formed by the precipitation of urine constituents such as calcium phosphate and uric acid, a process that is dependent in part on the pH of urine. Drugs that modulate urine pH and thereby reduce mineral precipitation are used in the treatment of renal stone disease.

Specific gravity

Specific gravity (SG) is a measure of the concentration of solutes in a solution. The SG of water is 1; urine SG can range from 1.001 (a very dilute urine) to 1.035 (a very concentrated urine). The actual level indicates state of hydration. A dehydrated patient should appropriately excrete urine of high SG, whereas a patient receiving too much fluid should excrete urine with low SG. Failure to concentrate urine appropriately when fluid is restricted can be an early signal of renal disease and diabetes insipidus.

References

1. Aycock, R. and Kass, D. (2012) Abnormal urine colour, *South Med J*, 105: 36–42.
2. Cone, T. (1968) Diagnosis and treatment: some syndromes, diseases and conditions associated with abnormal coloration of the urine or diaper, *Pediatrics*, 41: 654–8.
3. Tighe, P. (1999) Laboratory-based quality assurance programme for near patient urine dipstick testing, 1990–1997: development, management and results, *Br J Biomed Sci*, 56: 6–15.
4. Little, P., Turner, S. and Rumsby, K. (2010) Validating the prediction of lower urinary tract infection in primary care: sensitivity and specificity of urine dipsticks and clinical scores in women, *Br J Gen Prac*, 60: 495–500.
5. Deville, W., Yzermans, J. et al. (2004) The urine dipstick test useful to rule out infection. A meta analysis of the accuracy, *BMC Urology*, 4: 4–18.
6. Corwin, H. and Silverstein, M. (1988) Microscopic hematuria, *Clin Lab Med*, 8: 601–10.
7. Grossfield, G. and Carrol, P. (1998) Evaluation of asymptomatic microscopic hematuria, *Urol Clin North Am*, 25: 661–76.
8. Khan, M., Shaw, G. and Paris, A. (2002) Is microscopic haematuria a urological emergency?, *BJU International*, 90: 355–7.
9. Rao, P.K. and Jones, J.S. (2008) How to evaluate 'dipstick hematuria': what to do before you refer, *Cleveland Clinic J Med*, 75: 227–33.

Further reading

Topham, P., Jethwa, A. et al. (2004) The value of urine screening in a young adult population, *Family Practice*, 21: 18–21.
Viswanathan, G. and Upadhyay, A. (2011) Assessment of proteinuria, *Adv Chronic Kidney Dis*, 18: 243–8.

GLOSSARY OF SOME TERMS USED IN LABORATORY MEDICINE

Acidaemia	Abnormal increase in acidity of blood – reduced blood pH
Acidosis	Abnormal increase in the acidity of body fluids associated with reduced blood pH
Acetaminophen	Alternative name for the drug paracetamol
Aetiology	The cause(s) of a disorder/disease
Agranulocytosis	Complete or near absence of granulocytes in blood
Alkalaemia	Abnormal increase in alkalinity of blood – increased blood pH
Alkalosis	Abnormal increase in the alkalinity of body fluids associated with increased blood pH
Anaemia	The condition of reduced oxygen delivery to tissues that results from reduced haemoglobin concentration – many possible causes
Anisocytosis	Red cells vary in size
Antibody	A protein (immunoglobulin) that circulates in blood plasma. Binds specifically to the antigen that provoked its production
Antigen	A substance (protein or carbohydrate) present on the surface of cells that provokes specific antibody production
Anuria	Failure to produce urine
Atheroma	Disease of artery walls that leads to atherosclerosis
Atherosclerosis	Thickening and hardening of arterial walls reducing blood flow, a common chronic condition that is the cause of coronary heart disease, strokes and peripheral artery disease
B-Cells	One kind of lymphocyte. Matures to antibody producing plasma cell. One of many blood cells involved in the immune process
Bacteraemia	Presence of bacteria in blood
Bacteriuria	Presence of bacteria in urine
Basophil	One of five kinds of white blood cells – it is a granulocyte

Understanding Laboratory Investigations: A Guide for Nurses, Midwives and Healthcare Professionals, Third Edition. Chris Higgins.
© 2013 John Wiley & Sons, Ltd. Published 2013 by John Wiley & Sons, Ltd.

Benign tumour	Abnormal growth of tissue whose margins are well defined – it may grow large but does not spread beyond its local site
Biopsy	A sample of tissue removed for microscopic examination to diagnose disease
Blast cell	Immature white cell – not normally present in blood
Cancer	General term for all diseases associated with malignant tumours
Carcinoma	A specific term for malignant tumours that originate in epithelial cells anywhere in the body
Commensal bacteria	Bacteria that colonise the human body without causing disease
Dysplasia	Tissue in which there is evidence of increased cell division
Ecchymosis	Abnormal brown/red discoloration of skin caused by bleeding into tissues. A signal of coagulation defect or reduced platelet numbers
Endocervical cells	Epithelial cells that line the internal surface of the endocervical canal. One of the cell types normally seen in cervical smear
Endothelial cells	The cells that line the internal surface of blood vessels
Eosinophils	One of five types of white cell normally present in blood; it is a granulocyte
Erythrocyte	Red blood cell
Erythropoiesis	Process by which erythrocytes develop from bone marrow stem cell
Erythropoietin	Hormone produced by the kidney that regulates red cell production
Euthyroidism	Normal production of thyroid hormones by the thyroid gland
Exudate	Fluid produced during inflammatory tissue damage
Frozen section	Rapid technique for preparation of biopsied tissue prior to microscopical examination. Enables histopathological diagnosis within an hour or so
Factor V Leiden	Common inherited defect in blood coagulation due to mutation in Factor V gene
Gram Stain	A staining technique that allows classification of all bacteria to one of two groups: Gram-positive and Gram-negative. The first step in identifying bacterial species
Glycosuria	Abnormal presence of glucose in urine
Glycolysis	The metabolic process by which glucose is oxidised to produce energy
Granulocytes	White blood cells (neutrophils, eosinophils and basophils) that have granules in their cytoplasm
Haematuria	The presence of blood in urine
Haemoglobin	Oxygen carrying protein present in red blood cells

Haemoglobinopathies	A large group of inherited diseases caused by defect in haemoglobin structure or synthesis
Haemolysis	Rupture of red cell membrane, destruction of red cell. Increased *in vivo* haemolyis is the cause of one kind of anaemia – haemolytic anaemia. Can occur during blood collection (*in vitro*) rendering samples unsuitable for analysis
Haemolytic anaemia	See haemolysis
Haemophilia	A group of inherited disorders that result in increased bleeding due to a clotting factor deficiency
Haemopoiesis	Process of blood formation in bone marrow
Hepatitis	Inflammation of the liver
Hypercalcaemia	Raised plasma calcium concentration
Hypercapnia	Increased amount of carbon dioxide in blood – raised PCO_2
Hyperglycaemia	Raised blood glucose concentration
Hyperkalaemia	Raised plasma potassium concentration
Hyperlipidaemia	Raised blood lipid (cholesterol and/or triglycerides) concentration
Hypernatraemia	Raised plasma sodium concentration
Hyperthyroidism	Increased activity of thyroid gland
Hypocalcaemia	Reduce plasma calcium concentration
Hypocapnia	Reduced amount of carbon dioxide in blood – reduced PCO_2
Hypoglycaemia	Reduced blood glucose concentration
Hypokalaemia	Reduced plasma potassium concentration
Hyponatraemia	Reduced plasma sodium concentration
Hypothyroidism	Reduced activity of thyroid gland
Hypoxaemia	Reduced amount of oxygen in blood – reduced PO_2
Hypoxia	Reduced amount of oxygen in tissues
Infarction	Necrosis of tissue due to ischaemia
Ischaemia	Reduced blood flow to tissues usually the result of vessel blocked by thrombus and/or atherosclerotic plaque
Jaundice	Yellow discoloration of skin and sclerae due to abnormal accumulation of the pigment bilirubin
Kernicterus	Accumulation of bilirubin (unconjugated) in the brain which can cause permanent brain damage
Ketoacidosis	An abnormal metabolic state due to accumulation of ketoacids (ketones) in blood
Ketones	The collective name for three chemicals which accumulate in blood during increased fat metabolism
Ketonuria	The abnormal presence of ketones in urine
Lactic acidosis	An abnormal metabolic state that results from accumulation of lactic acid in blood
Leucopaenia	Reduction in white blood cell numbers

Leucocytosis	Increase in white cell numbers
Leucocytes	Alternative name for white blood cells
Lymphocyte	One of five main types of white blood cells. Two main kinds: B- and T- lymphocytes; both required for acquired immunity, they are cells of the immune system
Macrophage	A phagocytic cell present in tissues that is derived from a monocyte
Malignant tumour	A solid tumour that can spread (metastasise) to distant sites and grow
Megaloblastic anaemia	Anaemia caused by deficiency of B12 or folate
Metabolic acidosis	Acidosis caused by the accumulation of metabolic acids (e.g. lactic acid) in blood
Microcytosis	Red cells, on average, smaller than normal – reduced MCV
Microcytic anaemia	All those anaemias associated with reduced MCV
Monocyte	One of five types of white blood cell, matures to tissue macrophage
Necrosis	Death of cells or tissue due to disease or injury
Neuroglycopaenia	Reduced glucose in cells of the central nervous system (including the brain)
Neutrophil	The most abundant of five types of white blood cell. It is a phagocytic cell and a granulocyte
Neutropaenia	Reduced number of neutrophils in blood
Neutrophilia	Increased number of neutrophils in blood
Nocturia	The need to urinate during the night
Nosocomial infection	Hospital acquired infection
Oedema	Abnormal accumulation of fluid in the interstitial space of any tissue
Pathogen	A microbial species (bacteria, virus or fungi) that causes disease
Platelets	Formed particles present in blood – required for blood clotting
Pleural fluid	The fluid present in the pleural cavity that surrounds the lungs
Pleural effusion	Abnormal accumulation of pleural fluid
Poikilocytosis	Red cells vary in shape
Polyuria	Increased urine production
Polydipsia	Increased thirst
Proteinuria	The abnormal presence of protein in urine
Respiratory acidosis	Acidosis caused by failure to eliminate carbon dioxide from blood
Sepsis	Systemic inflammatory response to infection
Thrombocyte	Alternative name for platelets

Thrombocytopaenia	Reduction in platelet number
Thrombocytosis	Increase in the number of platelets
Thrombus	Blood clot formed inappropriately within blood vessels
Thromboembolus	A thrombus that moves through the bloodstream eventually causing blockage of small vessels

ABBREVIATIONS

AAFB	Acid-alcohol fast bacilli
ACD	Anaemia of chronic disease
ACE	Angiotensin converting enzyme
ACS	Acute coronary syndrome
AIDS	Acquired immune deficiency syndrome
AKI	Acute kidney injury
ALL	Acute lymphatic leukaemia
ALT	Alanine aminotransferase
AML	Acute myeloid leukaemia
ANF	Anti-nuclear factor
AP	Alkaline phosphatase
APPT	Activated partial thromboplastin time
AST	Aspartate aminotransferase
ATP	Adenosine tri-phosphate
CBC	Complete blood count
CHD	Coronary heart disease
CIN	Cervical intra-epithelial neoplasia
CKD	Chronic kidney disease
CLL	Chronic lymphatic leukaemia
CML	Chronic myeloid leukaemia
CRP	C-reactive protein
CSF	Cerebrospinal fluid
CSU	Catheter specimen of urine
DIC	Disseminated intravascular coagulation
DNA	Deoxyribonucleic acid
DVT	Deep vein thrombosis
ECF	Extracellular fluid
ESR	Erythrocyte sedimentation rate
FBC	Full blood count

Understanding Laboratory Investigations: A Guide for Nurses, Midwives and Healthcare Professionals, Third Edition. Chris Higgins.
© 2013 John Wiley & Sons, Ltd. Published 2013 by John Wiley & Sons, Ltd.

FT4	Free thyroxine (T4)
FT3	Free triiodothyronine (T3)
GFR	Glomerular filtration rate
GGT	Gamma glutamyl transferase
GH	Growth hormone
HAV	Hepatitis A virus
Hb	Haemoglobin
HBV	Hepatitis B virus
HCV	Hepatitis C virus
HIV	Human immunodeficiency virus
HPV	Human papilloma virus
ICF	Intracellular fluid
IDA	Iron deficiency anaemia
IF	Intrinsic factor
INR	International normalised ratio
IPT	Immunological pregnancy test
ITP	Immune thrombocytopaenic purpura
LFT	Liver function tests
MCHC	Mean (red) cell haemoglobin concentration
MC&S	Microscopy, culture and sensitivity
MCV	Mean (red) cell volume
MI	Myocardial infarction
MRSA	Methicillin resistant *Staphylococcus aureus*
MSU	Midstream urine
NSTEMI	Non ST segment elevation myocardial infarction
PA	Pernicious anaemia
PCV	Packed cell volume
PT	Prothrombin time
PTH	Parathyroid hormone
RDW	Red cell distribution width
RNA	Ribonucleic acid
SLE	Systemic lupus erythematosus
STEMI	ST segment elevation myocardial infarction
TATT	Tired all the time
TB	Tuberculosis
TFT	Thyroid function tests
TIBC	Total iron binding capacity
TSH	Thyroid stimulating hormone
TT	Thrombin time
UA	Uric acid
U&E	Urea and electrolytes
UTI	Urinary tract infection
VRSA	Vancomycin resistant *Staphylococcus aureus*
VTE	Venous thromboembolism
WBC	White blood count

ADULT REFERENCE RANGES

The column headed 'Local laboratory reference range' is left blank for you to fill in the precise reference range used at your hospital.

Test	Approximate reference range	Local laboratory reference range
Sodium	133–146 mmol/L	
Potassium	3.5–5.3 mmol/L	
Bicarbonate	25–30 mmol/L	
Urea	2.5–7.8 mmol/L	
Creatinine	55–105 µmol/L	
Fasting blood glucose	3.5–5.0 mmol/L	
pH	7.35–7.45	
Hydrogen ion	35–45 nmol/L	
$PaCO_2$	4.7–6.0 kPa	
Bicarbonate	22–28 mmol/L	
PaO_2	10.6–13.3 kPa	
Base excess	−2.0–+ 2.0	
Lactate	0.5–2.0 mmol/L	
Bilirubin	<21 µmol/L	
Alanine aminotransferase (ALT)	10–40 U/L	
Aspartate aminotransferase (AST)	10–40 U/L	
Gamma glutamyl transferase (GGT)	<50 U/L	
Alkaline phosphatase (AP)	30–150 U/L	
Albumin	35–50 g/L	
Amylase	<200 U/L	
Magnesium	0.7–1.0 mmol/L	
Calcium (total)	2.20–2.60 mmol/L	
Calcium (ionised)	1.15–1.30 mmol/L	
Phosphate	0.80–1.40 mmol/L	
Parathyroid hormone (PTH)	10–70 ng/L	

Understanding Laboratory Investigations: A Guide for Nurses, Midwives and Healthcare Professionals, Third Edition. Chris Higgins.
© 2013 John Wiley & Sons, Ltd. Published 2013 by John Wiley & Sons, Ltd.

(cont'd)

Test	Approximate reference range	Local laboratory reference range
Total cholesterol	NSF Target* <5.0 mmol/L JBS Target* <4.0 mmol/L	
LDL-Cholesterol	NSF Target* <3.0 mmol/L JBS Target* <2.0 mmol/L	
HDL-Cholesterol	>1.2 mmol/L	
Thyroxine–Free (FT4)	9–26 pmol/L	
Triiodothyronine–Free (FT3)	3.0–9.0 pmol/L	
Thyroid stimulating hormone (TSH)	0.3–4.5 mU/L	
Uric acid	150–400 µmol/L	
Cortisol (9.00am)	150–680 nmol/L	
(Midnight)	<100 nmol/L	
Adrenocorticotrophic hormone (ACTH) (9.00 am)	<50 ng/L	
Cardiac troponin T (cTnT)		
Cardiac troponin I (cTnI)		
CK(MB)		
Myoglobin		
Haemoglobin (Hb)	Male 13–17 g/dl Female 11 15 g/dl	
Red cell count	Male 4.5–6.5×10^9/L Female 3.9–6.5×10^9/L	
Packed cell volume (PCV)/Haematocrit	Male 40–52% Female 36–48%	
Mean cell volume (MCV)	80–95 fl	
Mean cell haemoglobin conc. (MCHC)	20–35 g/dl	
Red cell distribution width (RDW)	10–15%	
White cell count	Male 3.7–9.5 x 10^9/L Female 3.9–11.1 x 10^9/L	
Erythrocyte sedimentation rate (ESR)	Male 1–10 mm/hr Female 5–20 mm/hr	
C-reactive protein (CRP)	<10 mg/L	
Platelet count	150–400×10^9/L	
Prothrombin time (PT)	10–14 sec	
Activated partial thromboplastin time (APPT)	30–40 sec	

(continued)

(*cont'd*)

Test	Approximate reference range	Local laboratory reference range
Thrombin time (TT)	14–16 sec	
Iron	10–30 µmol/L	
Total iron binding capacity (TIBC)	40–75 µmol/L	
Ferritin	10–300 µg/L	
Vitamin B12	150–1000 ng/L	
Folate	150–700 µg/L	

*See text pages 139 and 145.

ALPHABETICAL INDEX OF TESTS

INDEX

*Understanding Laboratory Investigations: A Guide for Nurses, Midwives
and Healthcare Professionals,* Third Edition. Chris Higgins.
© 2013 John Wiley & Sons, Ltd. Published 2013 by John Wiley & Sons, Ltd.